AIDS:
Crisis in Professional Ethics

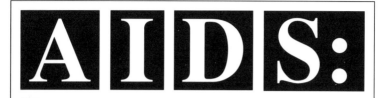

AIDS:
Crisis in
Professional Ethics

Edited by
Elliot D. Cohen and Michael Davis

Temple University Press
Philadelphia

Temple University Press, Philadelphia 19122
Copyright © 1994 by Temple University
Published 1994
Printed in the United States of America

The paper used in this publication meets the minimum requirements of American
National Standard for Information Sciences—Permanence of Paper for Printed Library
Materials, ANSI Z39.48—1984

Library of Congress Cataloging-in-Publication Data
AIDS : crisis in professional ethics / edited by Elliot D. Cohen and
  Michael Davis.
    p.   cm.
    Includes bibliographical references and index.
    ISBN 1-56639-164-4 (cloth). — ISBN 1-56639-165-2 (pbk.)
    1. AIDS (Disease)—Moral and ethical aspects.   I. Cohen, Elliot
D.   II. Davis, Michael, 1943–   .
RC607.A26A3457324   1994
174′.2—dc20   93-43171

Contents

AIDS:
Crisis in Professional Ethics

Introduction

Elliot D. Cohen
Michael Davis

This collection of original essays addresses some of the important problems we have come to group under the short name "AIDS." It differs from most works on AIDS in two related ways. First, its focus is on the moral choices of individual practitioners rather than no empirical research or social policy. Second, the practitioners whose problems are discussed include—besides the more usual physicians and nurses—dentists, counselors, preschool teachers, business managers, college administrators, lawyers, clergy, journalists, and politicians. This is a contribution to the literature on professions as well as to the literature on AIDS.

This collection began with the realization that, even in a hospital, many people with whom an AIDS patient might come in contact will be neither physician nor nurse but the psychologists, social workers, or clergy who now do much of the counseling in hospitals. As this fact sank in, we realized something else. Most people with HIV (the infection that causes AIDS)—indeed, most people with AIDS—are not in a hospital. They attend college, seek dental care, work at a job, or need legal advice. Some may even run for office or become the subject of a reporter's story.

With this second realization came a third. AIDS is a hyperbolic disease, an epidemic of ironic extremes. Among the easiest diseases to prevent, it carries with it the virtual certainty of a slow, ugly death. A disease associated with social pleasures, it carries a stigma that tends to leave those infected painfully alone. A new disease, it forces us, especially professionals, to face old questions, questions that have become harder for long neglect.

While the general reader will find much to ponder in this collection, it was designed for three more specific audiences: students (and teachers) of medical ethics, students (and teachers) of professional ethics, and practitioners (both those whose professions are actually represented here and those whose professions bear some analogy to these).

Many courses in medical ethics would, we believe, benefit from a second text allowing students to see medicine in the context of other professions. All too often courses in medical ethics are simply courses in moral problems arising in a hospital. Comparison with other professions may help students appreciate the distinctive commitment of their profession—indeed, to see their choice of career as a profession—and so prepare them to recognize that some with whom they will work have different commitments.

Another course that would benefit from supplementary use of this collection is contemporary moral problems. By examining the impact of AIDS on a number of professions (or semiprofessions), this collection provides a relatively comprehensive view of the moral ramifications of one of today's urgent social problems.

"Generic" courses in professional ethics could also use a second text like this one. Generic professional-ethics courses tend to be relatively general, drawing most of their illustrations from the two "paradigm professions," law and medicine. Other health professions, such as nursing and dentistry; professions without clients, like journalism; and "quasi professions," like management and politics, tend to be overlooked, impoverishing the student's understanding of professions. With its wide range of professions, this collection provides an antidote to that tendency—without producing the opposite (and more debilitating) tendency of generic courses, a mere parading of professions. AIDS puts each profession to much the same test, providing a structure for comparison.

We also believe that many practitioners, faced with the reality of HIV infection in a client, patient, parishioner, student, colleague, employee, or subject, will benefit from the thoughtful analyses of our contributors. Here are questions that, though crying out for discussion, have too often been answered with silence. Here too are answers that, whatever their ultimate merit, at least invite systematic and reasoned response. This collection should help practitioners carry on a useful discussion with both colleagues and public.

Finally, and most generally, because AIDS threatens us all, and because all of us in our lifetimes are likely to be consumers of many professional services, we believe this book should concern every informed member of society, layperson and professional alike.

The remainder of the Introduction is divided into three parts. The first offers a primer on AIDS. The next explains the connection between

AIDS and the field now generally known as "professional ethics." The last provides a critical survey of each of the book's chapters.

Some Facts About AIDS

"AIDS" is the acronym for acquired immune deficiency syndrome. During the 1980s, AIDS emerged as a leading cause of death among young adults in the United States. Using current trends, the Centers for Disease Control (CDC) predict that the disease will continue to spread rapidly during the 1990s.[1] While most reported deaths in the 1980s occurred among intravenous drug users and gay men, the number of reported AIDS cases is rapidly increasing in the general population.[2]

AIDS is caused by the human immunodeficiency virus (HIV). HIV's core consists of two strands of RNA, structural proteins, and an enzyme called "reverse transcriptase." When the virus enters the body, it attacks the T-cells of the immune system. These are white blood cells, manufactured in the bone marrow, whose central function is to stimulate the production of antibodies to fight infection. Once the virus has injected its core inside a T-cell, reverse transcriptase enables the viral RNA to be copied in the form of viral DNA, which replicates the virus's genetic information. These DNA genes are then integrated into the chromosomes of the host cell, taking genetic control. Protected in this way, the virus can lie dormant for a long time. Activation of the immune system stimulates the host cell to produce more of the virus, which is then released to invade more T-cells. As this process continues, the immune system loses its ability to fight infections.

Because the genetic structure of T-cells harbors the infection, developing a therapeutic option that destroys HIV without also destroying the immune system has proved difficult.[3] One drug that has had some success in slowing the rate at which the virus reproduces is azidothymidine (AZT). AZT works by interfering with the role of reverse transcriptase in producing viral DNA. While not a cure for AIDS, AZT seems to add significantly to the productive life of many patients with AIDS, especially if treatment is begun early.[4]

The most common test for HIV is the enzyme-linked immunoabsorbent assay (ELISA). This test indirectly confirms HIV by directly detecting HIV antibodies. Because of this indirectness, someone with HIV will (falsely) test negative on ELISA if the immune system has not yet produced enough HIV antibodies.

The test's indirectness can also produce the opposite result. Because a newborn baby carries the mother's antibodies, ELISA can give a positive result even if the baby is not actually infected with HIV. ELISA becomes reliable only after about eighteen months, that is, after the baby loses the mother's antibodies. Researchers are looking for a means of testing for HIV that will circumvent this waiting period.[5]

While ELISA is quite reliable, physicians generally do not consider it reliable enough to justify a diagnosis of HIV infection. To be "HIV-seropositive" (that is, for the HIV antibodies to be considered present in one's blood), one must test positive both on a second ELISA and on a more complicated and expensive test, the Western Blot.

To be HIV-seropositive is not necessarily to be sick. Many people with HIV are free of symptoms and may remain so for several years. Their T-cell count may even fall below the normal range of 600 to 1200 without giving them any reason to believe they are infected. Yet they can spread the disease to others in just the way those with symptoms can.

HIV infection is associated with a broad range of symptoms, including diarrhea, swollen lymph nodes, weight loss, fatigue, fever, night sweating, and tuberculosis. These are grouped under the name AIDS-related complex (ARC) rather than AIDS. People with ARC are generally able to carry on normal lives.

A diagnosis of AIDS is made if, and only if, an HIV-seropositive person has certain diseases associated with a severely compromised immune system. These include Kaposi's sarcoma (a type of cancer), *Pneumocystis carinii* (a rare pneumonia), and HIV encephalopathy (a brain disorder that causes cognitive or motor dysfunction). While some people with AIDS live relatively normal lives for a time, these "opportunistic" infections and cancers are eventually fatal.

Sexual intercourse appears to be the primary means by which HIV is spread. While there is evidence that oral–genital sex also transmits HIV, unprotected anal and vaginal sex are the most likely means of sexual transmission. Some studies have shown that latex condoms are effective in preventing the sexual transmission of HIV.[6]

Other confirmed means of transmission are the sharing of contaminated intravenous needles, accidental needle sticks in a medical context, transfusion of contaminated blood or blood products, organ or sperm donorship, and contact between an infected mother and her child during pregnancy or childbirth.

There have also been some case reports pointing to the possibility of other, less common modes of transmission. For example, some reports have suggested that the virus can be spread through contaminated breast milk fed to nursing children.[7] Other reports suggest that a child can infect its mother through breast feeding or through direct contact with the child's blood or feces.[8]

In general, the *frequency* of viral transmissions seems to be a major factor in determining the probability of infection. For example, each stick with a contaminated needle, or each act of unprotected vaginal or anal sex with an infected partner, increases the probability of contracting HIV. This is not, of course, to say that a single such act cannot produce infection. Reported cases of HIV infection include some in which, for example, only one act of sexual intercourse with an infected partner took place.[9] Every exposure to infected body fluids heightens the risk of infection.

HIV is now considered a "pandemic," that is, a disease simultaneously epidemic in more than one region of the world. "AIDS" names the climactic stage of that disease and (at the risk of confusion) the disease as a whole. Our use of the term "AIDS" in the title of this book reflects this double meaning.

AIDS and Professional Ethics

As the title suggests, this collection is about problems that AIDS (or, more precisely, HIV) poses for "professional ethics." But what is professional ethics? Since "ethics" has several different senses, let's begin with a discussion of these.

In one sense, ethics is the *descriptive study of morality*. Ethics (in this sense) might attempt to describe alternative ways that can be or have been used to deal with a particular moral problem, the arguments that have been marshaled on their behalf, and even the actual consequences of each alternative put into practice. Ethics of this descriptive variety does not attempt to justify any alternative (or even to explain why one is better than another). Ethics in this sense takes a hard but impartial view.

While this is not the primary sense in which ethics is used in this collection, it is nonetheless a part of many of the chapters. For example, much of what Al Gini and Michael Davis do in "AIDS in the Workplace" is to report the different policies employers have adopted to deal with their HIV-seropositive employees.

"Ethics" can also mean the *philosophical study of morality*. In this sense, ethics includes—along with the impartial description of alternatives—an attempt to show one (or more) of the alternatives to be morally permissible, morally required, or morally prohibited (or morally better or worse). "Philosophical" signals a focus on reasoning, the analysis of key terms, and the clarification of issues, all with the purpose of winning for one position the rational support of those concerned. "Moral" signals that those concerned are (at least) all the rational agents whom the decision might affect. It is in this sense, for example, that ethics would attempt to determine whether a nurse has a moral obligation to care for AIDS patients. This is the primary sense in which "ethics" is used in this book.

Ethics—as the philosophical study of morality—has two distinct but related branches. There is, first, *ethical theory*, the attempt to formulate and defend a general criterion (or set of criteria) for distinguishing the morally right from the morally wrong (or the morally better from the morally worse).

At least two historically important ethical theories (or, more exactly, two families of theory) may be relevant here. One has often been called "utilitarian ethics" (or "consequentialism"). According to this theory, an act is morally right if, and only if, doing it will do at least as much to maximize overall happiness or welfare as doing any alternative. The other theory is often called "Kantian ethics" (after its greatest defender, the German philosopher Immanuel Kant) or "deontologism." According to this theory, an act is morally right if, and only if, it treats human beings as "ends in themselves" (or "autonomous" beings) rather than as "mere means." To treat human beings as ends in themselves is to treat them as rational agents who, being capable of following standards they themselves endorse, must always be treated in accordance with such standards.[10]

The second branch of the philosophical study of morality is now commonly called *applied ethics*. Applied ethics is concerned not with general criteria of right conduct but with specific issues of right conduct (for example, whether abortion is morally permissible). Applied ethics is (in part) an opportunity to put ethical theory to work on practical problems. Insofar as professional ethics is concerned with moral issues of practical importance for professionals, professional ethics is a field of applied ethics. This book constitutes work in applied ethics.

The connection between ethical theory and applied ethics is controversial but important. Both utilitarianism and Kantianism may (and often do) have a role in applied ethics. Either may provide a framework for the justification (or criticism) of a course of action. For example, some of the contributions to this collection use the right to privacy to argue against mandatory HIV testing of health providers or patients. But why accept the premise that there is such a (morally defensible) right? Why suppose such a right could contribute to a decisive argument against mandatory testing? Both utilitarianism and Kantianism offer answers for these questions.

A utilitarian answer to the first question would be: privacy is a right because (and only because) recognizing privacy as a moral requirement serves the general happiness or welfare. The Kantian answer might be: allowing people to control personal information regarding their own health is a necessary condition of respecting them as "ends in themselves"; to force people to reveal such information would therefore treat them as "mere means" for the benefit of others; hence, people have a moral right to such control, a right to privacy.

Of course, neither the utilitarian nor the Kantian answer can be accepted as just stated. Each would require a defense turning (in part) on controversial factual assumptions (for example, for utilitarians, on claims about the effect of a certain policy on the general happiness; for Kantians, on claims about what it is rational to want). In general, ethical theories are not substitutes for empirical knowledge but tools for helping us make sense of what we know (and for identifying what we need to find out).

Ethical theories not only provide strategies for defending general rights, they also provide strategies for making exceptions to, overriding, or ignoring those rights in particular cases. For example, both utilitarian and Kantian theories suggest a justification for making an exception to the right to privacy.

Consider utilitarianism first. Assume that the health information in question could be shown to reduce substantially the probability of someone becoming infected with HIV. Considerations of general welfare might then justify overriding the right to privacy this time. Whether general welfare does in fact justify overriding the right would, of course, depend on other facts, for example, how such violations of privacy would affect the willingness of people to be tested for HIV and how that would affect the progress of the disease.

Though Kantian ethics tends to depend less on particular facts than utilitarian ethics does, it too must take the facts into account. Treating people with respect means taking their interests into account as they would at their rational best. Part of being at one's rational best is considering the consequences of any standard of conduct one is asked to endorse. So, even for Kantian ethics, the facts may sometimes justify making an exception to a general right. Rational agents may well prefer a standard of conduct allowing exceptions in certain cases (for example, to save a life) to an exceptionless standard (for example, "Respect privacy at all costs"). Morality is not a suicide pact. (Of course, showing that mandatory testing for HIV fits in—or does not fit in—under one of these exceptions also depends on facts as well as on theory.)

Not all facts relevant to how professionals should respond to HIV are necessarily facts about HIV. Professions are a social undertaking, so social facts may also be important. Three sorts of social fact seem especially relevant to professional ethics: first, facts about the individuals involved in a particular situation (for example, that this client is depending on this lawyer); second, facts about social roles, functions, or expectations (for example, the fact that the public expects lawyers to keep confidences in a situation like this); and third, the standards of conduct a profession has imposed on itself (for example, what the code of ethics requires of lawyers in a situation like this).

The first sort of social fact is common ground between professions, quasi professions, and ordinary occupations. Ordinary moral standards apply to everyone. Without them, there would be no reason to talk about ethics (and so no reason to talk about professional ethics). Several of the chapters in this book treat applied ethics in this way. While one might expect such a treatment in a discussion concerned with business, like that of Gini and Davis, it is also the way in which, for example, Albert Flores determines the obligations of physicians. The standards he appeals to (privacy, avoiding harm, and so on) are (or, at least, seem to be) standards binding on all of us, not simply on physicians.

The second sort of social fact, one's social role, does seem to impose special standards of conduct. For example, a physician may, by law, have the obligation to report to the public health department any occurrence of a certain disease, an obligation the ordinary citizen does not have. Such special obligations are, however, not unique to professionals. For example, a restaurant owner may also have special obligations concerning public health such as the obligation to make employees wash their hands before they handle food.

While some terms of a social role may be embodied in law, licensing regulation, or other formal statement, many may not be. For example, the public seems to expect more confidentiality from journalists than the law does. Social roles are generally ambiguous, that is, open to widely different interpretations. This ambiguity makes appeal to social role seem a deceptively easy form of argument. Those who appeal to social roles generally have two burdens to carry before they can consider their argument complete. One is to show that, indeed, the role in question does carry such an obligation. The other is that the obligation thus established outweighs other considerations. Appeal to social roles is a legitimate move in moral argument, not a substitute for such argument.

One way to think about a profession is as a group (but not the only group) from which we ("society") expect conduct morally better than we expect from ordinary people. If these (social) expectations are morally relevant, professionals may have moral responsibilities others in the same position would not have. The clearest example of such a role analysis is Howard Cohen's discussion of the quasi profession of university administrator.

The third sort of social fact likely to be relevant to discussions of professional ethics is the profession's own code of ethics. Such a code explicitly sets standards for members of the profession. Generally, such codes ask more of members than ordinary morality does. Thus, such standards should, it seems, impose moral responsibilities that members of the profession would not otherwise have. Interestingly, only five of the chapters—those by Michael Davis, Kenneth Kipnis, Elliot Cohen, Martin Gunderson, and Michael Pritchard—make explicit reference to a profession's code. Such references are strikingly absent from Flores's discussion of physicians and from Joan Callahan and Jill Powell's discussion of nurses. Is that absence an indication that codes of ethics are in fact not that important to professional ethics? Or an indication of something else (for example, the failure of the relevant codes to provide any guidance)?[11]

Survey of the Chapters

In "AIDS: Moral Dilemmas for Physicians," Flores examines three hard questions that AIDS has raised for physicians: Should the medical practice of HIV-seropositive physicians be restricted? Should there be mandatory HIV testing for physicians? Should HIV-seropositive physicians disclose their HIV status to patients?

The questions are, of course, related. A policy of restricting the practice of HIV-seropositive physicians or forcing them to disclose their HIV status is likely to be ineffective without mandatory testing to determine who is HIV-seropositive. It is therefore significant that Flores finds much to object to in mandatory testing. First, from the perspective of law and ethics, mandatory HIV testing clearly violates a person's right to privacy. Second, mandatory testing implies a violation of informed consent. Physicians are forced to submit to medical tests on pain of losing their jobs. Third, HIV-seropositive physicians do not appear to constitute a serious health risk. This last claim is central to his argument.

Given the extremely low risk of an HIV-seropositive physician infecting a patient, Flores concludes, "It seems a gross overreaction to mandate HIV testing of all physicians without at the same time legitimizing wholesale violations of physicians' rights."

Flores's argument rests on at least three assumptions. The first is that universal precautions are diligently observed. The second is that mandatory HIV testing cannot be justified on a limited basis. The third is that the only risk to patients whose physicians are HIV-seropositive is from transmission of the virus itself and not from other factors related to HIV infection (for example, fatigue).

Callahan and Powell raise serious doubts about each of these assumptions in "Nurses and AIDS: Some Special Challenges," an examination of some of the ways the HIV epidemic has affected nursing. This examination leads them to consider, among other issues, whether nurses have a right to refuse to provide care for HIV-seropositive patients and whether there should be mandatory HIV testing of nurses (and other health-care providers).

Citing CDC statistics, Callahan and Powell argue that the risk of HIV transmission through occupational accidents such as needle sticks is significantly increased when hospitals (or others employing nurses) fail to establish mandatory safety procedures, fail to enforce them, or fail to provide the resources necessary to follow them. According to Callahan and Powell, nurses may then justifiably refuse to care for HIV-seropositive patients—but *only* as a means of forcing their employers to protect employees, practitioners, volunteers, and, ultimately, patients. Nurses are not otherwise entitled to refuse to treat patients with HIV. This position thus differs from that of Flores only for cases in which the hospital (or other institution) fails to maintain a reasonably safe working environment.

Callahan and Powell's position on mandatory testing of nurses for HIV is also somewhat more modulated than Flores's position on testing of physicians. While there are moral, medical, and fiscal reasons against such a general policy, mandatory testing may, they argue, still be justified in certain circumstances, for example, when a needle sticks a nurse and then a patient.

Callahan and Powell also discuss the case of David Acer, an HIV-seropositive dentist who infected at least six of his patients with HIV. According to CDC researchers, the transmissions may have been due to accidents during invasive dental procedures. (Acer frequently suffered HIV-related fatigue when working.) Callahan and Powell argue that Acer's failure to discontinue performing procedures he was no longer able to perform competently was largely due to a health-care system that fails to provide "reasonable accommodations" for competence-compromised HIV-seropositive providers.

Some may wish to draw a different conclusion from the idea of HIV-related incompetence. Since the professional competence of HIV-seropositive health-care providers, including both nurses and physicians, may be compromised by their illness, recipients of their health care may be placed at additional risk beyond that of HIV transmission. (For instance, an HIV-seropositive surgeon may suffer cognitive or motor impairments, magnifying the usual surgical risks as well as adding the risk of HIV transmission through accidents that expose the patient to the surgeon's blood.) Does the patient's right to informed consent require information regarding the HIV status of his or her health-care providers? Do health-care institutions, as part of their "special duties" to patients, have a duty to maintain surveillance on any factors that could substantially affect the quality of the patient's health care? These questions certainly suggest a possible justification for mandatory HIV testing.

Still, as Flores reminds us, the risk of harm to the patient must be weighed against the health-care provider's right to privacy. Since the competence of HIV-seropositive professionals may not be compromised by their illness (they may, for example, be asymptomatic), mandatory HIV testing could not reasonably be used as a decisive test of professional competence—and hence as a reliable indicator of risk to patients. To say otherwise opens the door to systematic abuse of the rights of HIV-seropositive health-care providers who are still competent.

In "The Dentist's Obligation to Treat Patients with HIV," Davis defends the position that, under the present dental-care system, dentists have a professional obligation to give dental care to patients with HIV. Beginning with an analysis of the general concept of a profession, Davis argues that, like other professions, dentistry is defined in part by its code of ethics. This code—the American Dental Association's Principles of Ethics, together with its Code of Professional Conduct and Advisory Opinions—calls for dentists to serve "the public," that is, anyone in need of dental care, including HIV-seropositive patients. Since the dental profession, as defined, is a morally good but burdensome practice (that is, one performing a morally good function by imposing special duties on dentists), dentists who refuse to treat patients with HIV are helping to undermine the practice while still voluntarily reaping the benefits it produces. They are, in effect, taking unfair advantage of those colleagues who still shoulder burdens as the code requires.

Davis's argument, unlike that of Callahan and Powell, does not depend on showing that the risk of HIV transmission from patient to practitioner is insignificant. According to Davis, even if, contrary to fact, the risk of an HIV-seropositive patient infecting a dentist were small, but still significant, the dentist would still have the same obligation. "The argument for treating a patient with HIV," he contends, "does not depend on such inherently changeable data [as that of risks]."

But what if (hypothetically speaking) an HIV-seropositive patient posed a serious and generally recognized risk of infection to other patients? Could a dentist then justly refuse to take HIV-seropositive patients (without first changing the dentists' code of ethics)? Undoubtedly, many patients would avoid dentists if they had good reason to think that the odds of becoming infected with HIV in a dentist's office were substantial (as high, say, as one in twenty). Indeed, except for very serious emergencies, it would then, arguably, be more rational to take one's chances without receiving dental treatment or to attempt home remedies instead. Then, unless dentists were prepared to relinquish their monopoly on the provision of dental care or to make special provisions for the care of patients with HIV, the goal of providing service to all in need would be defeated—notwithstanding that patients with HIV would receive dental care. It is, perhaps, at this juncture that Davis's argument does, after all, depend on facts about the risk of infection.

Or perhaps it does not. As Davis recognizes, differential dental care of patients with HIV presupposes the ability to identify and distinguish those with HIV from those without it. Unless mandatory HIV testing is made a prerequisite to dental care (testing capable of giving a definitive result on the day it is administered), how likely is it that dentists will be able to identify all patients with HIV? After all, as Davis points out, many patients with HIV may not know that they have the disease. Of those who do know, how many would tell their dentist if they thought the likely consequence of candor would be stigma, inferior care, or outright refusal of care? So, routine dental care of some (and perhaps many) HIV-seropositive patients will probably occur regardless of what other provisions are made.

What then should a dentist do about a patient who worries that the fingers about to be put in his mouth may just have been in the mouth of someone known to have HIV? Davis suggests that the patient be told that there is no significant risk of infection because the dentist uses proper infection control. Should that satisfy the patient? Why should a patient not worry that the dentist who protects herself by wearing rubber gloves may still fail to change those gloves between patients?

As Callahan and Powell note, nurses and physicians do not always follow universal precautions. The same may be true of some dentists. Since dentists typically have private practices, monitoring their infection control is harder than in large institutions such as hospitals. (For example, we still do not know whether Dr. Acer infected at least six patients by failing to follow proper infection control procedures or in some other way.) This suggests that patients may need to be more informed consumers of dental services.

"HIV and the Professional Responsibility of the Early Childhood Educator" shifts the focus from hospitals to preschools. Kipnis considers two questions: Should an HIV-infected child be permitted to attend preschool? If the child is permitted to attend, should the parents of the other children be informed?

Kipnis approaches the first question by considering two arguments for excluding HIV-infected children from preschool. Both rely on the Code of Ethical Conduct of the National Association for the Education of Young Children—a code Kipnis helped draft. The code (Principle 1.1) explicitly forbids any practice that harms or endangers children.

The first argument is "paternalistic." Since exposure to the disease-causing microorganisms common in preschools can be detrimental to an HIV-seropositive child whose immune system has been significantly compromised, admitting such a child to preschool risks harm to that child. So, HIV-infected children should be denied admission for their own good. To this argument, Kipnis responds that risks to the child from attending must be weighed against the benefits of attending, that the people best placed to do such weighing are the child's parents and physicians, and that therefore the decision is outside the purview of preschool administrators.

The other argument for excluding children with HIV is concerned with protecting children without HIV. If attendance of an HIV-infected child poses a danger to the other children in the preschool, the school's director has a professional obligation to disallow attendance. Noting that the argument clearly depends on the premise that the HIV-seropositive child poses a risk of infection to others, Kipnis considers whether the premise is true.

Carefully examining the evidence concerning both standard and nonstandard modes of transmission, Kipnis rejects this premise. He concludes that it is highly unlikely that the presence of an infected child could ever pose a significant risk to other children, so admitting HIV-infected children to preschool does not violate Principle 1.1.

(Kipnis does, however, qualify this conclusion with some recommendations for the reduction of any risks posed by biting behavior and bleeding.)

That makes answering Kipnis's second question easy: since the contact that children are likely to have in preschool is not associated with any known risk of infection, parents need not (and, therefore, for reasons of confidentiality, should not) be informed that their child has had contact with an HIV-infected child.

Unlike Davis's primary argument, Kipnis's arguments clearly depend on adequate risk assessment. Here, however, it might be well to recall Davis's caution that we have become suspicious of official evaluations of risk since risk is often underrated at first. Especially when the lives in question are those of children, who are not competent to decide for themselves, appeals to official reports concerning risks seem to lose some of their persuasiveness.

Nor is the matter resolvable by appeal to the facts alone. The conclusion that no significant risk exists is not a purely descriptive statement. What constitutes a significant risk is not a question that can be settled empirically. It includes an *appraisal* of the risk. Indeed, Kipnis explicitly makes such an appraisal: "I therefore propose that the dangers contemplated by Principle 1.1 must be supported, at the very least, by at least one anecdotal report." Kipnis also assumes that when the known risk fails to cross some very low threshold, early childhood educators may disregard it. Since Kipnis acknowledges at least some anecdotal evidence for HIV infection through biting, his argument must depend (in part) on whether the risks in question are appraised as negligible (that is, *properly* neglected) in a preschool context.

Unlike Flores (and unlike Callahan and Powell), Kipnis does not appeal to the rights of HIV-seropositive individuals (for example, their right to privacy or to self-determination). What are we to make of that? Does Kipnis simply believe that the risks of infecting other children are too small to worry about? Or is a rights argument left implicit, or made unnecessary by appeal to the profession's code? There must, it seems, be more to his argument. After all, unless the HIV-infected child has an overriding right to a preschool experience, any risk, however small, to other children would, it seems, invoke the right to be protected from harm and thereby override any mere interest a child with HIV has in attending preschool.

In "AIDS in the Workplace: Options and Responsibilities," Gini and Davis explore some key questions HIV raises for business managers: How should employees with HIV be treated? What should be done to promote employee awareness about AIDS and to insure safety and morale? How should a manager balance legal and moral interests of employees against business interests?

Gini and Davis are not primarily concerned to argue for any particular answer. Their goals are to describe alternative options and strategies for answering the above questions, to clarify the stakes, and to structure what originally might seem overwhelmingly complex.

Gini and Davis begin with the case of a manager of a hospital cafeteria who has just been told that a cook she is considering for promotion has AIDS. What, they ask, are the key issues for managers in this or similar contexts? The current lack of evidence that HIV can be spread through casual personal contact suggests, they argue, that although AIDS is a health issue, the issue is not one of contagion. Fear has prevented many businesses from formulating explicit policies for dealing with employees who have HIV. Fear makes poor policy.

On the positive side, Gini and Davis emphasize that, under the 1991 Americans with Disabilities Act (ADA), a legally sanctioned trend toward discrimination against employees with HIV has been reversed. Employees with HIV are now considered "disabled" and receive the same treatment under law as other disabled persons. Here we might wonder whether there is, nonetheless, some *relevant* difference between, say, an asymptomatic carrier of HIV and a paraplegic. Should HIV be legally classified as a disability in the first place?

Gini and Davis describe some possible options that businesses have adopted in dealing with employees with HIV. These options include guaranteeing full salary and benefits provided the employee does not return to work, relying on general health policies (rather than a specific HIV policy), and formulating a specific HIV policy.

Each of these options may raise moral, legal, and practical questions. Each has disadvantages as well as advantages. Managers need, therefore, to think carefully before adopting any particular option. For example, while paying salaries and benefits to employees with HIV if they do not come to work may relieve other employees of many of their fears, it also caters to the hysteria surrounding AIDS, encouraging discrimination against persons with HIV. The practice may also serve to undermine the dignity and morale of employees with HIV by ostracizing them and by depriving them of meaningful, productive activity. And, as Gini and Davis note, the legality of this option remains to be determined.

On the other hand, while relying on general policies instead of a specific AIDS policy may allow for greater "flexibility" in addressing HIV cases, it may also overlook important differences between HIV and such illnesses as cancer and heart disease. For instance, the hysteria surrounding AIDS has increased the need for AIDS education for all employees as well as for AIDS support groups or counseling for employees who have HIV or who know someone who does. A few major companies that have adopted specific HIV policies have included provisions for education and counseling.

Gini and Davis claim that, for managers, AIDS is not a contagion issue. Should their claim be construed to mean that company policy aimed at reducing the risk of HIV transmission to employees or to customers is unnecessary? Suppose, for example, that a restaurant were to require all food handlers to wear sanitized gloves or to cover with clean gauze any open, oozing wound on arm or hand. Would such a policy be unreasonable? If, as Gini and Davis say, "the real import of a carefully rendered AIDS policy" is to "[demonstrate] to workers, suppliers, and customers alike that management cares not only about the continued success of its business but also about the well-being of its employees and the people the company serves," should not such a policy include precautions of this sort?

While the manager of a hospital cafeteria may seem to have little in common with a senior administrator in a university, Howard Cohen's "Leading by Example: AIDS Policy and the University's Social Responsibilities" suggests otherwise. Cohen begins with three cases. In Case 1, the dean of a college considers whether to force an assistant professor with AIDS to go on disability rather than to continue missing classes. In Case 2, the president of a private, church-affiliated university must decide whether to accept a large gift for the reading program, a gift contingent on the university withdrawing recognition of a student group that has been distributing condoms on campus. In Case 3, a vice-president for student affairs must decide whether to help a student, fired from his job in a university cafeteria because he has HIV, bring a discrimination suit against the independent food service that runs the cafeteria under contract to the university.

Cohen, himself a senior administrator, takes considerable time pointing out how each of these cases pulls the decisionmaker in several different directions. None of the three cases seems to lend itself to a "creative" solution that would satisfy everyone. Each presents a genuinely hard choice among options each of which has both advantages and disadvantages. Indeed, each requires giving up something morally important. In this respect, Cohen's cases resemble the case Gini and Davis discuss. Yet, Cohen's discussion represents an important advance over that of Gini and Davis. Where Gini and Davis seem satisfied to clarify issues, Cohen offers a procedure for resolving them.

For each case, Cohen suggests, we should first identify all the relevant considerations, that is, all the various "tugs" or interests we feel, including the claims of our social roles. We should then categorize those interests. Which are merely personal? Which belong to our office? Which arise from the institution? Which arise from our status as human beings? Each successive category has priority over the one before because each is more "general." For example, applying his method to Case 3, we immediately see, according to Cohen, that the vice-president should ignore any personal distaste for, or admiration of, the student pressing for an investigation until the interests of the institution have been satisfied.

Though Cohen's method apparently leads to an attractive solution in each case he poses, we are left to wonder about both the method's generality and its defensibility. For example, will his method work in an ordinary business like Gini and Davis's cafeteria or in a professional context like Kipnis's preschool? Or is there something about universities in particular that makes it seem to work there? Could it be that the manager of a business is not morally required to satisfy the general interest before satisfying the interests of the business, or that a preschool administrator is morally required to protect the children in her care before paying heed to any other interest?

These questions suggest that Cohen needs to justify his method (as well as explain it), to show that general interests should always take priority over narrower interests (or, at least, to show that a certain class of such interests do).

While the chapters so far considered generally avoid such forays into ethical theory, the next does not. In "What Would a Virtuous Counselor Do?" Elliot Cohen develops a conception of the virtues of a counselor, defends it by appeal to a utilitarian argument, and then applies that conception to resolve some hard cases. Cohen thus relies on ethical theory in his method of reaching practical solutions.

Counselors learn much about their clients (in part) because the clients suppose that what they say will be kept confidential. Occasionally, however, counselors think they should reveal what they have learned, either to another individual (for example, the client's spouse) or to a public agency (for example, the police). Such disclosure may, in fact, be sanctioned by law and codes of ethics. In some cases, however, neither law nor code provides clear guidance. Cohen's discussion concerns three such cases. In one, a client with HIV tells a counselor that he is regularly having unprotected sex with his unknowing fiancée. In the second case, the client with HIV tells the counselor that he is having unprotected sex with anonymous (and unknowing) "pickups." In the third, the counselor is counseling both husband and wife. During one session, when the wife is not present, the husband informs the counselor that he has been having anonymous unprotected sex with pickups, that he has not told his wife (with whom he is also having unprotected sex), and that he has not been tested for HIV. What, Cohen asks, should the counselor do in each case?

Cohen begins his answer to that question by asking what virtues (fixed dispositions to think, feel, and act) counselors should embody. Cohen then considers what he calls the "fiduciary model," the "autonomy model," and the "welfare model" of the virtuous counselor.

The *fiduciary model* recognizes that counseling depends on trust. The good counselor should therefore have the virtues that justify trust. These are honesty (to the client), candor (to the client), competence (in treating the client), benevolence (to the client), diligence (for the client), loyalty (to the client), and discretion (concerning the client's affairs). While admitting that these virtues are necessary for a good (or virtuous) counselor, Cohen argues that they are insufficient. By themselves, they demand a kind of fanaticism, for example, benevolence toward the client even if the whole world suffers as a result. The American Counseling Association (ACA) has explicitly rejected this conception of counseling. The counselor is not to be a mere instrument of the client's interests.

The *autonomy model* (which Cohen attributes to psychotherapist Carl Rogers) selects the counselor's virtues by considering what dispositions a counselor needs to enable clients to become independent, autonomous persons. Cohen identifies three: congruence, unconditional positive regard, and empathetic understanding. He argues that each of these dispositions is needed to increase clients' self-understanding, freedom, self-reliance, and willingness to take responsibility for their own thoughts and feelings.

The *welfare model* departs from the other two by directly taking account of more than the client. According to this model, a disposition of a counselor is a virtue if counselors "as such" must have the disposition "to maximize human welfare."

This model is the one that most satisfies Cohen since it provides a criterion for limiting the virtues recognized in the other two models while still admitting them as virtues. So, for example, loyalty to the client is good insofar as it contributes to the trust on which successful counseling depends. (Counseling, after all, tends to improve human welfare.) But loyalty that knows no bounds tends to harm the general welfare more than it helps; therefore, such extreme loyalty is no virtue.

Having defined a set of virtues, Cohen attempts to show that they resolve (or help resolve) the hard cases with which he began. For the first case, for example, Cohen suggests that the counselor (out of concern for human welfare) first urge the client to inform his fiancée of the risk of HIV infection. If the client refuses to do as urged, the counselor should remind him of something the counselor said during their first meeting, that is, that the risk of serious harm to others is one of the grounds for violating confidentiality. If the client still refuses to inform his fiancée, the counselor should do it himself. But the counselor is to do all this in a way calculated to show respect for the client as a person and to avoid rupture of the relationship.

Does anything in this solution require appeal to the virtues of a counselor? Could the same result have been reached, for example, from an interpretation of the code of ethics of the ACA (in the manner of Kipnis or Davis)? Or by appeal to the most general interests (in the manner of Howard Cohen)? What advantage is there to Elliot Cohen's appeal to ethical theory? Is his method easier to use or more convincing?

Elliot Cohen argues that his virtues approach is appropriate to counseling ethics since it can deal effectively with emotional and attitudinal dimensions of counseling, such as those related to empathy, benevolence, congruence, and unconditional positive regard. In this respect, he considers a virtues approach to be more appropriate than one appealing primarily to rules found in codes of ethics. But if this is true of counseling, is it also true of other professions for which the professional–client relation is important, if not essential? For example, would a virtues approach be the best model for understanding nursing ethics? Would it work best as a model for understanding the physician–patient relation?

Martin Gunderson's chapter, "The Attorney, the Client with HIV, and the Duty to Warn," resembles Elliot Cohen's in at least three respects. First, it concerns counseling, though legal rather than psychological counseling. Second, Gunderson's lawyer, like Cohen's counselor, must resolve an apparent conflict between a duty to maintain confidences and a duty to warn. And third, like Cohen, Gunderson cannot resolve the conflict without thinking carefully about the purpose of the duties in conflict, especially about their role in defining a morally good (or at least a morally defensible) practice.

There are, however, important differences between the two chapters. Some of these differences are, no doubt, simply byproducts of the different interests of the two authors. For example, Gunderson, a lawyer (as well as a philosopher), takes some pains to define the legal liability to which a lawyer might expose herself both by revealing a client confidence to protect a third party and by failing to reveal the confidence if the third party is subsequently harmed because she failed to act. Cohen's counselor (and any other professional confronting a conflict between the duty to maintain confidence and the duty to warn) would, it seems, benefit from Gunderson's discussion here.

Other differences in the two chapters seem to be the product of something more fundamental than differences in interest. Gunderson never explicitly discusses virtues in the way Cohen does. His discussion of the attorney's role takes only a few pages, much of it concerned with comparing (and contrasting) the lawyer's role with that of physician or psychotherapist. Of special importance for Gunderson is that the lawyer alone belongs to an adversarial profession, that is, a profession that must always "work with an eye to adversarial proceedings" in which today's "third party" may be tomorrow's "other party." Once revealed, a confidence may not only harm the client but harm the very case on which the lawyer is working. (A disclosure of HIV infection might, for example, destroy any chance of winning custody of children after a divorce.) Is Gunderson assuming that a lawyer is necessarily a fiduciary (in Elliot Cohen's sense)? Or would a lawyer's situation be much the same even if we thought of lawyers along the lines of the human welfare model?

Instead of outlining the virtues a good lawyer should have Gunderson tries to identify, explain, and evaluate all the considerations relevant to a decision to breach confidence for the purpose of warning a third party. Gunderson begins with the lawyer's code of ethics (the American Bar Association's Model Rules of Professional Conduct). The code provides a framework for thinking about the duty to maintain confidences and the duty to warn. Unfortunately, while settling many questions, it does not settle Gunderson's.

Since (as Gunderson suggests) the law is also more or less silent about how to resolve Gunderson's question, a lawyer deciding whether to warn a third party of the risk of HIV infection has to take moral (and practical) considerations into account. She will not be able to treat disclosure as a "purely" legal question. Gunderson devotes most of his chapter to pointing out and explaining the moral (and practical) considerations a lawyer should take into account.

In this respect, Gunderson's chapter resembles that of Howard Cohen. Yet it differs from his in one important respect. Gunderson expressly denies that an obvious or mechanical way exists to weigh all of the factors against each other. General considerations do not necessarily take precedence over more parochial ones; (minor) moral considerations do not necessarily take precedence over (major) considerations of self-interest. In this respect, Gunderson's method is closer to that of Gini and Davis. Indeed, Gunderson observes: "It is still an open question whether any [ethical] theory [e.g., consequentialist or deontological] can succeed in finding a principle that can be used to weigh all of these factors against one another." What might Howard Cohen (or Elliot Cohen) respond?

In "AIDS: A Transformative Challenge for Clergy," Joseph Edelheit reminds us of another range of considerations. Like psychologists and lawyers, clergy act as counselors; and like psychologists and lawyers, they learn much in confidence and must sometimes choose between betraying a confidence and preventing harm. But ministers, priests, rabbis, pastors, imams, and other clergy must speak for more than mental health, legal rights, and other merely temporal concerns (the nature of this "more" varying somewhat from religion to religion). How can the clergy resolve the conflicts generated by the clash between religious tradition and the AIDS pandemic? How can they resolve the conflict between their tradition and secular morality?

Traditions are, by definition, behind the times. They are practices, teachings, and modes of feeling the past "hands over" to the present. They carry authority (in part at least) because they have passed through so many hands more or less unchanged. Yet all traditions, including religious traditions, either change with the times or die. How can a religious tradition both hand over the past and yet speak to the present? That in essence is Edelheit's problem. Though himself a representative of one religious tradition, Reform Judaism, Edelheit attempts an "ecumenical" answer, one good at least across Christian and Jewish traditions.

Edelheit begins by describing the many ways HIV has affected what clergy do or, more exactly, the choices they must make about what they do. What AIDS does, he argues, is present at particularly uncompromising challenge to certain traditional ways of dealing with "sin." Seldom has the clergy had as stark a choice between life and death. In this respect, AIDS resembles the holocaust.

Like several others in this collection, Edelheit does not argue directly for a particular resolution of the problems he discusses. Instead, he cuts off certain easy ways around the problem ("denials"), encourages the reader to get as close to the facts (and especially to the people involved) as circumstances allow, and then points out considerations that should weigh heavily in any decision the reader makes. He also suggests that choosing under such conditions will be "transformative," whatever the actual outcome.

In a collection in which abstract arguments play so large a part,

Edelheit makes a useful point about the role concrete actions have both in giving insight and in changing what we think. Virtue is as much the product of intelligent choice as right choice is the product of virtue. But for Edelheit, this point has a larger significance. It is the key to how religious tradition can change while handing over the past intact. If one chooses from "within" the tradition, confronting the sacred texts as well as today's facts, one's perception of the tradition (and of the rest of the world, too) may change. The old texts may yield new interpretations; old beliefs, new applications.

For those with religious commitments different from his, Edelheit's new perception of tradition may seem to abandon the sacred texts rather than reinterpret them. Yet these readers cannot challenge Edelheit without justifying their own interpretation of the texts. There are, it seems, only three methods of justification open to them, none without difficulty.

First, they could adopt Edelheit's method. They would then have to work with people suffering from AIDS (as Edelheit did) before saying anything more. Edelheit's method is demanding.

Second, those objecting to Edelheit's conclusions could appeal to "nature" to reveal God's intent when the sacred texts seem unclear. But then they would face the daunting task of explaining how we are to divine God's will in nature. After all, no one supposes black lung disease to be God's punishment for digging coal from the depths of the earth. Why then suppose that AIDS is God's punishment for engaging in anal intercourse or taking illegal drugs by syringe?

Third, those inclined to appeal to the "clear" language of the Bible face a similar problem making out an objection to Edelheit. What, for example, are we to make of the story of Lot at Sodom? The story has traditionally been considered a condemnation of homosexuality, so much so that "sodomite" has come to refer to one who engages in anal intercourse. Yet, as philosopher Richard Mohr suggests, the text itself seems to identify inhospitality as "the sin of Sodom."[12] In any case, whatever method is used to interpret the story of Sodom will have to be applied to other biblical stories, including the story of unpunished incest by which Lot's daughters begot Moab and Benammi upon a father whom they had made drunk for that purpose soon after they fled Sodom. If destruction of Sodom is proof that God condemns sodomy, why is the story of Lot's daughters not proof that God approves of incest or drunken sex?

For Edelheit, the sanctity of human life itself provides a common thread binding past religious traditions to future ones, thereby permitting a coherent transformation. But will those clergy who resist such a transformation find at least as compelling grounds for adhering to established traditions? Will they eventually be persuaded to yield to Edelheit's new perception?

This last question is fundamental since religious traditions require consensus. The answer may be the most important factor in determining whether many of those with HIV who would not now seek pastoral care will eventually find solace in established religion.

Perhaps Edelheit's clergy resemble Elliot Cohen's virtuous counselors in at least one respect: such clergy do not "stand on ceremony" when human life (human welfare?) hangs in the balance. It often takes courage to oppose authority, be it law or tradition. Yet when law or tradition seems to militate against doing what is right, morally concerned professionals of all kinds may find themselves confronting such hard choices.

We are accustomed to thinking of psychotherapists, lawyers, and clergy as counselors. We generally do not think of journalists that way although in many respects that is what they are. We rely on them for information (both straight news and investigative reporting), insight (interpretation and features), and advice (editorials). Their relation to us is, however, not personal as is the typical relationship of psychotherapists, lawyer, or clergy. We generally do not confide in journalists. Yet sometimes they know (or can find out) something about us we would not want made public. More often, they have information about others we would like to have. In "Journalistic Responsibilities and AIDS," Pritchard considers what journalists should (and should not) publish about HIV (and how they should do it).

At first, the media gave the AIDS story less coverage than similarly mysterious diseases, such as legionnaire's disease, that killed far fewer people. Next, having recognized the story, the media tended (out of a sense of delicacy) to conceal important information by euphemism (for example, "homosexual contact" for "anal sex"). Having given up euphemism, the media still often fail to present the information they have in a useful way. For example, journalists from Ann Landers to George Will seem to have trouble explaining the relative risk of various sorts of conduct (in part perhaps because they do not themselves understand relative risk very well). Pritchard's criticism is, however, mixed with examples of (relative) success and advice on how to do better.

Having devoted most of his chapter to the journalist's failure to inform adequately, Pritchard considers the danger of disclosing too much. He gives two examples. One concerns a (fictional) reporter who learns through friends that a surgeon is HIV-seropositive. Should the reporter publish the story? One reason for publishing the story is that it contains information that the surgeon's patients might want to have. A second is that the story would interest many others (boosting the medium's audience). A third reason is that the scoop would help the reporter's career (at the surgeon's expense).

Pritchard argues that the story probably should not be run. First, he claims, the public's right to know that the surgeon is infected is not clear. Second, even if the surgeon's HIV status did constitute a significant risk of harm to patients, the question would remain whether publicizing her status is the best way to protect her patients. Still, we might wonder (following Howard Cohen) whether the reporter should consider the harm the story will do to a few individuals of secondary import when the public's interest is involved. Shouldn't the public interest come first?

Pritchard's second example, Arthur Ashe, the tennis champion, makes an appealing case for sometimes not reporting a true story of interest to the public if reporting it would harm even one individual.

But Pritchard's examples fall well short of a decisive argument. "After all," a reporter might respond, "as a reporter, my job is to keep the public informed, not to protect people from harm—or, at least, not to keep them from the harm that comes from publishing a true story. True stories are almost always embarrassing to someone, often to many. My job is to inform the public and let the chips fall where they may."

Vincent Samar devotes much of his chapter "AIDS and a Politician's Right to Privacy" to refuting this argument. His reason is worth noting. Samar, himself a former candidate for Chicago's City Council, is concerned with what *politicians* should do about AIDS. One choice they face is whether to reveal their own HIV status. Does the public have a right to know? To answer this question, Samar considers in detail what the news media should (or should not) publish about politicians.

The media are often, it seems, the only way for the public to find out much about politicians; so, in a democracy, what the media tell us about politicians is likely to have a substantial impact on the kind of politicians we have. More information does not necessarily mean better politicians. (Who would run for office if, for example, every candidate had to publish a full-length color photo of him- or herself naked?) All of us, but especially journalists, need to make qualitative judgments about what information should be made public. Neither truth nor public curiosity, nor the two combined, is sufficient to justify publication. What then is? Samar offers a framework for answering that question. Having done that, he moves on to consider what those in office should do about AIDS.

Samar recognizes that information about a politician's life and conduct should be made available to the public—but only that part of the politician's life and conduct that "might bear on future policy decisions." The problem with this standard, argues Samar, is that it would still justify far too much intrusion into a politician's private life. The public's interest in knowing about a politician's life and conduct must be balanced against another public interest, the protection of privacy.

Samar argues that when rights protecting these two interests conflict, the conflict should be resolved in a way that maximizes autonomy. The public has a right to know not what it is merely curious about but only what will help it vote its interests. The politician has a right to keep private only those aspects of life whose exposure would threaten his autonomy more than it would serve the public's.

From these premises, Samar concludes that being HIV-seropositive is not, as such, something the public needs to know, while being in a late stage of AIDS might be. There is a general presumption against making HIV status public because publication of HIV status invites the public to probe too much into central aspects of a politician's life, aspects generally having only a weak connection with how he might vote. The presumption may be overcome in a late stage of AIDS because the public needs to know whether, for example, a candidate has much chance of serving out his term.

Are the premises from which Samar begins correct, however? Can autonomy—even taken to mean simply the right to vote one's interest—supply a satisfactory standard of conflict resolution? Will autonomy itself need on occasion to yield to some further standard, for example, the welfare of the citizens? Does Samar need some moral theory here? Would Elliot Cohen's human welfare model work here?

Samar's analysis of rights based on autonomy sets the stage for his attempt to define the *duties* of politicians with respect to AIDS. Autonomy is as central here as it was in defining politicians' rights. Samar argues that politicians are obligated to formulate policies that rationally and compassionately promote the fundamental rights of those with AIDS as well as those who are as yet uninfected. Furthermore, Samar argues, politicians as individual representatives (rather than as lawmakers) must provide the background expertise necessary for considering controversial public policy issues. They should speak out, helping to change the climate of opinion in which they must make decisions. On this point, Samar's politician seems rather like Edelheit's clergy.

Notes

1. Centers for Disease Control, "Mortality Attributable to HIV Infection/AIDS—United States, 1981–1990," *Morbidity and Mortality Weekly Report* 40, no. 3 (1991).

2. Centers for Disease Control, "Update: Acquired Immunodeficiency Syndrome—United States, 1981–1990." *Morbidity and Mortality Weekly Report* 40, no. 22 (1991): Table 1 (p. 362).

3. Margaret A. Hamburg and Anthony S. Fauci, "HIV Infection and AIDS: Challenges to Biomedical Research," in *AIDS and the Health Care System*, ed. Lawrence O. Gostin (New Haven, Conn.: Yale University Press, 1990), p. 173.

4. "A Ray of Hope in the Fight Against AIDS," *Time* (September 29, 1986): 60–61.

5. Marianne Burgard et al., "The Use of Viral Culture and p24 Antigen Testing to Diagnose Human Immunodeficiency Virus Infection in Neonates," *New England Journal of Medicine* 327, no. 17 (1992): 1192–1197.

6. William H. Masters, Virginia E. Johnson, and Robert C. Kolodny, *Human Sexuality*, 4th ed. (New York: HarperCollins, 1992), p. 156.

7. Jacquelyn Haak Flaskerud, *AIDS/HIV Infection: A Reference Guide for Nursing Professionals* (Philadelphia, Pa.: Saunders, 1989), p. 33.

8. Masters, Johnson, and Kolodny, *Human Sexuality*, p. 512; and Centers for Disease Control, "Apparent Transmission of Human T-lymphotropic Virus Type III/Lymphadenopathy-associated Virus from a Child to a Mother Providing Health Care," *Morbidity and Mortality Weekly Report* 35, no. 5 (1986): 76–79.

9. Masters, Johnson, and Kolodny, *Human Sexuality*, p. 507.

10. For a thorough discussion of these two theories, see Jeffrie Murphy and Jules Coleman, "Utilitarian and Kantian Ethics," in *Philosophers at Work: An Introduction to the Issues and Practical Uses of Philosophy*, ed. Elliot D. Cohen (New York: Holt, Rinehart and Winston, 1989), pp. 14–23.

11. For an extended analysis of professions, see Chapter 3 of this volume.

12. Richard D. Mohr, "Gay Basics: Some Questions, Facts, and Values," in *AIDS: Ethics and Public Policy*, ed. Christine Pierce and Donald VanDeVeer (Belmont, Calif.: Wadsworth, 1988), pp. 198–199.

1

AIDS: Moral Dilemmas
for Physicians

Albert Flores

Since its discovery a little more than a decade ago, acquired immune deficiency syndrome (AIDS) has been responsible for the deaths of over 130,000 Americans, with more than 200,000 currently diagnosed with clinical AIDS, a disease that no one has yet survived.[1] More than one million Americans are infected with the human immunodeficiency virus (HIV), a retrovirus identified in 1983 as the cause of AIDS. HIV destroys the immune system, leaving one vulnerable to opportunistic infections that are often lethal. Recently, the Centers for Disease Control (CDC) reported that AIDS is the second-leading cause of premature death among men ages 25 to 44.[2] The World Health Organization (WHO) estimates that worldwide 2.6 million persons have developed AIDS, and nearly 13 million more are infected with HIV; WHO predicts that by the end of the century up to 110 million of the world's population will be infected with the AIDS virus.[3] As Dr. Jonathan Mann of Harvard University's AIDS Institute and chair of the Eighth International Conference on AIDS said, "The global effort against HIV/AIDS has reached a dangerous impasse," leaving the world "more vulnerable to the spread of HIV."[4]

Given this context, it was not surprising that the public reacted with shock and panic when, in July 1990, the CDC reported the first known case of transmission from an HIV-infected health-care professional—a Florida dentist—to a patient (as a result of removing the patient's wisdom teeth).[5] It was eventually determined that this dentist, who later died of AIDS, had infected a total of six of his patients, although the means of transmission has never been established and still remains a mystery.[6] Kimberly Bergalis, the best known of these patients, who died of AIDS in 1992, became a powerful symbol of the "innocent victim" unknowingly infected by her dentist. Her desperate public pleas for mandatory HIV testing of all health-care professionals and steadfast demands for restrictions on those professionals who test HIV-positive stirred a hornet's nest of controversy that continues unabated today.[7]

Nowhere is this more evident than in the medical profession. The possibility that a patient might be infected by an HIV-positive physician raises important moral dilemmas for medicine that pits the public's right to be safe from harm against the competent physician's legal and professional rights to practice and moral right to privacy. It is well recognized that physicians are required by ethical and professional standards to put their patients' medical needs first, to do them no harm, to obtain their informed consent for medical treatment, and to maintain their trust by upholding high standards of honesty and integrity.[8] Each of these duties suggests a prima facie reason for wondering if restrictions on the clinical practice of HIV-positive physicians are needed to protect the public's health and safety.

While this is a legitimate public concern, it is equally important that we avoid the alarmist response that comes from an exaggerated reaction to the risk of AIDS. While emotionally appealing, calls for punitive social action aimed at restricting the liberty of those who are HIV-positive, including seropositive physicians, nonetheless invite discrimination and tolerate the sacrifice of important civil liberties. Demands for mandatory HIV testing and for restrictions on the liberty of seropositive physicians to practice may be justified only if it can be shown or reasonably inferred that these measures help reduce the risk of HIV infection.

The intensity of this debate suggests several important questions of interest to professional ethics and public policy, questions that will help to structure this discussion. Is there a serious risk of HIV-positive physicians transmitting HIV to their patients? Should the clinical practice of HIV-positive physicians be restricted, or are such restrictions discriminatory? Does the risk of HIV transmission require that physicians submit to periodic, mandatory HIV testing? Should physicians know their HIV status, and do they have an obligation to disclose this information to their patients? And finally, how should we balance the patient's right to know against the physician's right to privacy?

Estimating the Risk of HIV Transmission

Although six dental patients are known to have been infected by a single HIV-positive dentist, to date not one *medical* patient is known to have acquired HIV from a seropositive physician despite millions of clinical procedures and countless hours of physician–patient contact.

Since HIV is transmitted by an exchange of body fluids, the most likely way for a patient to contract HIV is during an invasive surgical procedure wherein transmission of blood occurs due to an accidental puncture injury to the HIV-positive surgeon. Nonetheless, there is a growing consensus that the risk of transmission from an infected practitioner may be exceedingly low, especially when the procedure is noninvasive and when universal precautions—infection control procedures—are scrupulously observed.[9]

In fact, the evidence shows that even in cases of invasive surgical procedures, the risk of contracting HIV remains extremely low. Researchers have conducted a number of so-called look-back studies of over 15,000 patients of thirty-two known HIV-positive physicians, the great majority of whom were surgeons, and no evidence was found that any of these patients were infected with HIV.[10] In another study of an HIV-positive surgeon in Nashville, Tennessee, only 1 of the 616 patients he had operated on tested HIV-positive, but this patient was found to be an intravenous drug user who was seropositive before his surgery; the authors of this study concluded that "the risks to patients operated on by HIV-infected surgeons are most likely quite low."[11]

While such studies are helpful and reassuring, they are far from conclusive, since only a few HIV surgeons have been studied in this way and not always systematically.[12] Look-back studies are also unable to tell us how many patients in a medical setting have actually been exposed to HIV. Moreover, it would hardly be surprising, given the use of universal infection control procedures, that there would be very few infections and then only in clusters, as in the case of the dentist's patients.

In response to the public's growing concern that the clinical activities of HIV-positive physicians might lead to a patient's infection, the CDC developed, early in 1991, a risk model that attempts to provide a more reliable estimate of the risk to patients of an HIV transmission. Estimating this risk is complicated by a variety of factors, including the type and length of the procedure, the number of surgeons participating, the kind of exposure, the size of the inoculum, and the stage of the HIV infection when exposure occurs. Despite these difficulties, the CDC has calculated the probability of transmission from a seropositive surgeon to a patient to be between 1 in 42,000 (or 0.0024 percent) and 1 in 420,000 (or 0.00024 percent).[13] The variation in risk probabilities is due, in part, to the different kinds of needles used for suturing: the hollow needle, unlike the solid version, will more easily transmit a greater quantity of contaminated blood, hence the increased risk. According to the CDC, a seropositive surgeon who continues to perform invasive procedures has a probability of between 0.8 and 8.1 percent of infecting at least one patient in a seven-year period; as of 1991, the CDC estimated that between three and twenty-eight patients may have been infected with HIV through surgery, though thus far no one has been identified.[14]

One helpful way to appreciate the magnitude of the risk of seroconversion is to compare it with more common risks that we readily accept each day. For example, for every 10,000 miles we drive our automobiles, we face a risk of 1 in 4,000 of dying in an accident. Conversely, while the statistical probability of being killed by a lightning bolt is more remote, with a probability of 1 in 2 million in any given year, it has been noted that the risk of a physician-induced HIV infection "is only one tenth the chance of being killed by lightning, one fourth the chance of being killed by a bee, and half the chance of being hit by a falling aircraft."[15] Clearly, then, by comparison, the risk of seroconversion is actually quite remote.

The normal risks we face in a medical setting also far exceed the risk of contracting HIV. Surgical patients have between four and forty times greater likelihood of dying from anesthesia than of being infected with HIV; the risk of death from a penicillin reaction is at least equal to, if not four times greater than, the risk of contracting HIV. Indeed, two decades of experience with hepatitis B virus (HBV), a blood-borne virus, shows that the risk of an HBV infection is one hundred to one thousand times greater than an HIV seroconversion. HBV is ten times more prevalent among health-care professionals than HIV is, and as many as 25 percent of health-care professionals have a residual HBV infection.[16] Nonetheless, the transmission of HBV has dropped off dramatically since 1987, when rigorous universal precautions were instituted.[17] Simply said, the risk of HIV is far less than most routine medical risks, and significantly less likely since adherence to universal precautions were mandated.

In fact, the CDC may have actually overstated the risk of seroconversion from exposure to an HIV-positive surgeon. The CDC's risk estimate is based in part on a comparative analysis of rates of HIV transmission from infected patient to a health-care professional, a risk calculated to be about 1 in 330; however, the CDC has acknowledged that this estimate has serious limitations because it is based on assumptions that are known to be faulty.[18] Alternative estimates suggest that the risks of a surgeon to patient HIV transmission are more reasonably somewhere between 1 in 100,000 and 1 in 1 million operations.[19] Others have estimated that when the HIV status of the surgeon is unknown the risk of infection is 1 in 21 million per hour of surgery; in contrast, when the surgeon is known to be HIV-positive the best estimate of the risk of infection is 1 in 83,000, with a lower and upper limit of 1 in 28,000 and 1 in 500,000.[20] The author of this study concludes that "the risks are clearly low and might have the same magnitude as fatal injury to the patient en route to the hospital."[21]

Should Physicians with HIV Be Restricted?

Despite the extreme rarity of becoming infected by an HIV-positive physician, the public's reaction was to call for restrictions on physicians who were HIV-positive. As an indication of the depth of concern, a recent public opinion poll showed that 94 percent of those surveyed wanted to know the HIV status of their physician; 63 percent said seropositive surgeons should be forbidden to practice; and slightly more than half wanted restrictions on all HIV-positive physicians.[22]

Clearly, the public's perception of the risk of seroconversion is influenced by factors other than the actual magnitude of the risk. This is obvious from the fact that the reaction to the greater risks of an HBV infection, which is more common among practitioners and may be as deadly, has not produced equivalent calls for restrictions on the practice of HBV physicians. Research on risk perception shows that familiar and voluntary risks are more readily accepted than risks that are unfamiliar and imposed without an individual's consent, which may explain why this issue is so controversial.[23] Moreover, the public appears to have some difficulty understanding the concept of risk probabilities and distrusts what it perceives as the self-serving assurances from the medical profession that the risk is low. In the context of uncertainty, assurances like these are seldom persuasive; this is especially true given the public's painful experience, early in the AIDS epidemic, when it was mistakenly assured that the transfusible blood supply was safe from contamination by the AIDS virus.

Responding to growing public concern about the risk of contracting an HIV infection from a clinician, in July 1991 the CDC issued its much-anticipated guidelines aimed at preventing the transmission of HIV and HBV in a medical setting.[24] The CDC recommended that all HIV-positive physicians voluntarily refrain from surgery involving "exposure-prone" invasive procedures and called on local medical review committees to identify those surgical procedures with the greatest risk of an HIV transmission. It defined an exposure-prone or "seriously" invasive procedure as one involving the use of a sharp instrument inside a highly confined anatomical site under conditions of poor visibility. The CDC recommended that all those who perform such procedures should know their HIV status, though it rejected calls for mandatory HIV testing, suggesting that the low risk of transmission did not warrant mandatory testing. It further recommended that HIV-positive surgeons could perform seriously invasive procedures only if they were authorized to do so by an expert review committee and they had informed their patients of their HIV status. Except for these restrictions, the CDC opposed all other restrictions of HIV-positive physicians, including restrictions of invasive procedures not considered exposure-prone. In sum, the CDC found that seropositive physicians who adhere to the use of universal precautions and avoid performing invasive procedures "pose no risk for transmitting HIV or HBV to patients."[25]

The CDC guidelines recommending restrictions on the practice of HIV physicians were supported by a number of leading medical organizations, including the 300,000-member American Medical Association (AMA), which had argued that "the health of patients must always be the paramount concern of physicians."[26] In anticipation of the CDC guidelines, the AMA had previously recommended HIV-positive physicians to stop performing invasive procedures that "pose an identifiable risk to patients" or to disclose their HIV status to their patients.[27] The AMA reaffirmed this position soon after the CDC guidelines were issued and reconfirmed its stated opposition to mandatory testing.[28] The American Academy of Orthopedic Surgeons concurred with the CDC recommendations, encouraging its HIV-positive members to "consider carefully the attributes of an exclusively office-based practice where less risk of HIV transmission would exist."[29] The Federation of State Medical Boards, a national licensing and disciplinary body, noted too that it would be professional misconduct for physicians to perform seriously invasive procedures without knowing their HIV status.[30]

Nonetheless, a surprising number of medical organizations rejected the CDC guidelines, including the American College of Surgeons, the American College of Physicians, the American College of Emergency Physicians, the American Academy of Pediatrics, the California Medical Association, the American Hospital Association, and the American Public Health Association.[31] In general, these professional groups opposed the guidelines because, given the remoteness of the risk of HIV transmission, there is no medically indicated reason to justify restricting the practice of HIV-infected physicians. They criticized the CDC for caving in to public pressure and for overreacting to a freak accident involving the dentist's transmissions by issuing guidelines that many thought would eventually prove to be an embarrassment. The American College of Physicians reaffirmed its 1988 policy statement, noting that HIV-positive physicians "present virtually no risk of HIV transmission to their patients."[32] Recommendations calling for seropositive surgeons to refrain from performing invasive procedures or to disclose their HIV status to their patients were widely characterized as "unwarranted, imprecise, and not in the public interest."[33] It was argued that physicians should not be required to disclose their HIV status if their clinical performance posed no significant risk of HIV transmission.[34]

Moreover, all of these groups unanimously rejected the concept of drawing up a list of so-called exposure-prone procedures. They argued that the very remoteness of the risk would make it nearly impossible to provide useful data to identify which procedures were exposure-prone. The American College of Surgeons concluded that any such list would be irrelevant since exposure-prone procedures "cannot be defined in any scientific or rational way."[35] Ironically, since the actual risk of transmission is dependent more on the skill and experience of the surgeon than on the type of procedure, the same procedure could both be, and not be, exposure-prone, depending on the surgeon's expertise, fatigue level, and so forth. In effect, the conclusion was that the CDC had focused its attention in the wrong place; the real problem of HIV transmission was not the infected practitioner but more precisely those activities that violate universal precautions and result in breaches of barrier protection.[36]

More surprising was the number of state health departments that refused to comply with the CDC recommendations, a position unheard of for a mandate from a federal agency such as the CDC.[37] States are required by legislation enacted by Congress to adopt the CDC guidelines or their equivalent within one year or face the loss of federal support for state health programs. By the end of 1991, only the state of Texas had done so, while Illinois had passed legislation requiring only that HIV-positive physicians notify patients who have had invasive procedures of the physicians' HIV status. In contrast, New York's State Department of Health issued regulations refusing to allow health-care facilities to disclose information to patients regarding the HIV status of hospital personnel, including physicians who perform invasive procedures.[38] In addition, the state health departments of Michigan and New York, despite the threatened loss of millions of dollars in federal aid, rejected the CDC guidelines, saying instead that they would issue alternative recommendations emphasizing strict adherence to infection control procedures.[39] Yet to be resolved is whether, after rejecting the CDC guidelines, these alternative state guidelines satisfy legal requirements that they be "equivalent" to the CDC guidelines.

The controversy over the CDC guidelines came to a critical juncture in mid 1992, when the National Institutes of Health (NIH) and, later, the National Commission on AIDS independently concluded that there is no medical or scientific justification for the CDC's restrictions on the practice of HIV-positive physicians.[40] The remoteness of the risk was once more offered as the principal reason for opposing the CDC guidelines. NIH officials also worried that restrictions on the practice of physicians infected with HIV might lead some physicians to refuse, in turn, to care for HIV-positive patients, leading to the creation of two classes of patient care depending on one's HIV status. Leaders of the National Commission on AIDS added that "to suggest that HIV-infected health-care professionals should be diverted to professional pursuits other than those for which they have been trained seems draconian and expensive, and it fans fear in the presence of a risk that so far is incalculably small."[41] The National Commission concluded that the best way to prevent HIV transmission is not through restrictions on practitioners but instead by increased adherence to strict infection control procedures. In the end, the CDC guidelines were viewed as an ill-considered response to the public's understandable but irrational desire for zero risk. As Dr. June Osborn, chair of the National Commission on AIDS, correctly observed, "This is not a world in which zero risk can be achieved by any means."[42]

The unremitting chorus of criticism and defiance from nearly the entire spectrum of the medical community eventually derailed the CDC guidelines; six months after issuing the guidelines, CDC officials conceded that the risk of HIV transmission is so small it would be impossible to provide data on "exposure-prone" procedures, so it withdrew its recommendation requiring that such a list be drawn up.[43] And while it still insisted that physicians should voluntarily be tested for HIV, the CDC acknowledged that the actual risk of transmission would depend more on the skill of the surgeon than on the nature of the procedure itself. Instead, the CDC would now emphasize more vigorously that physicians adhere to standard infection control precautions. Since the only logical explanation for the cluster of cases involving the Florida dentist suggested that infection control procedures had evidently broken down, this new policy seemed to satisfy the CDC's legally mandated concerns.

Are Restrictions Discriminatory?

From the perspective of professional ethics and public policy, what should we say about a policy that imposes restrictions on the practice of HIV-positive physicians? Can such restrictions be justified, or are they inherently discriminatory? As a means of answering these questions, three salient ethical considerations need to be addressed. Among the most important considerations is the need to protect the patient's health and safety, especially from preventable harms such as a physician-induced HIV infection. In addition, we cannot ignore concerns of justice and the presumptions of liberty that are equally relevant when considering restrictions on competent physicians' rights to practice. Finally, the social consequences of any proposed policy should satisfy the principle of utility so as to maximize the greatest good over evil for the greatest number. Accordingly, to justify restrictions on the practice of HIV-positive physicians we need first to show that patients face a significant risk of contracting an HIV infection, that proposed restrictions are fair limitations of liberty, and that such a policy promotes the greatest good for society.

Regarding the first consideration, members of the medical profession have recognized moral and social obligations to do no harm and to use their talents to promote the best interests of their patients.[44] Medical care that puts patients at risk of contracting an HIV infection as a result of a surgical intervention would obviously be in violation of these professional obligations. Indeed, the profession has as much interest in protecting patients from harm as patients have themselves; it cannot allow patients to become infected by HIV-positive physicians without at the same time contradicting the profession's own self-description as a "helping" profession. Moreover, the profession relies heavily on the public's trust and could not function effectively without it; hence, it cannot tolerate physician-induced HIV infections in patients without at the same time sacrificing the essential ingredient of trust on which the doctor–patient relationship depends. In short, the medical profession has equally good reasons to share the public's serious concern about the continued practice of HIV-positive physicians.

What divides the public from the medical profession, however, is a radically different assessment of the acceptability of the risk associated with HIV-positive physicians practicing, especially when performing invasive procedures. While there is admittedly a risk of infection to a patient during an invasive procedure, reliable estimates of the risk show that this is an extremely remote possibility, particularly when universal precautions are rigorously observed. In sum, based on this analysis of the risk, the great majority of the medical profession have concluded that there is no significant risk that a seropositive physician will infect a patient through general contact or during an invasive procedure.

Despite these assurances, calls by a concerned public for restrictions on the practice of HIV-positive physicians appear to be based on a refusal to accept any risk, no matter how remote. In effect, the public is demanding that medicine adopt a zero-risk standard. But if zero risk becomes the regulative standard for acceptable behavior in medicine, then *no* medical procedure will be deemed acceptable. Like all disciplines, medicine functions within the context of uncertainty such that there is always some risk that an injury or an untoward result may occur, even if every precaution is scrupulously undertaken by the most competent of practitioners. As in life, there can be no guarantees in medicine; hence, it is absurd to expect that physicians should be allowed to function only if there is no risk.

It may be objected that requiring *all* medical procedures to satisfy a zero risk standard is, of course, asking too much; instead, the demand for zero risk is only for procedures involving HIV-positive physicians. The rationale underlying this particular demand is fundamentally a fear of contracting AIDS. While the fear of AIDS is readily understandable, however, it is clearly an overreaction to demand that seropositive physicians refrain from practicing medicine when no good reason exists to believe that there is any significant risk to patients of becoming HIV-infected. Indeed, we must remember that not a single medical patient is known to have contracted HIV as a result of receiving medical care.

More important, to single out HIV-positive physicians in this way plays into the hysteria surrounding AIDS and that has resulted in widespread discrimination against those who are infected. The Federal Rehabilitation Act (1973) prohibits discrimination against persons with disabilities, and the recently enacted Americans with Disabilities Act (1990) recognizes HIV infection as a disability; thus, to restrict HIV-positive physicians from continuing their medical practice would necessarily involve actions that are legally proscribed because they are defined by statute as discriminatory. Moreover, not only would such restrictions be in violation of legal requirements aimed at protecting the disabled from discrimination, but they would only further fuel discriminatory attitudes toward those infected with HIV. Since the risk of physician-induced HIV infection does not appear to be significant, it seems reasonable to conclude that imposing restrictions on HIV-positive physicians may not be warranted.

This conclusion also helps resolve questions of whether restricting physicians with HIV is a fair limitation of their liberty. To justify restricting the liberty of HIV-positive physicians to practice, it must be shown that patients are harmed by the unrestricted practice of seropositive physicians. Violations of the "harm principle" have been the principal moral justification for restricting a person's freedom; as John Stuart Mill has eloquently argued, "The only purpose for which power can be rightfully exercised over any member of a civilized community against his will is to prevent harm to others."[45] But as we have seen, there is only a remote possibility that a patient will become infected; hence, it is very unlikely that any patient will be harmed. Under circumstances where there is no more than a remote possibility of harm, it is doubtful that this alone will be sufficient to justify abridging anyone's freedom. If it were sufficient, then a great deal of what we ordinarily do, such as driving an automobile, would be proscribed since there is always a possibility that it *may* have harmful consequences. An abridgment of freedom based on the mere possibility of harm would be an unfortunate expansion of the harm principle, and one that we could not rationally accept. As we have previously suggested, HIV-positive physicians should be granted the presumption of liberty to practice unrestricted, until it is proven or rationally presumed that they are unsafe to their patients.

We should note, too, that physicians, like patients, have fundamental moral rights that are intended to protect their legitimate interests from unwarranted intrusions and that society has a correlative duty to respect. Among the most important of these rights is the right of a licensed, competent physician to practice medicine without undue restriction; this right can be overriden only if another, more pressing moral consideration, such as a patient's right not to be harmed, can be shown or reasonably presumed to take precedence. But in this context the evidence seems clear that patients are unlikely to be harmed by their HIV-positive physician; hence, without convincing evidence of a significant risk, there appears to be no persuasive justification for overriding a physician's professional rights to continue clinical practice with no restrictions. In the end, actions aimed at restricting the practice of seropositive physicians do not seem to meet moral requirements that would reasonably warrant limiting physicians' liberties or setting aside their rights.

Finally, according to the "principle of utility," the consequences of imposing restrictions on HIV-positive physicians should be such that the restrictions contribute to maximize the overall good over evil in society. Indeed, one of the potentially beneficial consequences of restricting HIV-positive physicians is to increase the public's trust in the medical profession, while the reverse is likely if restrictions are not imposed. For this reason, the profession cannot ignore the problem of seropositive physicians, since medicine will be unable to function effectively if it loses the public's trust. On the other hand, imposing restrictions on HIV-positive physicians has a number of untoward consequences that we cannot ignore, namely, that the hysteria surrounding AIDS naturally will be increased; that physicians who are restricted would likely suffer from the loss of their professional life as well as become victims of discrimination; and that the medical profession would lose some of its dedicated members, not to mention the loss to society of their services. The severity of these consequences may be difficult to predict, and there may be other unanticipated consequences that we cannot now know. It may also be difficult to know whether maintaining the public's trust is comparatively more important than protecting the professional rights of HIV-positive physicians. Thus, from the perspective of maximizing social good, the consequences of imposing restrictions on HIV-positive physicians are equivocal at best.

Nonetheless, we may conclude that calls for imposing restrictions on HIV-positive physicians do not appear to meet basic moral requirements necessary to justify implementing those restrictions as a social policy. Not only does such a policy seem irrational given the extreme remoteness of the risk, but it seems to be based on an impossible requirement involving a zero-risk standard. In addition to its unreasonableness, the inherent unfairness of such a policy makes it unacceptable, for it would promote unwarranted restrictions of physicians' liberties, encourage discrimination, and lead to a direct violation of physicians' legitimate professional rights, all consequences that cannot be tolerated in any just society.

As the leaders of the National Commission on AIDS have eloquently argued, "A policy that removes HIV-positive professionals from duty without strong justification sends a dreadful message to doctors: Don't take care of HIV-infected people—to do so you run the risk of losing your professional life."[46]

Should HIV Testing Be Mandatory?

Another compelling reason for rejecting restrictions on HIV-positive physicians is that the only effective way to enforce such a policy would be to institute mandatory HIV testing of all physicians, including residents and possibly medical students.[47] In fact, frequent HIV testing would be required to assure the public that all infected practitioners are properly and routinely identified. Such a program would obviously be highly intrusive, and the cost would likely be enormous. More important, instituting mandatory HIV testing would also be ethically problematic because it directly violates informed consent requirements, undermines autonomy and privacy rights, and offends against justice given that those who are so identified will likely become the victims of discrimination.[48] In this context, to justify mandatory HIV testing, that is, testing without consent, we must show not only that such testing will protect the public from contracting an HIV infection but also that protecting the public good in *this* way takes precedence over individual and professional rights to privacy and freedom.

Both the CDC and the AMA have rejected mandatory HIV testing of physicians on the grounds that the low risk of transmission does not justify such testing or the use of scarce resources for such an expensive and cumbersome program.[49] The list of organizations that have rejected mandatory HIV testing also includes the American Hospital Association, the American Public Health Association, the American Dental Association, the National Association of People with AIDS, the AIDS Action Council, and the American Civil Liberties Union, among others. Many feared that requiring physicians to submit to HIV testing would not only adversely affect health-care delivery, especially for persons with AIDS, but that it would lead to testing of all hospital patients, resulting in widespread violations of privacy rights while further fanning the flames of public fear and panic.[50]

Interestingly enough, advocates of mandatory HIV testing reason that the only equitable approach is to test everyone in the health-care setting, including pregnant women and their newborns. While there is general resistance to this kind of screening,[51] we should note that perinatally acquired HIV is more common than phenylketonuria (PKU) or congenital syphilis, both of which currently require mandatory testing.[52] In fact, some hospitals routinely screen their patients for HIV, sometimes without their consent.[53] They defend testing patients for HIV because it will help health-care professionals to better know with whom they should take greater precautions, arguing that such testing is necessary because it is unrealistic to expect health-care professionals to be vigilant in exercising infection control precautions at all times.[54] Actually, early HIV testing may be highly desirable since new drugs such as the antiviral azidothymidine (AZT) can help delay the onset of AIDS as well as possibly prolong life. Nonetheless, although the CDC recently recommended that hospitals encourage patients to voluntarily be tested for HIV on admission, even when they may not be at high risk for AIDS, it rejected testing of patients without obtaining informed consent.[55]

This may not be enough, for some in the medical profession, including the *New England Journal of Medicine*, believe the time has come for routine HIV *screening* of all patients and physicians.[56] In fact, a hospital in Aspen, Colorado, is hoping to bolster public confidence in the quality of its services by being among the first to screen all its staff physicians with an annual HIV test as a requirement for those who wish to maintain their hospital privileges.[57] Still, the majority of physicians are reluctant to be tested themselves, though many appear to favor testing patients, not only for the welfare of patients but also as a means of self-protection.[58]

In any case, mandatory HIV testing, whether for patients or physicians, remains a highly controversial policy, one that may not achieve the end for which it was intended, namely, preventing the spread of AIDS. Mandatory testing by itself cannot prevent AIDS, nor will it prevent further infections from occurring.[59] In fact, no evidence has ever been offered to show that mandatory testing would control the advance of the AIDS epidemic.[60] More important, a negative test result does not guarantee that one is free of an HIV infection, since it normally takes six to eight weeks after the onset of infection before seropositivity is detectable. False-negative test results can promote a mistaken sense of security that ironically might increase the spread of HIV infection.[61] Conversely, because the overall incidence of HIV infection is relatively low, the likelihood of a false-positive test result will be proportionally higher.[62] Tragically, because we lack a sufficiently sensitive and specific testing procedure, there is no way at present to eliminate mistaken positive and negative test results, or the consequent harm those who are misidentified will suffer. In the end, any policy of mandatory HIV testing must be tied to an appropriate counseling program to help spare those who are identified as HIV-positive—either properly or mistakenly—from the excessive and untoward emotional consequences associated with such a diagnosis.

From the perspective of law and ethics, mandatory HIV testing is in direct violation of basic rights to privacy to which every individual is entitled. The right to privacy is fundamentally a negative right to be left alone that protects us from being forced to reveal information about ourselves that we may wish to keep secret and that might be embarrassing if it were made public.[63] By respecting the privacy of each individual, we create a context in which individuals can feel secure in their person without the unsettling scrutiny of others. More generally, the rights of individuals place moral and legal limits on societal actions, and these rights cannot be violated even if they are conducive to the public good. Actions intended to bring about some social benefit but that violate the rights of individuals do so only by sacrificing protections that are essential to a person's well-being and thus critical to a society's sense of justice.

Although concern about the spread of AIDS is a legitimate societal concern, it cannot warrant the wholesale abuse of privacy rights implicit in a program of mandatory HIV testing. By requiring physicians to submit to HIV testing against their will, we are forcing them to reveal information about themselves that they have a legal and moral right to keep private; to cite but one example, a positive test result may suggest that one has been engaged in activities that are socially disapproved of, despite honest claims to the contrary. In an imperfect world, where many who are HIV-positive become the victims of irrational discriminatory attitudes, it is clear that respecting privacy is an essential mechanism for protecting persons from intolerance and victimization.

Similarly troublesome is the degree to which mandatory HIV testing takes away people's freedom or autonomy to decide for themselves whether to be tested or not. It is sadly ironic that after more than a generation of commitment to the concept of informed consent, we would now contemplate instituting testing without consent. The concept of informed consent was specifically designed to protect individuals from being forced to undergo medical treatment or experimentation against their wills. Because mandatory testing as a policy directly contradicts informed consent protections, most states currently have specific legal prohibitions against such testing.[64] Moreover, since mandatory HIV testing programs proposed for prisoners, immigrants, and others involved in high-risk activities have also been rejected across the board, it is curious why such a program would be viewed as appropriate for physicians.[65] In sum, in a context where the risk of an HIV-positive physician infecting a patient is extremely remote, it seems a gross overreaction to mandate HIV testing of all physicians without at the same time legitimizing wholesale violations of physicians' rights.

Finally, a cogent argument against instituting a program of mandatory HIV testing for all physicians is that it would not be worth the cost either financially or socially. Even ignoring the social cost, if each test costs an average of $50, and we administer HIV tests but three times a year to the 300,000-plus membership of the AMA alone, the bill would total about $45 million annually; and many times that if residents, medical students, and other health-care professionals were also routinely tested. If we add the cost of counseling programs for all those identified as HIV-positive, the costs rise precipitously. We may wonder whether mandatory HIV testing is worth this cost given its penchant for trampling on individual rights and its undermining of social justice.

And if, as many have suggested, mandatory testing forces those who are infected to go underground to avoid detection, then it is clear that any benefit such a policy may have is far outweighed by its adverse societal consequences.[66] In sum, when the economic and social costs are compared with the limited benefits that mandatory testing is supposed to provide, we cannot avoid concluding that it would surely be an unwise policy to implement.

Nonetheless, for those physicians who regularly perform seriously invasive procedures in which admittedly there is a risk of HIV transmission, albeit remote, it is not unreasonable to suggest that they voluntarily ascertain their HIV status, if only to protect themselves from the consequences of their own carelessness. The rejection of mandatory HIV testing does not mean that physicians "have a right to willfully or negligently infect others."[67] Given the real, though remote possibility, that a puncture wound could result in a physician's blood mixing with a patient's, no physician who puts the patient's best interests first can fail to recognize the importance of knowing his or her own HIV status. If we accept the view that knowledge is good, then only an informed physician can rightfully decide whether or not to continue performing seriously invasive procedures. A proper sense of professional integrity would dictate that physicians take appropriate steps to reduce the risk of transmitting HIV during routine medical procedures, and ascertaining one's HIV status can contribute to reducing the risk of a patient becoming infected with AIDS. Voluntary HIV testing by physicians that increases awareness of the importance of universal precautions and that results, in some cases, in an infected physician voluntarily refraining from performing risky procedures could go a long way toward lessening the public's obsession with mandatory testing.

Should the Patient Be Told?

Among the issues of greatest concern to the public is not knowing whether their physician is HIV-positive or not. As we previously noted, in a recent public opinion poll, 94 percent of those surveyed wanted to know the HIV status of their physician. Obviously, a phobic fear of AIDS is at work here, but in the context of medicine, something more important is at stake that explains the near unanimity of opinion in the public's wanting to know their physician's HIV status. To see what this is, we need only to recall that when the public seeks medical care, it is out of a need to overcome an inherent vulnerability created by an illness, injury, or a disease condition that they are incapable of resolving by themselves. The public assumes that trust in medical professionals is warranted, since the public sincerely believes that physicians are dedicated to using their knowledge and skills to assist others in recovering health.

However, the public would not normally entrust their health and welfare to a physician, or anyone else, unless they believed it was safe to do so. If routine medical attention puts patients at risk of contracting a deadly infection, then it is obvious that most people would prefer to avoid such a potentially lethal situation. Moreover, nobody should be put at risk without her consent, especially when she could take appropriate action to avoid the risk if she knew it existed. In fact, not knowing when a physician is HIV-positive can directly undermine the autonomy of patients by depriving them of knowledge that would allow them to exercise rightful control over their destiny; for example, patients would thereby be denied the opportunity to switch to an uninfected physician if they so desired. Under these circumstances, the public's investment of trust in the medical profession will be greatly diminished, if not destroyed, if physicians can keep their HIV status secret. Without this knowledge, patients have no option but to have this risk imposed on them without their consent and without their knowledge. Because of considerations such as these, patients believe they have a right to know their physician's HIV status.

Indeed, some in the medical profession have argued that physicians have a professional obligation to inform patients of their seropositivity at the earliest opportunity.[68] In effect, this would mean extending the duty of informed consent beyond its usual limits of informing patients of the risks and benefits of a medical procedure, to include disclosure of *personal* factors unrelated to the nature of the procedure itself. While it may seem desirable to do this, expanding the concept of informed consent to include disclosure of a physician's HIV status prompts the question: Why stop here? Does the patient's right to know also require that physicians disclose facts related to their emotional stability, stress management abilities, their drinking habits, drug use, grades in medical school, or whether they had a good night's sleep? Since these as well as a multitude of other personal factors could adversely affect the outcome of a medical or surgical procedure, should patients have a right to know all these details, too? And why limit disclosure to personal factors about the physician alone, when any number of other personnel, including nurses and laboratory technicians, could contribute to injury or an HIV infection.

Nonetheless, even if all of these considerations, and more, were disclosed to a patient, it does not mean that no one would become infected. Nor would it provide greater patient protection. Likewise, almost no one who needs medical attention would refuse it, even if fully informed of all these risks. They would normally have no other option but to hope that they were lucky enough not to be infected. Unfortunately, it is part of the tyranny of circumstances under which we must function that no matter how we strive to overcome uncertainty, we have nothing left but hope to sustain us when a difficult decision must be made. In short, to believe that full disclosure would significantly reduce the risk of infection amounts to believing that zero risk is still a realistic possibility.

Moreover, physicians have rights to privacy and professional rights to practice medicine that protect them from having to disclose information about themselves that is typically believed to be confidential. The public's interest in knowing the HIV status of their physician, while understandable and shared by many, does not, however, reasonably fit within the range of concerns normally covered by the public's right to know, since such a disclosure would violate physicians' legitimate privacy rights. In addition, given that we have no effective decision procedure for resolving a conflict of rights, we cannot simply assume that patients' rights automatically take precedence over the rights of physicians. And even if we could find some persuasive reason to set aside the rights of infected physicians in favor of full disclosure, does this also mean that infected patients should be required to disclose their seropositivity? Because the risk of transmitting HIV is far greater from patient to physician than in the opposite direction, there would seem to be more reason to demand patient rather than physician disclosure. But despite these arguments, we cannot forget that rights are intended to put limits on society, and they cannot be overriden simply because doing so serves some supposed social good. The injustice perpetrated in the name of promoting public safety reduces the protections that human rights provide to matters that are merely socially expedient.

In fact, the social consequences of requiring seropositive physicians to disclose their HIV status are not so good. If physicians were forced to disclose that they were infected, they would most likely lose most of their patients; most would switch to an uninfected physician rather than risk becoming infected. Norman Daniels calls this the "switching dilemma."[69] He asserts that while it is not irrational to switch to an uninfected physician, if we all switch, then overall each of us will be worse off. Switching produces a situation known as "the poverty of the commons," such that benefits and efficiencies normally gained from not expecting disclosure of confidential information will now be lost because of a breakdown of trust. The general result would not only foster mistrust, but resources that might be used for controlling the spread of HIV would now be used, instead, to remove and replace physicians who are infected. As a practice, switching will not only ruin many fine careers but it will aid and abet an increase of intolerance and the isolation of those infected with HIV. The overall consequences of full disclosure suggest that as a policy its benefits may not be worth its many adverse social effects.

In the final analysis, the demand to know the HIV status of physicians represents the kind of attack on individual rights that has been commonplace throughout the course of human history. It involves the same kind of fear mongering and repression of those who are different and the wholesale violation of their human rights that is so often justified by a twisted sense of the common good. If the confidentiality protection that privacy permits is lost here, then everybody will be worse off, for no one will be able to keep anything private. Until the risk of infection from HIV-positive physicians can be shown to be substantially greater than it is currently, calls for wholesale attacks on the privacy and professional rights of physicians seem seriously misplaced.

Notes

Acknowledgment: Earlier versions of this chapter were presented at the American Philosophical Association Pacific Division Meeting (March 1992) and to the Department of Philosophy, California State University, Fullerton (September 1991). Ronald B. Miller, M.D., Clinical Professor of Medical Ethics, University of California, Irvine, was also kind enough to provide helpful comments. I extend my appreciation to all those who have assisted me in this endeavor.

1. Centers for Disease Control, "The Second 100,000 Cases of Acquired Immunodeficiency Syndrome—United States, June 1981–December 1991," *Morbidity and Mortality Weekly Report* 41 (January 1992): 2; idem, "The HIV/ AIDS Epidemic: The First 10 Years," *Morbidity and Mortality Weekly Report* 40 (June 1991): 22; and idem, "Mortality Attributable to HIV Infection/AIDS— United States, 1981–1990, *Morbidity and Mortality Weekly Report* 40 (January, 1991): 3.

2. "AIDS the No. 2 Cause of Death for Young Men, Report Shows," *Los Angeles Times*, January 25, 1991. See also Centers for Disease Control, "Increased HIV/AIDS Mortality Among Residents Aged 25–44 Years, Baltimore, MD, 1987–1989," *Morbidity and Mortality Weekly Report* 41: 38.

3. "New Study Boosts Forecasts of AIDS Infection," *Los Angeles Times*, June 4, 1992.

4. "Progress, Pessimism Confront AIDS Experts," *Los Angeles Times*, July 19, 1992.

5. "Possible Transmission of Human Immunodeficiency Virus to Patient During Invasive Dental Procedure," *Morbidity and Mortality Weekly Report* 39 (1990): 489–493.

6. "Update: Transmission of HIV Infection During an Invasive Dental Procedure—Florida," *Morbidity and Mortality Weekly Report* 40 (January, 1991): 2.

7. "Panel Opposes Restricting Health Workers with AIDS," *Los Angeles Times*, July 31, 1992.

8. "Principles of Medical Ethics," American Medical Association, 1984.

9. B. Mishu, W. Schaffner, J. M. Horan, et al., "A Surgeon with AIDS: Lack of Evidence of Transmission to Patients," *Journal of the American Medical Association* 264: (1990) 467–470.

10. J. J. Sacks, "AIDS in a Surgeon," *New England Journal of Medicine* 313 (1985): 1017–1018; F. P. Armstrong, J. C. Miner, and W. H. Wolfe, "Investigation of a Health Care Worker with Symptomatic HIV Infection: An Empidemiologic Approach," *Milit Med* 152 (1987): 414–418; J. D. Porter, J. G. Cruickshank, P. H. Gentle, et al., "Management of Patients Treated by Surgeon with HIV Infection," *Lancet* 335 (1990): 113–114; R. N. Danila, K. L. MacDonald, F. S. Rhame, et al., "A Lookback Investigation of Patients of an HIV-infected Physician: Public Health Implications," *New England Journal of Medicine* 325 (1991): 1406–1411; "Panel Opposes Restricting Health Workers with AIDS," *Los Angeles Times*, July 31, 1992; "Little Risk of Getting AIDS from Doctor: Three Studies Find No HIV Transmission," *Chicago Tribune*, April 14, 1993.

11. Mishu et al., "Surgeon with AIDS."

12. L. Gostin, "The HIV-infected Health Care Professional: Public Policy, Discrimination, and Patient Safety," *Archives of Internal Medicine* 151 (1991): 663–665; idem, "HIV-infected Physicians and the Practice of Seriously Invasive Procedures," *Hastings Center Report* 19 (1989): 32–39.

13. Centers for Disease Control, *Estimates of the Risk of Endemic Transmission of Hepatitis B Virus and Human Immunodeficiency Virus to Patients by the Percutaneous Route During Invasive Surgical Procedures* (Atlanta, Ga.: Centers for Disease Control, 1991).

14. Ibid. See also J. L. Geberding, C. Littel, A. Tarkington, A. Brown, and W. B. Schecter, "Risk of Exposure of Surgical Personnel to Patient's Blood During Surgery at San Francisco General Hospital," *New England Journal of Medicine* 322 (1990): 1788–1793.

15. N. Daniels, "HIV-infected Professionals, Patient Rights, and the Switching Dilemma," *Journal of the American Medical Association* 267 (1992): 1368–1371; R. Wilson, "Analyzing the Daily Risks of Life," *Technology Review* 81 (1979): 41–46.

16. R. E. Rogers, and J. E. Osborn, "Another Approach to the AIDS Epidemic," *New England Journal of Medicine* 325 (1991): 806–808.

17. Centers for Disease Control, *Estimates of Risk*, p. XX.

18. B. Lo and R. Steinbrook, "Health Care Workers Infected with the Human Immunodeficiency Virus," *Journal of the American Medical Association* 267 (1992): 1100–1105. See also S. Landesman, "The HIV-positive Health Professional: Policy Options for Individuals, Institutions, and States: Public Policy and the Public—Observations from the Front Line," *Archives of Internal Medicine* 151 (1991): 655–657.

19. R. S. Rhame, "The HIV-infected Surgeon," *Journal of the American Medical Association* 294 (1990): 507–508.

20. A. B. Lowenfels and G. Wormser, "Risk of Transmission of HIV from Surgeon to Patient," *New England Journal of Medicine* 325 (1991): 888–889.

21. Ibid.

22. Barbara Kantrowitz et al., "Doctors with AIDS," *Newsweek*, July 1, 1991.

23. D. Nelkin, "Communicating Technological Risk: The Social Construction of Reality," *Annual Review of Public Health* 10 (1989): 95–113; P. Slovic, "Perception of Risk," *Science* 236 (1987): 280–285; C. Hohenemser and J. X. Kasperson, eds., *Risk in the Technological Society* (Boulder, Colo.: Westview Press, 1982).

24. Centers for Disease Control, "Recommendations for Preventing Transmission of Immunodeficiency Virus and Hepatitis B Virus to Patients During Exposure-prone Invasive Procedures," *Morbidity and Mortality Weekly Report* 40 (1991): 1–9.

25. Ibid.

26. "Halt Surgery, HIV-positive Doctors urged," *Los Angeles Times*, January 18, 1991.

27. American Medical Association, *Statement on HIV-infected Physicians* (Chicago: American Medical Association, 1991); "AIDS Infected Doctors and Dentists Are Urged to Warn Patients or Quit," *New York Times*, January 18, 1991.

28. American Medical Association, House of Delegates Resolution 84H, October 1991; "Surgeons Undergo Test for AIDS Virus," *Los Angeles Times*, March 7, 1991.

29. American Academy of Orthopedic Surgeons, *Advisory Statement on Orthopedic Surgeons Who Test Positive for Immunodeficiency Virus (HIV)* (Park Ridge, Ill.: American Academy of Orthopedic Surgeons, 1991); S. Staver, "HIV-infected Orthopedists Urged to Curtail Surgery," *American Medical News* (April 1, 1991).

30. Federation of State Medical Boards of the United States, *Formal Policy Statement on the Prevention of HIV/HBV Transmission to Patients* (Fort Worth, Tex.: Federation of State Medical Boards of the United States, 1991).

31. "Don't Bar Doctors with HIV, NIH Says," *Los Angeles Times*, June 11, 1991; S. Staver, "Opposition Mounts Against CDC Plan for Exposure-prone list," *American Medical News* (October 28, 1991). See also Lo and Steinbrook, "Health Care Workers."

32. American College of Physicians, *Statement of the American College of Physicians Before the CDC* (Philadelphia, Pa.: American College of Physicians, 1991).

33. N. M. Lederman, and M. J. Mehlman, "Physicians Infected with HIV," *Journal of the American Medical Association* 265 (1991): 2337–2338.

34. S. Frandzel, "Organizations Defend Their Position at CDC Conference on HIV-infected Health Care Workers," *AIDS Patient Care* 5 (1991): 129–133.

35. American College of Surgeons, *The Surgeon and HIV-infection: A Statement* (Chicago: American College of Surgeons, 1991).

36. D. M. Price, "What Should We Do About HIV-positive Health Professionals?" *Archives of Internal Medicine* 151 (1991): 658–659; E. S. Wong, J. L. Strotka, V. M. Chinchilli, et al., "Are Universal Precautions Effective in Reducing the Number of Occupational Exposures Among Health Care Workers?" *Journal of the American Medical Association* 265 (1991): 1123–1128; K. R. Courington, S. L. Patterson, and R. J. Howard, "Universal Precautions Are Not Universally Followed," *Archives of Surgery* 126 (1991): 93–96.

37. "Physicians Disregard CDC Rules on AIDS," *Los Angeles Times*, October 1991.

38. New York State Department of Health, "Policy Statement and Guidelines, Health Care Facilities and HIV-infected Medical Personnel," January 1991.

39. Rosner et al., "Ethical Considerations Concerning the HIV-positive Physician," *New York State Journal of Medicine* 92 (1991): 151–155. See also "Don't Bar Doctors with HIV."

40. "Don't Bar Doctors with HIV."

41. Rogers and Osborn, "Another Approach."

42. Ibid.

43. "Panel Opposes Restricting Health Care Worker with AIDS," *Los Angeles Times*, July 31, 1992; "Doctors with HIV Won't Face Curbs," *Los Angeles Times*, December 4, 1991.

44. President's Commission for the Study of Ethical Problems, *Making Health Care Decisions* (Washington, D.C.: Government Printing Office, 1983).

45. John Stuart Mill, *On Liberty* (New York: Bantam Books, 1961), p. 263.

46. Rogers and Osborn, "Another Approach."

47. Gostin, "HIV-infected Health Care Professional"; R. F. Jones and D. Green, "Students and Residents Confront New Era of Occupational Risk," *American Association of Medical Colleges Reporter* 1 (1992): 1–3; "Caring for Medical Students as Patients," L. W. Lane, G. Lane, et al., *Archives of Internal Medicine* 150 (November 1990). See also "Recommendations and Reports for HIV Testing Services for Inpatients and Outpatients in Acute-Care Hospital Settings and Technical Guidance on HIV Counseling," *Morbidity and Mortality Weekly Report* 42 (January 15, 1993).

48. K. R. Howe, "Why Mandatory Screening for AIDS Is a Bad Idea," in *AIDS:Ethics and Public Policy*, ed. C. Pierce and D. VanDeVeer (Belmont, Calif.: Wadsworth, 1988); R. Weiss and S. O. Their, "HIV Testing Is the

Answer: What's the Question?'' *New England Journal of Medicine* 319 (1988): 1010–1012; T. C. Quinn, "Screening for HIV Infection: Benefits and Costs," *New England Journal of Medicine* 327 (1992): 486–488.

49. American Medical Association, Council on Ethical and Judicial Affairs, "Ethical Issues Involved in the Growing AIDS Crisis," *Journal of the American Medical Association* 259 (1988): 1360–1361; Centers for Disease Control, "Recommendations."

50. "Health Care Workers Resist Taking AIDS Test," *Los Angeles Times*, February 22, 1991.

51. L. M. Hardy, ed., *HIV Screening of Pregnant Women and Newborns* (Washington, D.C.: National Academy Press, 1991).

52. M. Angell, "A Dual Approach to the AIDS Epidemic," *New England Journal of Medicine* 324 (1991): 1498–1500. See also K. Nolan, "Ethical Issues in Caring for Pregnant Women and Newborns at Risk for Human Immunodeficiency Virus Infection," *Semin Perinatology* 13 (1989): 55–65.

53. C. E. Lewis and K. Montgomery, "The Testing Policies of US Hospitals," *Journal of the American Medical Association* 264 (1990): 2764–07; J. M. Lombardo, P. C. Kloser, B. R. Pawel, R. C. Trost, R. Kapila, and M. E. St. Louis, "Anonymous Human Immunodeficiency Virus Surveillance and Clinically Directed Testing in Newark, NJ, Hospital," *Archives of Internal Medicine* 151 (1991): 965–968.

54. Angell, "Dual Approach," 1500.

55. "HIV Tests for All Hospital Patients Urged," *Los Angeles Times*, January 18, 1991; J. L. Baker, G. D. Kleen, K. T. Silvertston, et al., "Unsuspected Human Immunodeficiency Virus in Critically Ill Emergency Patients," *Journal of the American Medical Association* 257 (1987): 2609–2611.

56. Angell, "Dual Approach," 1499.

57. "Hospital's Doctors Must Get AIDS Test," *Los Angeles Times*, December 30, 1991. See also M. Barnes, N. A. Rango, G. R. Burke, and L. Chiarello, "The HIV-infected Health Care Professional: Employment Policies and Public Health," *Law, Medicine, and Health Care* 18 (1990): 311–330.

58. M. S. Schwartz, "AIDS Testing and Informed Consent," *Journal of Health Politics and Policy Law* 13 (1988): 607–621; G. D. Kelen, T. DiGiovanna, L. Bisson, D. Kalainov, K. T. Sivertston, and T. C. Quinn, "Human Immunodeficiency Virus Infection in Emergency Department Patients: Epidemiology, Clinical Presentations, and Risk to Health Care Workers: The Johns Hopkins Experience," *Journal of the American Medical Association* 262 (1989): 516–522; F. S. Rhame and D. G. Maki, "The Case for Wider Use of Testing for HIV Infection," *New England Journal of Medicine* 320 (1989): 1248–1254; B. Lo, R. L. Steinbrook, M. Cookie, T. J. Coates, E. J. Walters, and S. B. Hulley, "Voluntary Screening for Human Immunodeficiency Virus (HIV) Infection, Weighing the Benefits and Harms," *American Internal Medicine* 110 (1989): 727–733; T. A. Brennan, "Transmission of the Human Immunodeficiency Virus in the Health Care Setting: Time for Action," *New England Journal of Medicine* 324 (1991): 1504–1509; R. S. Janssen, M. E. St. Louis,

G. A. Satten, et al., "HIV Infection Among Patients in U.S. Acute Care Hospitals: Strategies for the Counseling and Testing of Hospital Patients," *New England Journal of Medicine* 327 (1992): 445–452.

59. Rogers and Osborne "Another Approach,"

60. "Mandatory HIV Testing of Youth: A Lose–Lose Proposition" (editorial), *Journal of the American Medical Association* 266 (1991): 2430–2431.

61. R. Knopp, et al., "The HIV-infected Emergency Health Care Professional," *Annals of Emergency Medicine* 20 (1991): 1036–1040.

62. E. M. Sloand, E. Pitt, R. J. Chiarello, and G. H. Nemo, "HIV Testing: The State of the Art," *Journal of the American Medical Association* 266 (1991): 3861–3866.

63. W. A. Parent, "Recent Work on the Concept of Privacy," *American Philosophical Quarterly* 20 (1983): 341–358.

64. M. A. Field, "Testing for AIDS: Uses and Abuses," *American Journal of Law and Medicine* 16 (1990): 33–106.

65. Gostin, "HIV-Infected Health Care Professional."

66. A. Novick, "At Risk for Aids: Confidentiality in Research and Surveillance," in Pierre and VanDeVeer, H. Aoun, *AIDS*; "When a House Officer Gets AIDS," *New England Journal of Medicine* 321 (1989): 693–696.

67. F. Rosner, P. P. Sordillo, J. R. Wolpaw, et al., "Ethical Considerations Concerning the HIV-positive Physician," *New York State Journal of Medicine* 92 (1992): 151–155.

68. E. H. Kluge, "Ethical Issues Concerning the HIV Status of Physicians and Patients," *Canadian Medical Association Journal* 145 (1991): 518–519; Letters in reply [to "Ethical Issues", *Canadian Medical Association Journal* 146 (1992): 811–813.

69. Daniels, "HIV-infected Professionals."

2

Nursing and AIDS: Some Special Challenges

Joan C. Callahan
Jill Powell

AIDS is not merely a killing disease, it's a psychological, moral, and legal minefield because it forces us to confront three taboo subjects—contagion, homosexuality, and death.—J. Allen McCrutchan

The pandemic of HIV infection has challenged society generally and the health-care system in particular. If statements such as Allen McCrutchan's are true in general, they are particularly true of health-care practitioners, and most true of nurses, who must provide constant, complex, and intimate physical and emotional care for persons with AIDS, and who have far more extended contact with these persons than do any other professionals.

As the rate of HIV infection has continued to rise, so has the demand for effective nursing care for persons who are HIV positive and persons with full-blown AIDS. Given the stunning increase in need for care, nurses, regardless of their practice areas, must now assume that the care of persons with HIV infection and AIDS will be a part of their professional lives. As we move deeper into the 1990s, virtually all nurses must expect to have to care for persons with AIDS, person with AIDS-related maladies (or AIDS-related complex [ARC]), and persons who are symptom-free but who are known to be positive for HIV. The issue, then, is no longer whether all nurses will be needed to care for these persons, but how effective that care will be.

This chapter focuses on several issues arising from the AIDS crisis that pose special challenges for individual nurses and nursing as a profession. These include (1) nurses' risk of HIV infection resulting from occupational exposure, and special complications in assessing these risks and how these risks relate to questions about the right to refuse to provide care; (2) mandatory testing of nurses for HIV and the conditions under which mandatory testing might be justified; (3) hiring and managing the work of nurses and nursing students who are HIV positive; (4) the demand for unremitting, complex, and often highly technical nursing care as the shortage of nurses continues to rise, coupled with the special psychosocial and emotional challenges nurses face in caring for persons with AIDS; and (5) how all these issues combine to present special challenges to nursing as a profession and how the profession can help to ameliorate some of the burdens associated with caring for persons with AIDS.

The Risk of Exposure and the Right to Refuse to Provide Care

The fear of contracting HIV through occupational exposure has been among the chief stressors for nurses since the beginning of the AIDS crisis. It is difficult to generalize about the level of nurses' fear of contagion and their reluctance to care for persons with AIDS, but some of the literature suggests that many nurses are unwilling or reluctant to provide care to HIV-positive individuals because of fear of occupational exposure (Blumenfield et al. 1987; Van Servellen, Lewis, and Leake 1988). Other researchers hold that such worries vary among groups of nurses, with those caring exclusively for persons with AIDS tending to be the least concerned about contagion and those who have cared only for a few persons with AIDS (or none at all) tending to be the most concerned (Hurley 1992). Still other studies suggest that even though there is significant fear of contagion among nurses, nurses are firmly committed to caring for persons with AIDS throughout the person's illness and dying (e.g., Wallack 1989).

Before taking up the question of the right to refuse to provide care, it is necessary first to identify as clearly as possible the actual risk nurses face in caring for persons who are HIV-positive. In 1988, the Centers for Disease Control (CDC) documented 18 cases worldwide of seroconversion of HIV resulting from occupational exposure since the onset of the AIDS crisis in the early 1980s (see Centers for Disease Control 1989, 32). Of these 18 cases representing all health-care workers, 5 involved nurses. Four of the 5 nurses contracted HIV through accidental needle sticks. The remaining nurse contracted the virus through a mucosal spray with HIV-contaminated blood. Of the five nurses reported, one was from the United States. Roughly 2,000,000 nurses are licensed to practice in the United States, of whom approximately 1,670,000 were actually practicing in 1988 (National League for Nursing 1992). On the basis of these figures, in 1988, the probability of a nurse's contracting AIDS through occupational exposure in the United States was, then, roughly 1 in 1,670,000.

It might be objected, however, that as the cases of HIV infection continue to multiply, the risk of occupational exposure to nurses increases. Thus, figures from 1988 tell us too little about the actual risks to nurses as we press into the 1990s. Indeed, as of September 1992, the CDC had documented 32 cases of occupationally acquired HIV infection among U.S. health-care workers, 12 of them nurses, with another 14 suspected cases involving nurses.[1] The risk of exposure is greatest at facilities caring for high numbers of HIV-positive patients. As just one example, Kelen et al. (1989) reported that at Johns Hopkins University Hospital, the rate of HIV positivity in persons admitted to the emergency room and who required emergency surgery was 13 percent. In such contexts, the most meaningful statistic for nurses is that of the official CDC estimate of seroconversion rate following needle-stick exposure to HIV-positive blood at 0.5 percent—1 in 200—a much higher probability than the 1 in 1,670,000 that was the general probability in 1988, or the roughly 1 in 139,917 in 1992.[2]

Still, the probability of a nurse contracting and dying from AIDS through occupational exposure is far less than the probability of her or his contracting and dying from hepatitis B virus (HBV) through occupational exposure. The CDC estimates that each year 12,000 health-care workers are infected with HBV, that 500 to 600 of these persons are hospitalized, that 250 of them will die as a result of the infection, and that 700 to 1,200 of them will become HBV carriers. Serologic evidence of current or past HBV infection is shown by 10 to 30 percent of health-care workers (Centers for Disease Control 1989, 5).

The rate of transmission of HIV is estimated to be 100 times less than the rate of transmission of HBV (Centers for Disease Control 1991b), probably because HIV is less concentrated in the blood than HBV is and because HBV is far hardier a virus than HIV. In general, then, all health-care workers run a considerably greater risk of death resulting from HBV contracted through occupational exposure than of death from AIDS contracted through occupational exposure. It is of no little interest that despite this fact, concern about contagion and reluctance or unwillingness to provide care arises with AIDS but not with HBV, a point we take up shortly. For now, we merely want to point out that just as the general possibility of contracting HBV from a patient would not be an acceptable reason for a nurse's refusal to provide care, the general possibility of contracting HIV from a patient is not an acceptable reason for refusing to provide care.

That much said, however, it needs to be realized that one of the problems that complicates the issue of risk for nurses and auxiliary health-care personnel is that HIV infection is believed to be fatal and that protection from exposure is not entirely in their own hands. Nurses and auxiliary personnel are particularly dependent on institutions and, to a significant degree, on physicians to insure their safety against exposure to communicable diseases, including AIDS. At least two of the known cases of nurses and nurses' assistants seroconverting after occupational exposure were caused by physicians. In one, a nurses' assistant seroconverted after being stuck by a needle discarded by a physician in some gauze on a bedside table; in another, a nurse and a physician were assisting a heart attack patient, when an uncovered needle held by the physician stuck the nurse in the forearm. Both cases have gone to court, and at this writing, the first has been decided in the nurses' assistant's favor ("AIDS Risk Reduction Strategies" 1990).

Furthermore, despite the emphasis on universal precautions given by the CDC, the Occupational Safety and Health Administration, and scores of researchers, institutions often make these precautions difficult to practice, for example, by not making latex gloves readily available (e.g., Doebbeling and Wenzel 1990, 2083).[3] Even worse, in some places nurses have been stridently discouraged from practicing universal precautions. For example, until recently at least one blood collection center known to us urged its technicians (roughly 10 percent nurses) to refrain from wearing gloves when working with donors. Despite the fact that great sensitivity is called for to avoid adding to the national near-panic over AIDS, precluding practitioners from exercising universal precautions when they are dealing with body fluids is, flatly, inexcusable.

Just as inexcusable is failure on the part of an institution or other corporate provider to make employing universal precautions maximally efficient and comfortable and maximally possible by ensuring not only that the appropriate safety supplies are readily available but also by ensuring as fully as possible that everyone in the institution's or provider's employ or practicing in its facilities is maximally protective of others. This can be accomplished only if institutions write policies, such as that of San Francisco General Hospital, that make it clear that people who do not comply with infection control precautions simply will not work (Eubanks 1992). On the other hand, if institutions are not scrupulous about protecting their practitioners, other workers, and clients, they invite resistance and refusals to treat that may well be justified.

In sum then, although a nurse's refusal to care for a person because that person is HIV-positive is no more acceptable than refusing because a person has some other potentially contagious fatal illness (or because a person is homosexual or black or female or Jewish), if an institution or other provider fails to do all it can to insure the safety of its practitioners, employees, and volunteers, including sanctioning those who deliberately, recklessly, or negligently place others at risk, then nurses may well have a morally acceptable ground for refusing to provide care, since such failure raises not only legitimate concerns about nurses' safety but also about the safety of persons who are dependent on that institution or provider for care. Thus, a nurse's refusal to provide care for persons who are HIV-positive cannot be justified on the basis of a general concern about risk of infection. But such a refusal might well be justified when institutional disregard or negligence makes the risk to the nurse (and others) unreasonable. Nurses may, then, be justified in refusing to treat persons who are HIV-positive as a way of pressing their employers to attend appropriately and quickly to the protection of employees, practitioners, volunteers, and, ultimately, clients.

Mandatory Testing

Off and on since the AIDS crisis began, there have been calls for mandatory testing of all health-care providers and, in some cases, all patients. In 1991, the death of Kimberly Bergalis led to renewed and vigorous calls for mandatory, generalized testing. Bergalis pleaded for mandatory testing of health-care providers after it came to light that she was infected with HIV while receiving care from her dentist, David Acer of Stuart, Florida, who died of AIDS in 1990.[4]

Molecular biologic and epidemiologic studies make it virtually certain that the infection began with Acer and was passed to his patients, although the manner of passage remains uncertain (Ciesielski et al. 1992, Ou et al. 1992). Researchers from the CDC suggest that Acer passed the virus to his patients in accidents during invasive procedures, since he frequently suffered fatigue while working (Ciesielski et al. 1992, 803). The same researchers point out, however, that the "dental practice had no written infection control protocol or consistent pattern for operatory cleanup and instrument reprocessing," nor was there any procedure for reporting occupational accidents, such as needle sticks (Ciesielski et al. 1992, 802). Other procedures in the practice raise serious concerns about sterile and infection control techniques, which were not consistently exercised (Ciesielski et al. 1992, 802). Another study suggests that failure to heat-sterilize high-speed drills may lead to the transmission of blood and tissue from one patient to others, which might explain transmission of the virus in the Acer case (Lewis and Boe 1992). This is a controversial suggestion, but it does cohere with one of the CDC's initial speculations on the passage of HIV in Acer's patients, namely, that the virus could have been passed through instruments contaminated with the dentist's blood or the blood of a patient already infected by the dentist (Centers for Disease Control 1991c).

Whatever the exact mechanism of transmission in Acer's dental practice, the critical point is that the Acer case is the single known case of transmission of HIV from a provider to patients. Despite this, calls for mandatory, generalized testing have continued to be put forward by both providers and potential patients. The arguments for testing in each case are grounded in the individual's right to determine what risks he or she will assume and in the individual's right to knowledge relevant to protection of his or her legitimate self-interest.

The moral problems with mandatory testing that are generated by considerations of the privacy, autonomy, and well-being of health-care providers are discussed elsewhere in this volume, so we shall not take them up here.[5] There are, however, some empirical facts that merit emphasis, as they help illuminate why mandatory testing makes neither moral, medical, nor fiscal sense. First, foremost, and again, the *only* documented cases of seroconversion in persons exposed to HIV by a provider are the six cases involving Acer's dental patients. Why this is not more widely realized and emphasized in discussions of mandatory testing of providers and why it seldom appears in media stories on AIDS is extremely puzzling.

Second, calls for generalized mandatory testing assume that testing will be accurate. But testing is not accurate unless it is extended. The initial test that is done is called the enzyme-linked immunoabsorbent assay (ELISA or EIA). The ELISA has an extraordinary sensitivity—99.7 percent. Thus, out of 1,000 people who have developed HIV antibodies, 997 will test positive on the ELISA. (False negatives are more likely to be the result of an individual testing too soon after exposure than the result of an inaccurate ELISA). A serious problem, however, is that the ELISA is not as specific as it is sensitive, and out of 1,000 people who have not been infected, only 970 (97 percent) will test negative, leaving 30 false positives. Ruling out false positives requires repeating the ELISA. The true positives will remain positive, and as many as one-third of the false positives will be negative when the test is repeated. Thus, even after repetition of the test, false positives will remain. To weed these out, another test, the Western Blot, is used. Like the ELISA, the Western Blot is extremely sensitive, but it is also quite specific. Blood testing positive on both the ELISA and the Western Blot is assumed to be a true positive.

It is important to realize that the ELISA was initially developed to insure a safe blood supply. If donated blood does not test negative on a single ELISA, it is discarded, even though the results may be incorrect. Using the ELISA to ascertain an individual's HIV status is quite another matter, however, and currently a minimum of two ELISAS or an ELISA and a Western Blot are necessary to conclude reasonably that a subject is HIV-positive. And all of this, of course, costs money. It is estimated that a single testing of all health-care workers would cost between $250 million and $1.5 billion (National Commission on AIDS 1992, 3).[6] And there still would be a number of false negatives.

This leads to the third problem with generalized mandatory testing, namely, that even if testing were 100 percent accurate, results showing a negative HIV status are outdated the minute the blood is drawn. That someone tests negative today in no way guarantees that she or he will test negative tomorrow. Thus, those who believe they can rely on test results to tell them who will and who will not place them at risk of HIV infection make not only a false but a very dangerous judgment, since taking less care to protect oneself from exposure through a provider or patient one believes is HIV negative could be a lethal mistake.

Generalized mandatory testing, then, makes neither moral, medical, nor fiscal sense. Not only is there simply no justification for it, it would be positively wrong to undertake it, because doing it would pointlessly deflect resources from other areas where they could be effectively used (e.g., in research on AIDS-related problems) and would encourage patients and providers alike to assume a false sense of security that would put them and others at increased risk.

But mandatory testing need not be general, and there have also been more moderate calls for testing only those providers who engage in care-providing tasks thought to have a high probability of resulting in HIV exposure—so-called invasive procedures. This may seem like a straightforward proposal, but it is not. The first question, of course, is what counts as an invasive procedure. Does bandaging a wound count? Does hand-feeding a patient with open mouth sores count? Even if we set aside these questionable examples, testing all providers who do procedures that are uncontroversially invasive would require testing all dentists (since virtually nothing dentists do is not invasive), all nurses who are qualified to give injections, all technicians who draw blood, and so on. Thus, the real question is Who would be left out of such testing? And, of course, the problems of false positives and false negatives, incalculable expenses, and false sense of security arise again. Thus, proposals for generalized testing limited to those who perform so-called invasive procedures run into the same problems as proposals for mandatory testing more generally. We see, then, no justification for generalized mandatory testing here either.

What, though, of cases involving an occupational accident where a nurse has exposed a patient or coworker to her or his blood—for example, those rare cases in which a needle falls, first puncturing a nurse, then puncturing a patient? Can a nurse rightly be required to undergo testing in such cases?

There are three good reasons for HIV testing when a person has been exposed to the body fluids of another. First, the relief of any form of suffering always serves as a strong reason for taking a certain course of action. Anxiety is a form of suffering, and concern about potential exposure to a life-threatening disease can create acute anxiety. If an appropriate series of tests shows that the person to whom one has been exposed is not positive for a life-threatening disease, then a good deal of anxiety will be relieved. Second, there is the question of additional transmission. If the person to whom one has been exposed tests positive, one who might otherwise have every reason to believe she or he has not been exposed to the virus will be in a position to protect others from possible exposure until it is known that she or he has not been infected. Third, there is the matter of early treatment. Persons now diagnosed with HIV are living much longer and much higher-quality lives than those who were diagnosed at the beginning of the AIDS crisis. This is in great measure a result of early treatment regimens. What is more, it is not yet known whether treatment given as soon as the virus is detected might preclude the virus from establishing itself. Thus, prophylactic treatments may well be effective for those known to have been exposed to HIV but who have not yet seroconverted.

These reasons combine to provide a strong justification for requiring providers who expose others to their body fluids to undergo testing. Now, of course, we do not mean "requiring" in the sense of seizing a dissident and physically forcing her to have her blood drawn. Such draconian measures would be far more morally repugnant than allowing whatever harm they might prevent. However, an institution would be justified in refusing to continue to employ or otherwise support a practitioner who refuses to undergo testing in the kind of case we are discussing. If one, even innocently, might be placing another at risk, there is a moral obligation to do all that one can to minimize that risk. In the context of health-care provision, this obligation is all the more stringent. Health-care providers are in a much better position to protect themselves from occupational exposure to HIV than are health-care recipients. Patients do not have the benefit of being able to practice universal precautions and are, for the most part, completely dependent on the conscientiousness of their providers. In assuming responsibility for that dependency, providers take on special duties of care, and these duties, combined with the ordinary obligation of moral agents to not harm others, issue in a stringent professional duty to undergo testing in the kind of case sketched above. In much the same way, providers (and other health-care workers) are dependent on the conscientiousness of others within the system, a dependency that likewise places a special moral burden on practitioners to see to the protection of others working in the system. These duties seem to us to be so strong that an institution not only may, but should, require that its providers undergo full testing when they might have exposed another practitioner or worker or a patient to any contagious disease, AIDS included. Thus, although mandatory blanket testing for HIV cannot be justified, we submit that testing should be required for certain individuals under these clearly circumscribed circumstances.

Hiring and Managing HIV-positive Nurses

Increasingly, questions are arising regarding the hiring and managing of providers who are HIV-positive. Some of the potential moral problems have been settled by law. For example, the Americans with Disabilities Act (ADA) precludes employment discrimination simply on the basis of HIV seropositivity or full-blown AIDS. We find this morally attractive, since the issue should not be whether someone is seropositive but whether someone is competent to safely perform the tasks associated with his or her position. Thus, it is inappropriate to inquire into an individual's HIV serostatus as part of an application for a position or as a condition for retaining a position. An individual might be HIV-positive yet have no handicap or diminution in competence resulting from her serostatus alone. If she is competent to perform the tasks covered within a given job description, she should be a viable candidate for hire; or if she is already employed, she should be able to retain her position and perform its tasks. What this means, however, is that individuals of questionable competence might justifiably be restricted from performing certain tasks, which raises some difficult questions about students.

Student professionals are in the process of acquiring competence, and if certain procedures are known to have a high rate of accidents involving potential transference of body fluids to patients when done by students, it would be legitimate to preclude HIV-positive students from participation in those tasks. But this again raises the question of blanket mandatory testing—if it is morally justifiable to exclude students from performing certain procedures, would it be morally justifiable to test all student practitioners for HIV positivity? The problems with blanket mandatory testing of students are quite the same as those with blanket mandatory testing of professional practitioners; and for all the same reasons, mandatory blanket testing of students is morally, medically, and economically a bad idea.

What is true, however, is that student practitioners, because of their relative incompetence, need to be especially scrupulous in attending to their HIV status and in reporting a positive status to their supervisors so that morally appropriate decisions can be made regarding their clinical work. In the same way, practitioners who know they are HIV-positive and who have even the slightest reason to believe that their competence is being affected by illness need to withdraw from performing procedures that present any danger to patients because of a diminution of competence.

One problem with such reporting and withdrawal is that students and practitioners alike are fearful of discrimination and of being prevented from practicing at all, that is, of not having available to them positions involving work that is meaningful for them. The case of Dr. Hacib Aoun illustrates the point. In 1982, the Baltimore cardiologist was infected with HIV after a test tube containing HIV-positive blood broke in his hand, piercing his thumb. In 1986, Aoun was diagnosed with AIDS. Administrators at Johns Hopkins University Hospital refused to renew his contract, precluding him from all clinical work in the hospital. Aoun was offered a faculty position, but his main interest was in providing patient care, and all opportunities for that work were closed to him (Kantrowitz et al. 1991; Navarro 1992).

Two problems arise in the Aoun case: (1) that Aoun's having AIDS was considered sufficient to justify barring him from all practice in the hospital and (2) that even though he was offered an academic position, he was unable to provide *any* patient care.

There is some hope that the ADA will alleviate such problems for practitioners working in corporate practices or institutions. The ADA requires that "reasonable accommodation" be made for persons with recognized disabilities. As we have just argued, a positive HIV serostatus alone should not provide a justification for limiting the tasks of competent practitioners. Thus, the question of reasonable accommodation should not even arise unless or until an individual's competence is compromised. In the case of HIV-positive providers whose competence is compromised and who want to be on the front lines of providing care, reasonable accommodation should be construed as including provision of care. This should include HIV-positive students as well as those professionals who are suffering competence-compromising effects of HIV infection.[7]

It is, however, crucial to realize that students and compromised practitioners are very unlikely to come forward to report their positive HIV status or failing competence unless their institutions make it absolutely clear that these students and practitioners will not be discriminated against and forced out of what, for each, is meaningful work. Administrators and others in authority in institutional settings need to be unequivocally committed to creating "safe places," and they need to back up that commitment with uncompromising policies that state explicitly that they will not do blanket testing of their practitioners and students and that they will accommodate them as fully as possible to maximally insure the safety of those served by and serving in the institution or practice. Since blanket testing is, for all the reasons we have seen, out of the question, practicing universal precautions, adopting safer technologies (an issue we take up in the last section), and creating this kind of safety and support for practitioners must become unwavering commitments in all health-care provision settings.

Finally, independent practitioners, including self-employed certified nurses, need to be supported as well. We have mentioned that CDC investigators believe that Dr. Acer infected his patients during invasive procedures he performed after his competence was compromised. As long as independent practitioners have no place to turn to for meaningful work and support that sustains their dignity and integrity as persons and professionals, we can expect that at least some who are competence-compromised by the effects of HIV will continue to perform procedures from which they should withdraw. The moral failures in these cases cannot be attributed to individuals alone—more at fault is a system that has systematically abandoned persons with AIDS.

Special Physical, Intellectual, Psychosocial and Emotional Challenges for Nurses

AIDS is known for its physical and emotional devastation. As a consequence, caring for persons with AIDS places enormous stress on nurses, who are in constant contact with their patients, unlike other providers who see their patients only intermittently. Since HIV involves the progressive destruction of the immune response, caring for affected individuals requires constant vigilance and response to maladies that are of little threat to immunocompetent individuals. The physical complications of the disease tend to be multiple, concurrent, and unpredictable, and they are often confusing. For example, persons with AIDS frequently suffer from opportunistic infections, secondary cancers, changing nutritional deficits, quick alterations in fluid volumes, various motor weaknesses, and the physiological consequences of the human immunodeficiency virus itself, all of which call for ceaseless close monitoring and constant decisions regarding what physical care is needed.[8]

What is more, persons hospitalized for AIDS-related maladies are generally placed on floors that already tend to be among the busiest in inpatient facilities, namely, general medical and surgical units. The physical and intellectual challenges of providing the complex and constant nursing care needed by persons with AIDS are further exacerbated by the current state of critical shortages in the profession and by the unique and particularly intense psychosocial and emotional burdens that nurses face in providing this care.

We have pointed out that in the past decade of AIDS surveillance, the only known cases of transmission of HIV from a provider to patients are those of six patients of a single dentist who performed invasive procedures while compromised and whose practice frequently failed to exercise sterile and infection control techniques. And we have pointed out that, in the same decade, deaths to health-care providers from AIDS are far below the number of deaths each year resulting from occupational exposure to HBV. Yet the fear of AIDS transmission in health-care settings remains pronounced, just as the fear of AIDS throughout the wider society remains pronounced. Motivated by fear, providers continue to refuse to provide care for persons with AIDS, and calls for generalized mandatory testing of providers and patients alike continue to be heard.[9] Why does the sense of panic hang on so tenaciously?

No small part of the answer to that question has to do with the groups with whom AIDS was initially associated and with whom it continues to be associated in our social consciousness, despite the fact that AIDS is now occurring at the highest rates among heterosexual teenagers. That is, as the AIDS crisis unfolded in the early 1980s, the primary victims were, from the dominant social point of view, *personae non gratae*—prostitutes, intravenous drug users, and most of all, homosexuals. AIDS came on us as a disease of "others" and, in particular, as a disease of "others" who were widely perceived as guilty, drawing disease as "penance" for their "sins."

Being part of the culture, nurses are not immune from dominant social views. We said at the beginning of this chapter that the real question of caring for persons with AIDS is no longer one of whether all nurses will have to care for these persons, but how effective that care will be. Effectiveness of care can easily be compromised if the persons responsible for providing care are in any way hostile toward or otherwise rejecting of their patients. Since nurses are the providers most in contact with persons with AIDS and most responsible for the hands-on provision of this care, it is crucial that they look carefully at their own value assumptions regarding persons with AIDS, clearly and deliberately coming to terms with whatever fragments they find in themselves of the socially dominant attitudes toward AIDS patients who are members of "hated groups"—attitudinal fragments that might compromise the quality of care they are responsible to provide these persons.

Many of the widespread, deeply negative attitudes toward prostitutes, intravenous drug users, and homosexuals rest on the view that persons in these groups act immorally. This easily leads to the punishment concept of AIDS, which can easily undermine fair and compassionate treatment of persons with AIDS (Kopelman 1988, 49). Although we cannot offer here even a partially adequate evaluation of moral views on prostitution, intravenous drug use, and homosexuality, a few things really should be said about these matters at every opportunity, even at the risk of oversimplification.

First, it cannot be emphasized strongly enough that nurses need to be very clear about the value judgments on the issues they bring with them when caring for persons with AIDS. Second, they need to realize that the deeply imbedded moral rejection of persons in these groups is not as easily justified as some might think.

For example, prostitutes often fall into prostitution because little (if anything) else is available to them in the way of well-paying jobs. It has been argued by social theorists since Marx and Engels that if all working-class women were provided with jobs that gave them meaningful work and a living wage, prostitution would wither away (Ericsson 1980; e.g., Tong 1984, chap. 2). Blaming the prostitute seems to many (who know what the world and "choices" of prostitutes tend to be like) to be among the most egregious instances of blaming the victim.

Victim blaming can be seen, too, in the condemnation of intravenous-drug users and needle sharing in the drug community. Not only are there serious (and complicated) questions about addiction here, there are also questions about the social conditions of those within the drug subculture. In a perceptive discussion of so-called voluntary victims, one ethicist points out that " 'washes'—the small amount of drug left in the syringe after injection—are often offered by one addict to others in need of a fix as a way of establishing or expressing friendship and loyalty in an environment which often constitutes the sole benign social world for the addict" (Kasachkoff 1992, 10). Refusing to use one's partner's "works" or to offer one's own "works" to a partner experiencing withdrawal would be to violate important standards within a culture that may be the only meaningful link an individual has to others (see Jarlais, Friedman, and Strug 1986, cited in Kasachkoff 1992).

Of these three groups of persons, homosexuals often present the greatest psychological difficulty to persons generally and health-care providers in particular. Prostitution and intravenous drug use are considered bad, but homosexuality is considered by some to be an unnatural perversion, a badness different in kind from and worse than prostitution and intravenous drug use. When it is treated as a crime, it is treated as the most heinous and bewildering kind of crime—a crime against nature itself.

There is, however, no plausible argument for the claim that homosexual behavior as such is immoral. The claim that homosexual behavior is wrong because it is unnatural is either incoherent, begs the question, is based on religious commitments that are not universally shared and are wrongly imposed on those who do not share them, or is not a genuinely moral claim at all, but merely the expression of an ingrained bias.[10]

It is morally incumbent on providers to carefully examine any biases they might have against persons with AIDS and, where they find biases, to acquaint themselves as fully as possible with the literature and other resources that provide an antidote to the biases in the dominant cultural attitudes that can so easily lead to unfair compromises in providing care for persons with AIDS.

Struggling with the cultural values that affect us all is one of the special challenges for nurses, for again, nurses more than any other providers are called on to provide unremitting care for their patients with AIDS. But even if a nurse has no biases of her or his own to manage in caring for persons with AIDS, other intense psychological stressors are placed on nurses in caring for these patients. Given that AIDS seems to be fatal and that it is riddled with recalcitrant social stigmas, persons with the disease often face terminal illness in relative isolation. The diagnosis of AIDS often carries with it the exposure of an individual's sexual orientation, intravenous-drug use, or sexual promiscuity, leaving the individual vulnerable to disapproval, warranted or not. Family members often respond with extreme detachment or outright hostility. For example, parents often "disown" sons or daughters because of their newly revealed association with feared or disapproved lifestyles or behaviors.

Our communities have not come forward to provide substantial help with all of this. Agencies providing specific services to persons with AIDS are sparse and, in general, poorly funded. Not only does this lack of community support add to the fear, guilt, and suspicion commonly experienced by those who are HIV-positive, it adds substantially to the sense of isolation of these people, who are usually young and recently vital, and may have had little (and sometimes virtually no) time to adjust to their diagnosis and long-term prognosis.[11] All of these factors combine to place enormous psychological burdens on nurses, who must grapple with their own responses to these facts while attending to the psychological devastation these patients so frequently experience.

That nurses are doing this well is clearly indicated by the frequency with which nurses are being asked by their AIDS patients to take on durable powers of attorney for them. That this is happening suggests not only that nurses in fact *are* providing critical and effective psychological support for their most isolated AIDS patients but that nurses' relationships with their AIDS patients are often on a level of intimacy that is much more profound than the relationships these persons have with any other providers, including physicians. Such deeply personal relationships make it virtually impossible for a provider to fully detach from "the job" when away from work. And these burdens are added to the provision of unremitting and highly complex physical care, as we have already seen. All this suggests that the profession of nursing and institutions and practices that employ nurses need to do all that they possibly can to provide nurses with the support needed to continue providing high-quality, effective physical and psychological care for persons with AIDS.

Challenges to Nursing as a Profession

The elements covered in this discussion all point to a number of special challenges for nursing as a profession. There is an unavoidable political dimension to professional ethics, and nursing leaders need to be unceasingly active in pressing for certain institutional arrangements (Callahan, in press). The burdens of care just discussed point to a critical need for support for nurses working with persons with AIDS, such as release time from floors for nurses to meet in support groups or to attend other kinds of meetings with colleagues caring for persons with AIDS.

The issue of contagion raises equally compelling challenges. We have argued that emphasis needs to be placed on creating a safe place for practitioners and students and on the exercise of universal precautions. Nursing needs to do all that it can to see that these goals will be achieved. This means that nurses need to be involved in continuing education efforts on HIV positivity and AIDS, on constructing policies and procedures that will make practitioners and students comfortable withdrawing from tasks they are not adequately competent to perform, and in doing all that is possible to see that institutional administrations are absolutely rigorous about exercising universal precautions. And nurses need to do all that they can to help transform the system in a way that will let it accommodate independent practitioners who need to withdraw from areas of their practices because of competence-compromising effects of HIV infection.

Unhappily, nurses have traditionally had relatively little power in the health-care setting. The relative powerlessness of nurses vis-à-vis administrators and physicians in health-care provision serves none of us well. In recent years, as nursing has pressed forward in professionalizing, much has changed. For example, hospital programs, which used to be the exclusive training arenas for nurses, have virtually vanished as nursing has moved its preparation programs to universities. Nurses are now urged by the profession to seek B.S.N.'s, M.S.N.'s, and Ph.D.'s, as well as certification. And the profession has worked hard to move away from the portrait of the nurse as physician handmaiden to an understanding of the nurse as client advocate. Indeed, the very term "patient" is replaced by "client" in the most recent revision of the American Nurses' Association Code for Nurses (1976). And the term "physician" doesn't even appear in the code.

Still, it is undeniable that nurses continue to fear for their positions if they "buck" powerful physicians or are too outspoken with administrators. This, too, serves none of us well. Nurses simply are in the best position in the health-care system to serve as recognized advocates of the rights and well-being of those in their care. As potential patients, we are all worse off for nursing's relative lack of power within health-care provision. As we face the dilemmas and burdens associated with AIDS, this is clearer than ever. If the actions of individuals or the policies of institutions in any way threaten the safety of those involved in the provision of health care or of those who receive health care, nurses are generally in a good position to see this, and they need to be in a good position to do something about it. That means that the nursing leadership, not just in general, but in every particular health-care setting, needs to insist on increasing the authority of nursing. The less forceful nursing leadership is in this regard, the less blameworthy individual nurses are for not functioning as advocates of those in their care. Conversely, the more forceful nursing leadership is in this regard, the more blameworthy individual nurses are for not functioning fully as advocates (see Muyskens 1982).

Advocacy must take place, however, not only on the level of particular issues, but on that of policy, as well. Much of the discussion in this chapter has focused on the issue of HIV transmission and the associated question of testing. By far the greatest danger of transmission of HIV in the health-care setting lies with needle sticks. It is estimated that over a million needle-stick accidents occur annually and are sustained by health-care workers ranging from surgeons to laundry personnel.[12] Given existing insurance arrangements in this country, a worker who contracts a disease as a result of one of these accidents will not receive Worker's Compensation benefits unless the disease can be shown to have been contracted in an occupational accident. Although many health-care workers do not report needle-stick accidents (perhaps largely because they are not aware that their Worker's Compensation benefits are contingent on reporting and subsequent testing), it still costs the health-care system roughly $750 million annually just to test injured workers after the needle sticks that are reported, with the average costs of a needle-stick injury falling at about $405, exclusive of prophylactic administration of azidothymidine (AZT) following needle-stick exposure to HIV (Jagger, Hunt, and Pearson 1990; House of Representatives 1992). Added to this are months of unimaginable worry until a worker can be confident that he or she has not contracted a communicable disease from a needle stick. This continues to occur even though needles are unnecessary for a number of uses (e.g., accessing intravenous equipment), and conventional needles could be replaced immediately with self-sheathing needles. If this were done, it is estimated that 90 percent of the needle-stick injuries from hollow-bore needles (which pose a greater risk than solid-bore needles) could be eliminated (Jagger 1992). The technology is available, yet institutions continue to resist adopting it.

Nurses, however, can make and have made a difference. For example, after a medical student on her floor was exposed to HIV through a needle stick, Janet Christensen brought a grievance against San Francisco General Hospital for not making available throughout the hospital the self-sheathing needles that were used in the hospital's emergency and ambulance areas (Christensen 1992). The grievance was settled in her favor. The hospitalwide introduction of self-sheathing devices at San Francisco General was slower than she would have liked, and practitioners have had some complaints about the particular devices put into place. But the critical point is that the insistence of a nurse in this case has made the important difference of beginning the introduction of safer devices throughout the hospital. What is more, San Francisco General has now developed a set of policies that are considered by many (including the CDC) to provide excellent models for other institutions preparing similar policies (Eubanks 1992).

Safer devices are more expensive than conventional devices, there is no question about that. But the costs of needle sticks are exorbitant, both financially and in terms of the illness, emotional devastation, and death that result from them. Since nurses constitute roughly two million of the roughly five million health-care workers in this country, it is not surprising that nurses as a health-care provision group sustain the greatest number of needle-stick injuries and have sustained the most occupationally acquired HIV seroconversions.[13] Nurses, therefore, have a particularly strong interest in minimizing the number of needle-stick injuries.[14] The profession as a whole needs to follow the lead of nurses like Christensen (and a number of other individual nurses), using every available tactic, from formal grievances to lawsuits to lobbying, to press for the quick adoption of safer instruments. And if this effort were organized by nursing on the national level, it would be much more effective.

Because of the nature of nursing care, AIDS raises both general issues that are exacerbated in the nursing context and issues that present special challenges to individual nurses and nursing as a profession. By pressuring institutional administrations, individual nurses and the nursing profession can do much to dispel some of the burdens created by AIDS. Where burdens cannot be dispelled, they can often at least be alleviated by policies that are uncompromisingly committed to maximizing safety and security for everyone in health-care settings and that provide needed support for those contending with the multifarious challenges that AIDS has brought to the health-care arena.

Notes

1. Of these 32 reported cases, there were 12 nurses, 11 clinical laboratory technicians, 4 physicians, 1 nonclinical laboratory technician, 1 maintenance

worker, 1 respiratory therapist, 1 surgical technician, and 1 health aide. At that time, the CDC suspected another 69 cases involving 14 nurses, 12 clinical laboratory technicians, 7 paramedics, 7 nonsurgical physicians, 6 dental providers, 5 health aides, 5 housekeeping/maintenance staff, 3 morgue technicians, 3 unspecified technicians/providers, 2 surgeons, and 2 from other "health related occupations" (Centers for Disease Control 1992, 824).

2. Henderson et al. (1990) estimate the rate of HIV seroconversion following occupational exposure through a needle stick involving HIV-positive blood to be 0.3 to 0.4 percent.

3. Universal precautions are measures that are to be taken by health-care workers to protect themselves from occupational exposure to blood-borne pathogens, including HIV. Precautions vary according to procedure or task, but the rationale for their implementation is the assumption that exposure to the blood of any patient (or any coworker) could result in transmission of a blood-borne pathogen; thus, precautions appropriate to the procedure or task are to be taken. For rules and recommendations regarding universal precautions, see Centers for Disease Control (1989) and Occupational Safety and Health Administration (1991).

4. Bergalis made a short but emotionally charged and highly publicized plea for mandatory testing of providers to the House Subcommittee on Health and the Environment as it heard testimony on a bill introduced by William E. Dannemeyer (R–Calif.). This bill would have required that HIV-positive health-care providers be prohibited from doing invasive medical procedures and would have allowed physicians to test patients for HIV infection without their consent.

5. See Chapter 1, for example.

6. In 1993, verifying that an individual is HIV-positive cost $100 to $150. If we go back to the number of practicing nurses in 1988 (1,670,000), it takes little to see that blanket testing of nurses (not to mention other health-care providers) would be prohibitively expensive. Assume that a single ELISA costs $45 (Jagger, Hunt, and Pearson [1990] record the cost of an ELISA at $46.20). A single test at $45 on all practicing nurses, using the 1988 figure, would cost $75,150,500. Out of every 1,000 nurses who have never been infected, 30 will be false positives. Even if we make the unlikely assumption that no practicing nurse is infected, an initial testing would yield at least 50,000 false positives, which would then require retesting, with the (minimum) cost of retesting alone being $2,254,500. That is a total cost of $77,404,500 to find that no practicing nurse is positive. Of course, in reality, there would be some true positives, which would only increase the cost.

7. The policy at San Francisco General Hospital makes fitness for duty the single consideration in regulating the work of HIV-positive providers: "If he or she is deemed fit, the worker may perform invasive procedures, regardless of his or her HIV or other blood-borne–pathogen status, provided appropriate infection control is maintained" (Eubanks 1992, 29).

8. For more detailed discussions of the sorts of physical maladies that commonly affect persons with ARC and AIDS, see Joshi (1990).

9. In November of 1992, *Lear's* magazine reported that the results of a survey of roughly 6,000 readers, which indicated the following percentage of respondents and the categories for which they believe mandatory testing should be required: 59 percent for dentists; 58 percent for marriage license applicants; 56 percent for physicians; 53 percent for prostitutes; 48 percent for health-care workers generally; 47 percent for nurses; and 40 percent for all hospital patients (Rubenstein 1992, 65). Furthermore, 13 percent of the respondents also indicated that they request that a new lover be tested for HIV positivity before having sex; and 9 percent indicated that they would have themselves tested before engaging in sex with a new partner (Rubenstein 1992, 64). All these figures suggest that the general public continues to think that testing can provide assurances that it simply cannot provide.

10. For a fuller discussion of the unnaturalness argument and its problems, see Callahan 1988, 15–17. For a discussion of what constitutes a genuine moral position as opposed to a mere bias or learned visceral response, see Dworkin 1977, 250, and Callahan 1987, 347.

11. For more detailed discussions of the emotional needs of persons who are HIV-positive, see Cohen and Weisman 1986.

12. For example, Gwyen Spruill, who works in a laundry facility that provides laundry services to eight hospitals in the Detroit area, indicates that "it is not unusual to pull up to a dozen needles, scalpels, and other [contaminated] surgical instruments out of the laundry every month" (Spruill 1992, 9).

13. See n. 1.

14. Nurses are outranked only by housekeeping staff in numbers of needle-stick injuries among all groups of health-care workers, including providers and ancillary personnel. See, for example, National Commission on AIDS 1992, 11.

References

"AIDS Risk Reduction Strategies Urged for Health Care Workers." 1990. *Hospital Risk Management* (June): 77–80.

Bartlett, J. G. 1992. "HIV Infection and Surgeons." *Current Problems in Surgery* (April): 199–280.

Blumenfield, M., J. Smith, J. Milazzo, S. Seropain, and G. Wormser. 1987. "Survey of Attitudes of Nurses Working with AIDS Patients." *General Hospital Psychiatry* 9:58–63.

Callahan, Joan C. 1987. "On Harming the Dead." *Ethics* 97:341–352.

———. In press. "Professions, Institutions, and Moral Risk." In *Professional Ethics and Social Responsibility*, ed. Daniel E. Wueste. Totowa, N.J.: Rowman and Littlefield.

———. 1988. *Ethical Issues in Professional Life*. New York: Oxford University Press.

Centers for Disease Control. 1989. "Guidelines for Prevention of Transmission of Human Immunodeficiency Virus and Hepatitis B Virus to Health-Care and Public-Safety Workers." *Morbidity and Mortality Weekly Report* 38(S6): 3–37.

———. 1991a. "Process for Identifying Exposure-Prone Invasive Procedures." *Morbidity and Mortality Weekly Report* 40: 565–566.

———. 1991b. "Recommendations for Preventing Transmission of Human Immunodeficiency Virus and Hepatitis B Virus to Patients During Exposure-prone Invasive Procedures." *Morbidity and Mortality Weekly Report* 40 (RR-8): 1–9.

———. 1991c. "Update: Transmission of HIV Infection During an Invasive Dental Procedure.' *Morbidity and Mortality Weekly Report* 40:21–33.

———. 1992. "Surveillance for Occupationally Acquired HIV Infection—United States, 1981–1992." *Morbidity and Mortality Weekly Report* 41:823–825.

Christensen, Janet. 1992. Testimony. *Healthcare Worker Safety and Needlestick Injuries*, pp. 12–15. Hearing before the Subcommittee on Regulation, Business Opportunities, and Energy of the Committee of Small Business, House of Representatives. Serial no. 102–50. Washington, D.C.: Government Printing Office.

Ciesielski, C., D. Marianos, C. Y. Ou, R. Dumbaugh, J. Witte, et al. 1992. "Transmission of Human Immunodeficiency Virus in a Dental Practice." *Annals of Internal Medicine* 116:798–805.

Cohen, M. A., and H. W. Weisman. 1986. "A Biosocial Approach to AIDS." *Psychosomatics* 27:245–249.

Doebbeling, B. N., and R. P. Wenzel. 1990. "The Direct Costs of Universal Precautions in a Teaching Hospital." *Journal of the American Medical Association* 264:2083–2087.

Dworkin, Ronald. 1977. "Liberty and Moralism." In *Taking Rights Seriously*, pp. 240–258. Cambridge, Mass.: Harvard University Press.

Ericsson, Lars O. 1980. "Charges Against Prostitution: An Attempt at Philosophical Assessment." *Ethics* 90:335–366.

Eubanks, Paula. 1992. "Infection Control Is Core of HIV-positive Worker Strategy at San Francisco General." *Hospitals* (September 20): 28–30.

Goldsmith, M. F. 1992. "Critical Moment at Hand in HIV/AIDS Pandemic: New Global Strategy Proposed." *Journal of the American Medical Association* 268:445–446.

Henderson, D. K., B. J. Fahey, M. Willy, J. M. Schmitt, K. Carey, et al. 1990. "Risk for Occupational Transmission of Human Immunodeficiency Virus Type 1 (HIV-1) Associated with Clinical Exposures: A Prospective Evaluation." *Annals of Internal Medicine* 113:740–746.

House of Representatives. 1992. *Healthcare Worker Safety and Needlestick Injuries*. Hearing before the Subcommittee on Regulation, Business Opportunities, and Energy of the Committee of Small Business, House of Representatives. Serial no. 102-50. Washington, D.C.: Government Printing Office.

Hurley, Patricia. 1992. Personal communication.

Jagger, Janine. 1992. Testimony. *Healthcare Worker Safety and Needlestick Injuries*, pp. 12–15. Hearing before the Subcommittee on Regulation, Business Opportunities, and Energy of the Committee of Small Business, House of Representatives. Serial no. 102-50. Washington, D.C.: Government Printing Office.

Jagger, Janine, Ella H. Hunt, and Richard D. Pearson. 1990. "Estimated Cost of Needlestick Injuries for Six Major Needled Devices." *Infection Control and Hospital Epidemiology* 11(11): 584–588.

Jarlais, Don C., Samuel R. Friedman, and David Strug. 1986. "AIDS and Needle Sharing Within the IV-Drug Use Subcultures. In *The Social Dimensions of AIDS: Method and Theory*, ed. Douglas A. Feldman and Thomas M. Johnson, New York: Praeger. Cited in Kasachkoff, "Voluntary Victims," pp. 10–11.

Joshi, Vijay V. 1990. *Pathology of AIDS and Other Manifestations of HIV Infection*. New York: IGAKU-SHOIN.

Kantrowitz, Barbara, Karen Springen, John McCormick, Spencer Reiss, Mary Hager, Lydia Denworth, Clara Bingham, and Donna Foote. 1991. "Doctors and Aids." *Newsweek* (July 1): 48–57.

Kasachkoff, Tziporah. 1992. "Voluntary Victims." Unpublished typescript. New York: Graduate Center, City University of New York.

Kelen, G. D., T. DiGiovanna, L. Bisson, D. Kalainov, K. T. Silverton, et al. 1989. "Human Immunodeficiency Virus Infection in Emergency Department Patients: Epidemology, Clinical Presentations, and Risk to Health Care Workers. The Johns Hopkins Experience." *Journal of the American Medical Association* 262:516–522.

Kopelman, Loretta. 1988. "The Punishment Concept of Disease." In *AIDS: Ethics and Public Policy*, ed. Christine Pierce and Donald VanDeVeer, pp. 49–55. Belmont, Calif.: Wadsworth.

Lewis, D. L., and R. K. Boe. 1992. "Cross-infection Risks Associated with Current Procedures for Using High-Speed Dental Handpieces." *Journal of Clinical Microbiology* 30:401–406.

McCrutchan, J. Allen. 1986. "What You Can Do to Stop the AIDS Panic." *RN* (October): 18–21.

Muyskens, James L. 1982. *Moral Problems in Nursing: A Philosophical Investigation*. Totowa, N.J.: Rowman and Littlefield.

National Commission on AIDS. 1992. *Preventing HIV Transmission in Health Care Settings*. Washington, D.C.: National Commission on AIDS.

National League for Nursing. 1992. Personal communication with Research Department.

Navarro, Mireya. 1992. "Dr. Hacib Aoun, 36; Championed Rights of Health Workers." *New York Times*, February 18.

Occupational Safety and Health Administration. 1991. "Occupational Exposure to Bloodborne Pathogens: Final Rule." *Federal Register* 56(235): 64175–64182.

Ou, C. Y., C. Ciesielski, A. Meyers, G. Bandea, et al. 1992. "Molecular

Epidemiology of HIV Transmission in a Dental Practice." *Science* 256:1165–1171.

Rubenstein, Carin. 1992. "The *Lear's* Report: How AIDS Has Changed Our Sex Lives." *Lear's* (November): 62–67.

Spruill, Gwyen, 1992. Testimony. *Healthcare Worker Safety and Needlestick Injuries*, pp. 9–11. Hearing before the Subcommittee on Regulation, Business Opportunities, and Energy of the Committee of Small Business, House of Representatives. Serial no. 102-50. Washington, D.C.: Government Printing Office.

Tong, Rosemarie. 1984. *Women, Sex, and the Law*. Totowa, N.J.: Rowman and Allanheld.

Van Servellen, G. M., C. E. Lewis, and L. Leake. 1988. "Nurses' Knowledge, Attitudes, and Fears About AIDS." *Journal of Nursing Science and Practice* 1:1–7.

Wallack, J. J. 1989. "AIDS Anxiety Among Health Care Professionals." *Hospital and Community Psychiatry* 40:507–510.

3

The Dentist's Obligation to Treat Patients with HIV: A Patient's Perspective

Michael Davis

For Larry Rose, 1950–1990

I am not a dentist, dental hygienist, dental assistant, dental clerk, dental lab technician, or even a professor of dentistry. I am a philosopher whose work with professional ethics has focused on lawyering, engineering, and other nonmedical professions. Why then do I write about dental ethics? I am a dental patient.[1] Like other such patients, I might now unknowingly be carrying the HIV virus; and also like the others, I might face discrimination should my dentist learn that I am a carrier. That is the possibility that motivates this chapter. I hope to shape how dentists, their staff, and their patients respond to the knowledge that someone among them has HIV.

The chapter has three parts. The first is about professions in general (but with dentistry as the chief example). Most of what I say in this part should be familiar. My purpose is not to break new ground but to make explicit an analysis of professions I believe we all take for granted. The second part applies this analysis to some central questions concerning dentists, other dental professionals, and HIV-infected patients. Only dentists are likely to find much of this part familiar.

These first two parts are best thought of as introducing (or defending) the third part, the argument I would make to my dentist if I had HIV and he were inclined to refuse to treat me for that reason. I regard this as the heart of the chapter. As I reviewed the literature on HIV and dentistry, I found much about the patient's interests, needs, and rights, but nothing about the patient as an active person with a case to make to her dentist. Something important is missing. Putting yourself in the other person's place is a potent means of gaining moral insight. Many clever arguments, or artful dodges, don't look nearly so good once you look at them from the other person's perspective. I therefore call your attention to the form of the argument in the chapter's third part. Whatever its substantive merits, it should provide a model for presenting other arguments.

Professions, Professional Obligations, and Ethics

The dentist's obligation to treat patients infected with HIV is, it is said, a professional obligation. But what are professional obligations? How does one come to have them? Why should professional obligations have a substantial place in a decent person's deliberations? To answer these questions, we must have a general analysis of professions.

The word "profession" has at least three different uses. "Profession" can, of course, be used to mean no more than those sharing a certain occupation. According to this usage, the dental profession would be all those persons who earn their living by providing a certain service. The dental profession in this sense has existed ever since someone made a business of pulling teeth.

"Profession" can also refer to those occupations defined by esoteric knowledge, high prestige, high pay, or some combination of these. According to this usage, dentistry is less of a profession than, say, medicine, because dentistry takes a year or two less to learn, dentists are paid less than physicians, and dentists have less prestige than physicians. In this sense, the profession of dentistry is a mere byproduct of technology, special market conditions, changing social perceptions, or some combination of these.

Though these two uses of "profession" are common, especially among sociologists, neither seems to me to capture what most professionals have in mind when they talk about "their" profession. A third use of "profession" does. "Profession" can also refer to an occupational group *organized* to provide its distinctive service (in part at least) *for the public good.* "Profession" in this sense distinguishes an occupational organization committed (at least in part) to public service from similar organizations (or collections of individuals) with only the purpose of recreation, making a profit, protecting members from exploitation, or the like.

Part of creating a profession is setting standards of skill and conduct its members are to meet. So, for example, the American Dental Association's (ADA) first Principle of Ethics declares that the dentist's primary professional obligation is "service to the public" and then identifies the primary component of that obligation as "competent and timely delivery of quality care within the bounds of the clinical circumstances . . . with due consideration being given to the needs and desires of the patient."[2] "Competence" is a standard of skill; "timely delivery," a standard of conduct.

Part of creating a profession is, I said, setting standards of skill and conduct. But not any standards will do. If the would-be members of a profession can agree to do only what market, law, and ordinary morality would exact even if they did not organize, they cannot organize as a profession (though they could of course still form some other organization). Public service is not simply serving the public. Every honest business does that—by providing a useful service at a fair price to those who want it. Rather, public service benefits the public in ways neither market nor law nor ordinary morality demands. Public service is service beyond what is necessary to make a living, stay within the law, and do nothing immoral. In this respect at least, public service is always voluntary. So, since professions are defined by their purpose of serving the public, a profession must, by definition, set standards of skill and conduct that go beyond what would otherwise be required.

These standards must, of course, be more than window dressing. Paper standards create only a paper profession. So, another part of creating a profession is taking reasonable steps to assure that the standards of skill and conduct will generally be met. Among these steps might be adopting a clear statement of standards, that is, a code of ethics. Other possible steps are setting educational requirements, instituting competency tests, providing interpretations of the code, investigating complaints, and disciplining members who do not conduct themselves as they should. "Profession" (in this third sense) almost necessitates an active professional society.

This sense of "profession" is the one invoked when, for example, someone claims that the ADA is a professional society, not just a trade association or union. It is, I think, also the sense usually invoked when a dentist says, "Dentistry is a profession, not just another trade or business."

To say that a profession (by definition) undertakes to provide a public service is not to say that members of a profession are public servants in the sense that public officials are. Public servants are government agents or employees. Some professionals, for example, public school teachers, are also public servants. But most professions, including dentistry, are nongovernmental organizations, the members of which are (mostly) either self-employed or employed by private organizations. Their public service is given directly to individual members of the public in the market (without government direction).

There is no contradiction between public service of this sort and being a member of a "free profession."

Given this sense of "profession," how does one come to be a member of a profession? If a profession is defined by its standards of skill and conduct, then, ideally, I should be a member of the profession in question if I satisfy those standards. In a few professions, for example, philosophy, this ideal is approached. You are a philosopher if you do philosophy reasonably well. But in any profession in which the risk of immediate harm to users is much greater than in philosophy—that is to say, in almost any other profession whatever—human organization should intervene to protect the unwary from harm. There should be letters of recommendation, tests of knowledge and skill, certification, and the like. Most professions have some formal means of admitting members. Since formal means are subject to error, every profession will sometimes admit people who should not be members and sometimes fail to admit people who should be. Since people can also change once admitted, losing the skill or good intentions they once had, the fit between the profession's declared standards and a professional's actual skill and conduct can be quite poor.

So, that someone is a professional, that is, a member of a certain profession, entails nothing more than that she satisfies the formal requirements of membership. She may in fact not now have the skill a member of that profession should or may not now be conducting herself as a member of that profession should. Someone is a dentist, for example, if she is licensed to practice dentistry, however incompetent she may be and however badly she behaves. She leaves the profession and becomes a former dentist only once she loses or gives up her license. A former dentist's connection with dentistry is merely historical. A former dentist is not a dentist at all.

Not so a retired dentist. By "a retired dentist" I mean a dentist who maintains his license but ceases to hold himself out as a dentist. He is a dentist, at least potentially, and has only to return to practice to be a dentist in the full sense. But, though a dentist, the retired dentist is no longer an active member of the profession. Since our concern here is only the practice of dentistry, we may hereafter ignore retired members of the profession.

If that is what a professional is (an active member of a profession), professional obligations must be those obligations one has because one *is* an active member of the profession. One's professional obligations must be to have the skills that members of one's profession are supposed to have and to act as members of that profession are supposed to act. Since by definition the obligations of a profession must, as a whole, exceed what market, law, and ordinary morality require, the profession must impose obligations ordinary people do not have. We have now reached the central problem for any theory of professions. Given that being an active member of a profession means having special obligations, why would any rational person want to be a professional? Why voluntarily take on special burdens?

The answer must be that the professional benefits in some way, for example, by being able to perform a service he could not otherwise perform, by being able to attract business he could not otherwise attract, or by appearing wiser than he would otherwise appear. Whatever the benefit in view, he must gain it by holding himself out as a member of the profession in question. His ability to do that ordinarily depends on what the clientele of that profession expects of those who hold themselves out as members of that profession. What determines what they expect? In large part at least, their expectations are determined by what other members of the profession have done (and are doing). If the other members have been skillful and honest, holding oneself out as one of them will be beneficial. If, however, they have too often proved incompetent or untrustworthy, holding oneself out as one of them would be pointless. Why identify oneself as a charlatan, quack, or shyster?

There is, then, a clear sense in which no member of a profession practices alone. To hold oneself out as a member of a particular profession is to make oneself a participant in a larger practice in which all other (active) members of that profession also participate. To claim to be a dentist, for example, is in effect to claim to have the skills dentists have formally undertaken to have and to conduct oneself as dentists have formally undertaken to conduct themselves. That claim is worth little unless dentists have undertaken to be more skillful than market, law, and ordinary morality require and to conduct themselves better. And, even so, that claim would be worth little unless dentists generally live up to their professional standards.

We call a practice "cooperative" insofar as the benefit making it rational for each participant to do her part depends in substantial part on the other participants doing theirs. A cooperative practice helps people achieve what they want by getting them to "operate together." Part of any cooperative practice is giving up some freedom one would otherwise have, in particular the freedom to operate in disregard of the rules governing the practice. Those voluntarily participating in a cooperative practice are thus involved in something like a contract with the other participants. While they have made no explicit promises to each other to do their part in the cooperative practice, they are morally in exactly the same condition as if they had. As long as the practice itself is morally permissible, anyone failing to do her part while claiming the benefits of a participant treats the other participants unfairly. She takes advantage of their work without doing her share to produce those benefits. She cheats her fellow cooperators of benefits they have worked for in part at least in expectation that she would do the same. She takes unfair advantage of them.[3]

So, if a dentist asks why she should do as her profession requires, we can answer: Dentistry is a morally permissible practice, indeed, a morally good one. You claim the benefits of that practice by holding yourself out as a dentist. Dentistry is a cooperative practice. If you claim the benefits while failing to do your part to generate those benefits, you help to undermine the practice on which those benefits depend. You cheat the other members of your profession. No morally decent person would want to do that.

I have so far said nothing about state licensing. That was no oversight. I think it important to recognize that professions are usually organized *before* they are licensed. Licensing is not part of what makes an occupation a profession but is instead part of the strategy professions adopt to protect the public against impostors. I don't think state licensing is morally significant.

I have also said nothing about the monopoly some professions have on the provision of certain services. In particular, I have said nothing about the fact that only dentists (and those working under them) are now permitted to offer to clean and repair teeth. I have said nothing so far because monopoly is not part of what makes an occupation a profession. But I need to say something. Unlike state licensing, the state-granted monopoly dentists have does seem morally significant. Rarely, if ever, would government impose a monopoly on an unwilling profession. The profession must first seek the monopoly, ordinarily as part of a strategy to protect the public from incompetents who do not hold themselves out as members of the profession. The strategy is frankly paternalistic. The state will ordinarily go along only if the profession in question has proved to be relatively good at what it does and the market has proved relatively bad at preventing abuses by others. The state grants the monopoly as a means of protecting the public.

Whatever the reason for a professional monopoly, the monopoly itself imposes a special moral burden on a profession. If clients or patients have no place else to go for help of the kind the profession provides and if the profession has helped to arrange things in that way, the profession has helped to arrange things so that the client cannot get help except through the profession's members. If its members now refuse to help, the profession makes some of the public worse off than they would have been without the profession. The profession is in effect harming some of the public.

Such an outcome could, I think, be justified only under unusual conditions, for example, when the only alternative is to harm other members of the public. Each profession with a monopoly should therefore include within its code of ethics provisions to protect the public from having the profession's monopoly make them worse off. The legal profession does this in part by urging a lawyer to take on a fair share of clients who could not otherwise find legal counsel. The dental profession does something similar. It allows individual dentists only "reasonable discretion" in selecting patients. Dentists are not allowed to refuse a patient simply because he is in some way undesirable.

That is not to say that, unless it has a monopoly, a profession has no reason to require its members to take a fair share of undesirable clients or patients. If the members of a profession want to serve the public better than the market requires, one obvious way to do that is to make its (superior) service available to all who can benefit from it. Professions therefore often impose such an obligation on their members even when they do not have a monopoly.

Nonetheless, once a profession has a monopoly, the obligation to serve all is of a different moral order. Once a profession has a monopoly on a service, the question is no longer whether a part of the public will be served better but whether it will be served at all.

HIV and the Dental Professions

That, I think, is enough about professional obligation in general. We are now ready to consider the obligations dentists in particular have to treat HIV-infected patients. Let me begin by putting aside until the next part some relevant considerations favorable to convincing dentists to do what they are supposed to do.

First, I give up for now any benefit to my argument that might come from the inability to identify all those carrying the HIV virus. I agree that this inability helps to make refusing to treat known carriers seem arbitrary. I shall nonetheless ignore the point for now because I think that dentists would have the same obligation to treat even if we could identify every carrier (without misidentifying any noncarriers) by, say, a red mark on the forehead. I want to establish the obligation to treat as clearly, and with as few assumptions, as possible.

Second, I give up for now any benefit I could derive from the fact that (except in one case) HIV does not seem ever to have been transmitted in a dental office following standard sanitary procedures. I will instead assume that the risk of HIV infection is, though small, still significant even in an office following standard procedures. I think it important to do this for three reasons: First, we have all come to be suspicious of official evaluations of risk. Our experience is that risk is often underrated at first. Second, debate over the data detracts from the main point. The argument for treating a patient with HIV does not depend on such inherently changeable data (though I certainly agree that such data makes it easier for a dentist to do what he should in any case do). Third, even if HIV cannot be transmitted in a dental office following standard procedures, other infectious diseases may be. Since we seem to be entering a new age of plagues, we will probably do more good in the long run if we begin now to talk in terms general enough to apply to the disease HIV might have been.

Last, I give up for now any benefit to be derived from what the law happens to require of dentists. I shall assume—again, contrary to fact—that any dentist can legally refuse a new patient because he carries HIV and, indeed, can even abandon a longtime patient for that reason. My focus is entirely on the *moral* obligation of dentists (though I shall assume that dentists have a legal monopoly on providing dental services).

I give up for now the benefit of any legal requirement for three reasons: first, I believe the law will sooner or later approximate what morality requires. While law and morality are not the same, law seldom strays far from significant moral considerations. Moral arguments are therefore more reliable in the long run. Second, emphasizing the legal arguments simply invites people to try to get around the law or change it. For any decent person, the central question is not whether the law happens to require something but whether what the law requires is right or at least reasonable. Third, legal arguments can be just as distracting as arguments about evidence of risk. We need, I think, to keep our attention squarely on the moral considerations. Hence, I shall avoid all legal distractions for now.

This said, the *basic argument* for treating HIV-infected patients is simple. Let me begin with dentists. Dentistry, like any other profession, is defined in part by its code of ethics. This code is to be found in the ADA's Principles of Ethics, Code of Professional Conduct, and Advisory Opinions. The principles state that the dentist's primary professional obligation is "service to the public."[4] According to the Code of Professional Conduct, service to the public allows only "reasonable discretion in selecting patients."[5] And an advisory opinion declares that the fact that an "individual has AIDS or is HIV seropositive" is irrelevant to the selection of patients.[6] Refusing to treat an HIV-infected patient is therefore clearly unethical.

A similar argument applies to dental hygienists. Hygienists have their own Principles of Ethics. One of these requires the hygienist to "serve all patients without discrimination."[7] Dental assistants also have a code of ethics, but theirs provides no guidance on this subject.[8] As far as I can tell, neither dental lab technicians nor dental clerks have a code of ethics (or even a professional association). So, we cannot make the same professional argument to them. Morally, they are a class apart.

Indeed, even the professional employees of a dentist are not in the same moral position as the dentist they work for. Dental hygienists and dental assistants can serve the public only under the supervision of a dentist, but the dentist could do what they do without them. The special skills of these auxiliaries are part of general dentistry. So if all dentists refuse a patient, the patient will not be able to get good dental care (or, at least, not be able to get it legally). If, however, all dental hygienists and dental assistants refuse to care for a certain patient, he can still get the dental care he needs from a dentist. Dentists guard the door to dental care. With this control must come a moral burden other dental professionals—and so, of course, ordinary employees—do not bear. Let us then approach these other professionals and employees through the dentist. And let us begin by considering what a dentist could say in response to the basic argument for treating the HIV-infected patient.

Since we have already explained the moral authority of any argument resting—as the basic argument does—on the dentist's professional obligations, we need now consider only those responses that *accept* the professional obligation. The only interesting ones I have encountered might be summarized this way:

> Yes, I have a professional obligation to treat HIV-infected patients. Yes, that is a moral obligation. But to say I have such an obligation is not necessarily to say that I am bound in conscience to fulfill that obligation. Special circumstances can excuse one from fulfilling one's professional obligation. The present circumstances are special. If I serve this HIV-infected patient, I will risk my own life. I will endanger my employees. I will also risk transmitting the disease to my family and to other patients. There are limits to what a profession can justly demand of its members. Risking one's own life, the life of one's employees, or the life of

members of one's family is beyond the limit. Certainly, risking the life of another patient is. Therefore, I have the right to refuse this patient.

This response may be divided into three parts. One concerns the dentist herself. Another concerns her employees and family. The third concerns other patients. Let us begin with the first part, the claim that professions cannot justly demand that a member risk her own life. That claim is certainly false. Police and firefighters are obliged to risk their lives in performance of their duty. We see no injustice in such an obligation. That is, as we say, "just part of the job."

Of course, police and firefighters generally enter their profession aware of the risk. Dentists generally have not. That is a failure of contemporary dental education the AIDS epidemic has helped to remedy. Still, dentists have no cause to complain. On the one hand, no one deliberately withheld information about the risk of HIV infection from them during their education. Their professors were as ignorant of the risk as they were. HIV is a new problem. On the other hand, nothing in the dentist's code of ethics guarantees that dentistry will not be life-threatening. And the history of dentistry contains ample warning. In the days before antibiotics, less than half a century ago, dentistry was probably as dangerous a profession as policing is today.

Most dentists would, I think, find much of what I have just said beside the point. The strength of the response we are now considering is risk a dentist would impose on others. Here, I think, it is important to point out that dentists are not drafted into their profession. They enter voluntarily and remain there only as long as they wish. A dentist can retire when she wishes. The choice a dentist faces when an HIV-infected patient walks into her office is not the morally difficult dilemma *either* to refuse the patient *or* to risk infecting family, employees, or patients. The dentist always has a third choice: to give up holding herself out as a dentist.

This is morally a much less difficult choice. Giving up dentistry ends the dentist's professional obligations (at least once she has helped her patients find a new dentist). Giving up dentistry also ends the risk to her employees, family, and patients. They will no longer have to worry about being infected because of what goes on in her office. Giving up dentistry may mean that her employees will have to find other employment, but that is a risk one takes whenever one enters employment. Just as an employee is free to quit his job when it suits his plans and provided he gives due notice, so an employer is free to retire when it suits her plans and provided she gives her employees due notice or adequate severance pay.

So, the dental profession does not force the dentist to choose between risking the life of others and turning away an HIV-infected patient. The dentist forces herself to make that choice when she decides that she wants the benefits of being a dentist so much that she is unwilling to retire.

Of course, if retiring meant starvation or penury for the dentist or her family, we might still hesitate to require her to retire rather than turn away an HIV-infected patient. But that is not what retiring means. Dentists are well enough educated that most could easily find other jobs. Quitting dentistry may well mean giving up the personal independence dentistry gives. It may also mean having to accept a lower standard of living. But that is about the worst it is likely to mean.

The dentist who pleads such consequences hardly deserves our sympathy. What she is pleading for are the luxuries she and her family derive from dentistry. She pleads for these luxuries while renouncing one of the burdens that dentists as a profession have undertaken. If she does not carry her fair share of that burden, other dentists will have to. She wants to be treated differently from other dentists even though she differs from them in no significant way. In effect, she wants to ride free on their backs. Surely, if that is what her plea comes to, the only honorable course of action open to her if she chooses to remain in the profession is to take her fair share of HIV-infected patients.

Much more sympathetic is the dentist whose concern is for her other patients. She certainly has a professional obligation to protect them. Shouldn't that professional obligation override any professional obligation to one patient with HIV? The answer is that it cannot. The dentist's code of ethics defines her professional obligations. She cannot plead her professional obligation to her other patients as an excuse for ignoring her professional obligation to the HIV-infected patient. Her profession specifically includes an obligation to take HIV-infected patients. Her profession protects other patients not by allowing her to discriminate but (in part at least) by imposing on her the additional obligation to take every reasonable precaution to prevent infection.

The dentist's profession may also impose another obligation relevant here, the obligation to explain to each patient the risks (and benefits) of receiving dental care from a profession that has undertaken not to discriminate against patients on the basis of HIV infection. This seems to me a reasonable interpretation of Rule 1-J of the Code of Conduct: "Dentists shall not represent the care being rendered . . . in a false or misleading manner."[9] A patient should not be given the impression that the risks of dentistry are less than they in fact are. He should be given the opportunity to avoid any risk of infection associated with getting dental care from a profession that refuses to discriminate against patients infected with HIV.[10]

The patient might also be told that he is free to try to do away with the profession's monopoly so that he can get dental care from a profession or trade that does discriminate in the selection of patients on the basis of HIV infection. He should, however, also be asked to consider how he would feel if he were infected with HIV, as he might well be, and could not find a competent person willing to look at his aching tooth. The dentist's nonselectivity is a kind of insurance against the worst, but it is a form of insurance that probably would not exist long in a market that allowed nondentists both to compete with dentists and to leave dentists with all the undesirable patients. Like other forms of insurance, this "dental insurance" may seem a poor bargain until the worst happens.

So the dentist has an obligation to accept HIV-infected patients and no valid excuse for doing otherwise. What then can the dentist tell her employees should any of them object to working on an HIV-infected patient? To her hygienist, she can say, "You claim to be a professional. Your code of ethics imposes the same obligation of service that mine does. You have the same choice I have: to serve this patient or renounce your profession. Choose." If this appeal does not work, the dentist can still tell her hygienist what she can tell any other employee who gets in the way of her meeting her profession's standards of skill and conduct: "You must either help me do what my profession requires of me or go elsewhere. There's work to be done. If you won't do it, I must find someone who will—or do it myself."

This may seem to end the matter, but it does not quite. One question remains: Why should dentists not change their code of ethics? This is, after all, a real possibility. Codes of ethics are not written in stone like the Ten Commandments, nor are they, like those tablets, the work of a god. Codes of ethics are human inventions for a human purpose. If some provision of a code turns out to demand too much of the profession's members, nothing would be more reasonable than for the profession to change the provision. Indeed, doing so would be wise. A code that demands more than most members of a profession can reasonably do will never be more than empty words accusing those who endorse them. We must, then, consider what reasons dentists have not to reduce what is required of them. Why should the dental profession not allow its members to turn away HIV-infected patients?

Here, of course, would be a good place to bring in all the data about risk. But I promised not to do that in this part. What other arguments can there be for letting the dental code remain as it is? The answer may seem plain: on the evidence we have, we are asking dentists to do no more than what we can reasonably expect of them. Other occupations such as policing or firefighting seem to accept greater risks. Dentists have in the past actually accepted the risk of life-threatening infection as part of their profession. So unless dentists have changed radically for the worse in the last fifty years, we do not seem to be asking the impossible of them.

Still, the question remains: Why should the dental profession not take the easy course and reduce risk to themselves by allowing a dentist to refuse patients who carry HIV? While I don't think there is a decisive reason to answer one way or the other, I do think two reasons ought to carry great weight with any dentist considering how to answer. The first reason concerns the ideal around which dentistry is organized; the second, the monopoly dentists treasure.

We might put the first reason this way. The ideal of service to the public seems to include trying to assure dental care to all who need it. If individual dentists are allowed to refuse to accept, or even allowed to abandon, patients because they are infected with HIV, the dental profession must either make some special provision for the care of HIV-infected patients, for example, special clinics, or give up trying to assure dental care to all who need it.

If there are to be special clinics, dentists would have to staff them. If enough dentists could be found, then all would be well. But if not enough dentists could be found, other dentists would have to share the burden according to some fair procedure. We would be back to something like the arrangement we now have.

I think it reasonable to assume that not enough dentists would be found to staff those clinics. Few dentists are already infected with HIV. These are not likely to be numerous enough, or distributed evenly enough geographically, to serve all, or even most, patients who would have to be served in the special clinics we are imagining. Many healthy dentists would have to serve in those clinics for all those needing dental care to have it. For these healthy dentists, serving in the clinics would not (we are assuming) be a professional requirement but an act of charity—indeed, on the assumption that led us to consider this alternative, an act of heroism. Whatever diffuse risk of infection exists in ordinary practice would now be concentrated in one place. Dentists who suggest this approach are therefore hoping for courage in others far beyond what they can find in themselves. They should not be allowed to give up their present obligations on the mere promise that enough such heroes would take their place.

A dentist could respond to my demand that he first find enough heroes by saying that there is no need of that. If there are not enough heroes, then HIV-infected patients will just have to do without a dentist. This possibility brings me to the second reason against changing the Code of Ethics to allow dentists to refuse patients infected with HIV: dentists' monopoly on dental care. Renouncing the ideal of universal service would leave the public with only two choices: to condemn some HIV-infected people to do entirely without dental care or to allow nondentists to fill the gap in service the dental profession has left. Surely the second choice is the more reasonable. But once the public has allowed nondentists to fill the gap, why should they leave dentists a monopoly over the choicer patients? A profession that prefers its own safety even when doing so means turning the needy from their door looks more like a trade association than a profession. Hence, if only for symbolic reasons, dentists would be well advised to preserve their code as it is, even if doing so means making members share the risks of treating patients with HIV.

This completes my discussion of arguments dentists might use to try to get out of their professional obligation to serve patients with HIV. While these may not be all the arguments, they are, at least, the major ones. We are now ready to hear an HIV-infected patient make a case for treatment to his dentist, who would rather send him elsewhere.

What I Would Say to My Dentist

Dr. B., I have been your patient for seven years. Our relationship began when my tooth abscessed while my former dentist was on vacation. You did a root canal. I have not heard from that tooth since. Because you were there when I needed you, I became a regular patient, coming to you for a routine checkup and cleaning twice a year, as well as for an occasional filling and that one crown. I have never missed an appointment or failed to pay a bill on time. I have, as you admit, been a good patient. Why then do you now refuse even to let me sit in your dental chair? I have come on time. I am still able to pay. I am due for a checkup and cleaning. I am the same person I was before—except that I have now been diagnosed as having HIV (and will, in all probability, some day develop AIDS).

I told you that I had HIV because you asked whether my medical history had changed. I thought you were asking *as my dentist*. I told you because I thought knowing that I had HIV might some day help you with a diagnosis. I certainly would not have told you had I thought you would react like this. You have nothing to fear from me. You run a good office. Both you and your dental hygienist wash up before and after seeing me. You have always worn rubber gloves when working in my mouth. Your hygienist even wears a white coat and surgical mask. You do the same when you do anything more than look into my mouth. You are meticulous about your instruments. You have told me more than once that they are first bathed in two different disinfectants and then autoclaved overnight. The counters around your dental chair are always clean when I come. More than once I have noticed your assistant begin to clean them as I leave. I found all that reassuring when I thought only other people got HIV. I still find it reassuring. You need take no more precautions with me now.

Who made me an expert in dentistry? No one, of course. I have, however, done my homework. My first reaction on learning that I had HIV was complete desolation—as if I had been diagnosed with leprosy in the days when lepers were sent to special colonies. I was afraid that I would have to be quarantined. I didn't know much about HIV then. Like most people, I suppose, I had all sorts of misconceptions. But I had the sense to go to a good library. I was surprised at what I found. What I had thought a highly contagious disease turns out to be very hard to transmit. You cannot catch HIV by touching the skin of an infected person or breathing in what he breathes out. The virus can be carried only by blood or semen. Air or water will kill it. Hepatitis is much more infectious.

I got this information from reports issued by various dental societies, including the American Dental Association.[11] There was remarkable agreement among them. Not only did they agree on the risks of HIV infection, they agreed as well on how a dentist should treat a patient with HIV. Discriminating against a patient because he has HIV is against your own code of ethics. Dr. B., you have a professional obligation to treat me just as you would any other patient.

I should tell you one more thing I learned at the library. Both federal and state laws prohibit discrimination against the handicapped in public accommodations. Under applicable federal and state law, your office is a public accommodation and having HIV is considered a handicap. So you can no more legally refuse to treat me than you can refuse to treat someone because she walks with a limp or is blind. Should you refuse me treatment, I can sue you, asking both for money damages and for an order forcing you to take me back. Since the calculation of damages would include all pain and suffering denial of treatment causes, the damages could be quite large. The awards routinely run into the thousands of dollars.[12]

Yes, you say, ideally you should not discriminate, but you have to be practical. You have employees who are afraid of AIDS; a wife, two children, and several hundred patients who may not accept the medical evidence—people who were once told that nuclear power is safe and have since learned that it is not. Patients who have heard of Kimberly Bergalis may not want to hear anything more. You understand that I can take you to court. But you hope I won't because I can see that you have no choice but to be "practical." Would I act any differently if you were the one with HIV instead of me?

If you had just informed me that you had HIV (and I believed I did not), would I stick with you or desert you as perhaps many other patients would? Honestly, Dr. B., while I hope I would stick with you, I don't know what I would do. But that seems to me beside the point. I am not a professional patient. You are a professional dentist.

Anyway, I have to be as practical about this as you want to be. I have teeth that need a dentist's regular care. All you have offered me is a reference to a clinic across town about which I know nothing. At a minimum, going there would be an expensive inconvenience. My time is valuable. Going there might also turn out to be a mistake. I may not like the way that clinic operates. More to the point, if you can abandon me because I have HIV, what assurance can you give that they will not do the same? Surely, they too must be "practical."

I can see that I have not yet changed your mind. Let's then really try to be practical. Let's try to think how you might handle your staff, your family, and your other patients. How much do you have to fear from them? Let's begin with your staff.

Your hygienist is, like you, a professional. Like the ADA, her professional society, the American Dental Hygienists' Association, forbids discrimination in the selection of patients. So you can tell her that she has a professional obligation to work on me whether she likes it or not. You can tell her that if she's unwilling to work on me, she might as well stop calling herself a dental hygienist.

If that doesn't change her mind, you can always tell her to start looking for another job. But if you don't want to lose her, you might add that she won't be much safer anywhere else. My physician now thinks I contracted the virus nine years ago from a blood transfusion I had during an appendectomy. Those were the days before blood banks tested for HIV. The infection has been undiagnosed all this time. I would still not know that I had HIV if my physician had not begun to check for it as part of every physical (and if she had not told me what she found). Undiagnosed HIV is now sufficiently common in the general population that few dentists do not have at least one undiagnosed carrier among their patients. So you can tell your hygienist that she will not be significantly safer if she quits you for another dentist. You can also remind her that she is today no more in danger of getting HIV from me than she was last year or the year before last.

You can make the same point to your receptionist, lab technician, and dental assistant. None of them will be safer working for any other dentist. They will not even be safer if they go into some other line of work. Dentistry is not without its special risks to health, but HIV is not one of them.

What then of your family? We are agreed that objectively I present no danger to them. We are now concerned only with what they will think if they find out you are treating a patient with HIV. Here I must admit some disappointment in you. You have a professional obligation to keep all sensitive facts about your patients confidential. You certainly should not tell your family anything about your patients that might lead them to interfere with the dentist–patient relationship. Yet they are not likely to learn that you treat patients with HIV unless you (or your staff) tell them.

But, yes, we're trying to be practical now. There's just so much you can keep from your family when they want to know. All right then, what can you tell them when they ask whether any of your patients have HIV? Here's what I would tell them if I were you:

> Given the size of my practice, the answer is, Almost certainly. You just can't practice dentistry in this city without taking that risk. I run a good office, so I am in no danger of infection there. And so neither are you. To make you any safer, I'd have to give up dentistry. Do you want me to do that? Think hard before you answer. Look around at what you have because I am a dentist. You might have to give up a lot of it if I start a new career. And in my professional opinion, you would give it up merely to calm an unfounded fear.

That is what I would tell your family if I were you. What about your patients? Here, I admit, you must be more careful. Your patients can easily find a new dentist. They can decide to leave you without consulting with you. They can leave on the basis of rumor or mere suspicion. On the other hand, individual patients can be replaced. What you need to keep your practice is not any particular patient but about the same number of patients. You can afford to lose one now and then. Indeed, you are constantly losing some as they move away, marry into a family with a dentist, or die. You are also always making up those loses as people see your advertisement in the phone directory or hear one of your patients say how good you are. So what you need to think through is how to explain to your patients what you are doing in such a way as not to scare them off. You probably should not bring up the matter yourself. But you should be ready to answer any questions they might ask.

What might a patient ask? One question we have already talked about: Do you treat anyone with HIV or AIDS? The answer you give your patients could be the same as that you would give your family. HIV is now so common here that some of your patients must have the disease. Any other dentist in town is in exactly the same situation.

What if the patient presses you, asking whether you know of any patients with HIV? Here you need to begin by pointing out the importance of keeping health information confidential. How would this patient like to have you telling some other patient about what she has told you in confidence?[13] You also need to add that the patient should not conclude from what you just said that you know of any patient with AIDS. You are stressing the importance of keeping the patient's confidence to make clear why you cannot answer the question.

You should, however, not let the matter end like that. You do not want to sound like you are hiding something. You should therefore offer to answer her question "hypothetically." What would you do *if* you learned one of your patients had HIV? That is a question you can answer. Your answer should be, Nothing. You are already doing everything your profession believes reasonable to prevent contagion. You also have no choice but to treat an HIV-infected patient the same as any other. That's the law. That's also what your profession requires. Any dentist who tells a patient he does anything else is either lying or engaged in illegal and unethical conduct. Would you want a dentist like that?

That is what I would say if I were you and one of your patients asked whether you treated patients with HIV or AIDS. I would also hand him an educational brochure from the ADA just to show you know what you are talking about. I don't see how you could be much more practical than that. You will have given your patient no reason to go elsewhere. Indeed, you may have given him a good reason to stay where he is. You have been candid. You have been knowledgeable. You have behaved like someone he can trust.

You will also have done one thing more. If you take the course I have suggested, you will not have it on your conscience that you abandoned a loyal patient in need, abandoned him against the dictates of reason, law, and profession because you were afraid of what an employee, a member of your family, or another patient might ignorantly think. You are a decent person, Dr. B. Now is a time to show it.

Notes

1. This chapter began as a presentation to the Dental Curriculum Meeting, Midwest AIDS Training and Education Center, University of Illinois at Chicago, December 9, 1988. I would like to thank Dr. Erick Hars for inviting me, providing a long reading list, and otherwise encouraging me to participate as an intelligent outsider in a meeting consisting mostly of deans of major dental schools. Staff at the American Dental Association, hearing of that paper, invited me to contribute what became "Dentistry and AIDS: An Ethical Opinion" (*Journal of the American Dental Association Supplement* [November 1989]: 9–11), a much-revised version of the second section of the conference paper. That piece provoked more letters than any other I have written. Although about half of the letters objected to my views, I might have let matters go at that if the California Dental Association had not invited me to participate in its Symposium on Dental Ethics in Sacramento, September 21, 1990. I read a later version of the Sacramento paper at the National Meeting of the Professional Ethics in Dentistry Network, in Rosemont, Illinois, November 11, 1990. Thanks to the encouragement and criticism I received at those two events, that paper eventually became "Treating Patients with Infectious Diseases: An Essay in the Ethics of Dentistry" (*Professional Ethics Journal*, forthcoming). That paper attempted to respond to many of the objections I had by then come across, mostly in letters (or in articles pointed out to me). These conferences and publications constitute the sum of my nonpatient relationships with dentistry. They are, I believe, not enough to weaken significantly my credentials as a patient.

2. Rena A. Gorlin, ed., *Codes of Professional Responsibility* (Washington, D.C.: Bureau of National Affairs, 1990), p. 87. Beside the ADA's Code of Ethics, some related documents (including some ADA Opinions) are conveniently reprinted on pp. 85–96 of this volume.

3. This paragraph summarizes a theory of professions I have defended more fully elsewhere, most recently in "Do Cops Really Need a Code of Ethics?" *Criminal Justice Ethics* 10 (Summer/Fall 1991): 14–28.

4. Gorlin, *Codes of Professional Responsibility*, p. 85.

5. Ibid.

6. American Dental Association, "Report of Council on Ethics, Bylaws and Judicial Affairs Regarding Ethical Ramifications of Refusing to Treat Patients with AIDS or Patients Who Are HIV Seropositive." Unpublished paper (1988), pp. 4–5. See also "Policy Statement on AIDS, HIV Infection, and the Practice of Dentistry, as approved by the [ADA's] House of Delegates, October 12, 1988."

7. American Dental Hygienists' Association, *Principles of Ethics* (revised, 1975). The ADHA is now completely revising this code.

8. American Dental Assistants Association, *Principles of Ethics and Code of Professional Conduct* (1980).

9. This seems to me to be a reasonable extension of (the new) paragraph 1-K of the Code of Profession Conduct (Patient Involvement): "The dentist

should inform the patient of the proposed treatment, and any reasonable alternatives, in a manner that allows the patient to become involved in treatment decisions.''

10. What if a dentist herself has HIV? Until the Bergalis case is cleared up, the dentist has a professional obligation to inform her patients of her infection. For more on this point, see my "Treating Patients with Infectious Diseases."

11. See, especially, *Journal of the American Dental Association* supplement *Facts About AIDS for the Dental Team*, 3d ed. (American Dental Association: Chicago, July 1991).

12. That was true even before the Americans with Disabilities Act began to take effect January 1992 (assuming HIV status alone to be a "disability"). The act, does, however, add new federal remedies to the state and local remedies already available in many states.

13. What if my dentist asked, "What if she responds that she is not asking for a name, only for general information? Surely, confidentiality does not protect that." My answer is that, under the circumstances, it certainly does; but space does not allow me to say more here.

4

HIV and the Professional Responsibility of the Early Childhood Educator

Kenneth Kipnis

From 1984 to 1989, I served as a consultant to the National Association for the Education of Young Children (NAEYC). Working with Stephanie Feeney, a leading scholar in early childhood education (ECE), our task was to develop a code of ethics for the field in a way that would generate a sense of ownership among its 60,000 members. Questionnaires were used, workshops were conducted throughout the United States, articles were published in *Young Children* (NAEYC's journal), and drafts of the code were circulated for comment and review. In late 1989, the Governing Board of NAEYC approved its Code of Ethical Conduct (CEC).[1]

At one level, this chapter represents merely my view of how ECE practitioners should understand their responsibilities regarding HIV-infected persons. But because the work I have done over the last eight years has had a significant impact on how the field itself understands these responsibilities, this chapter should not be read as the commentary of an ivory-towered bystander.

I should also add that, since 1984, as a rare specialist in legal philosophy and medical ethics in Hawaii, I have been involved in the legal and ethical issues that have been generated by HIV infection. I have worked with physicians, epidemiologists, social workers, legislators, judges, attorneys, public officials, and others in an effort to craft appropriate ways of addressing this phenomenon.[2] I have had to become conversant with the scientific and medical literature that has been generated as the disease has progressed. This discussion is an effort to bring together what I have learned about professional responsibility in early childhood education with what I have learned about AIDS.

Illness and Early Childhood Education

It is common to distinguish between the biological processes by which disease-causing microorganisms establish themselves in persons and spread through populations, and the social activities that represent distinctively human responses to illness. Governments, businesses, unions, educational institutions, hospitals, military organizations, families, and organized religions have had to respond to the phenomenon of HIV infection, arguably the most significant pandemic of this century.[3]

So AIDS has challenged ECE: the emerging profession that takes as its core responsibility the provision of "safe, healthy, nurturing, and responsive settings for children."[4] In their own ways, preschools and early childhood centers can be affected by HIV-spectrum disease. The impact can be direct, as when a staff member or a child is discovered to be infected, becoming ill and dying, or, perhaps, when he or she is merely suspected of being infected. Or the impact can be more indirect, as when a member of a child's family becomes ill, or someone close to a staff member sickens, perhaps without any suspicion that the child or the staff member might be harboring the virus as well. The impact of any illness is heightened by ignorance and by the fear of catching the virus from someone at the center.[5]

Some of these problems are not unique to AIDS. Difficult issues can arise whenever serious illness or death touches the lives of the staff, the children, and the children's families. The assassination of an American president, the demise of the classroom hamster, or the unexpected death of a small classmate will likely raise important questions for children and create important responsibilities for those who care for them.

Early childhood educators have distinctive background responsibilities when managing the social, emotional, and cognitive issues that arise for children in connection with serious illness and death. It is widely appreciated that the information disclosed to children should be determined by what the child needs to know: early childhood educators need to be clear about the questions children are asking before proffering answers. And it is also understood that privileged information (information entrusted to early childhood educators) about the diagnosis or the cause of death should be disclosed to others— children and staff—only to the extent that confidentiality has been explicitly waived.[6] As set out by the CEC in Principle 2.9: "We shall maintain confidentiality and shall respect the family's right to privacy, refraining from disclosure of confidential information and intrusion into family life."

At a much less dramatic level, common diseases and the dangers these impose present familiar issues in ECE.[7] In addition to those conditions that seem to distinguish childhood (chickenpox, measles, and mumps), there are other infections (sore throats, colds, head lice, ear infections, etc.) that are especially common among children. It is not much of an exaggeration to describe illness as a daily preschool event.

Children who become ill or who show symptoms of contagious illness are routinely sent home. Their parents are asked to keep them home until the risk of spreading infection has passed. Other parents are informed when their children are exposed to an infectious condition at the center and are at risk of contracting the illness. The CEC says (Principle 2.5): "We shall inform the family . . . of risks such as exposures to contagious disease that may result in infection." Teachers advise parents, often in writing, to be alert for, say, the early signs and symptoms of chickenpox or head lice, so they can help to stem the spread of these illnesses and minimize adverse effects.

But unlike chickenpox and sore throats, HIV-spectrum disease is an infectious, fatal condition. The effects of HIV on daily life at a child-care center are of greater ethical complexity. Given the seriousness of this disease, given questions that have been raised about modes of transmission, given widespread ignorance and misinformation, and given the fears and pressures that have surrounded it, how are preschool teachers to understand their responsibilities to fellow staff members, to the infected person (child or staff member), to the other children and staff at the center, and to the families of the children? These are the questions addressed in this chapter.

The central questions are those regarding the child who has the AIDS virus.[8] We can imagine the director of a preschool finding out that a particular five-year-old is infected. On these facts alone, the following issues might arise:

1. The Attendance Question: If a child who is infected is currently applying to or attending the preschool, is the infection a reason for exclusion? Similar questions can arise in relation to staff.

2. The Information Question: If the decision is made to admit the child, should the families of the other children be informed that an HIV-positive child is attending the school? Similar questions can arise in relation to staff.

Directors may be pressured by school owners or parents to behave in ways that violate professional responsibilities. But one function of a professional code—especially when there is strong professional consensus on how it should be applied—is to provide a basis for resisting improper suggestions. Parents may fear for the safety of their children, and center owners may be concerned about maintaining positive relationships with their clientele. As strong as the obligations may be to defer to employers and parents, they are not strong enough to require early childhood educators to violate the professional standards of their field. The crucial question for this chapter regards the professional obligations that arise for ECE in relationship to children with the virus. Parental fears and the concerns of center owners, when they are reasonable, need to be responded to with appropriate cautionary measures. When they are unreasonable, they need to be answered with sympathy and understanding, and the best information available. It is the aim of this chapter to set out the best information currently available and to delineate the dimensions of appropriate caution.

Arguments for Excluding Children Infected with HIV

Since the question of informing families about the presence of HIV-positive children arises only if such children are present, it makes sense to take up the question of attendance first. What then are early childhood educators' responsibilities toward infected children and toward other children? As it happens, the discussion of the attendance question illuminates the information question.

Two types of reason are commonly advanced for excluding infected children from participation in programs. One rests on a paternalistic concern about the ill effects on the infected child.[9] The second is predicated on the responsibility to prevent healthy children from being harmed by those who are infected. These are taken up in order.

The Paternalistic Argument

Contact with other children and participation at the center can have bad effects on some infected children. With a damaged immune system, children with AIDS may be gravely threatened by disease-causing microorganisms that would be of little or no consequence for healthy children. But while this concern is real, it seems that any decision to discourage attendance by HIV-positive children should be made by the child's parents in consultation with the child's physician. The significance of the risk is a function of the status of the child's immune system and the magnitude of the risks that are imposed by the preschool setting itself. Exposure to the droppings of pets, to active herpes lesions, and to certain childhood diseases—notably measles and chickenpox—can pose grave health risks to children with suppressed immunity. But these risks need to be weighed against the benefits to the child from participation in center activities, considering the reduction in quality of life that would follow from exclusion.

Notwithstanding the professional background of the director, it would appear that the technical issues here are medical ones, outside of the professional knowledge base of the early childhood educator. While it would be reasonable for the director to consult with the family and the child's physician[10] so that information can be shared and all can be informed about the risks to the child from daily life at the preschool, the decision to prohibit the child from attending the center, for reasons having to do with the health-related interests of the child who is infected, would seem to be a decision that only the parents, working with a well-informed physician, can make.

In the background is the familiar balancing of the length of a life against its quality. Every time we engage in high-risk activities, we weigh concerns about the quality of our lives against concerns for longevity. These same issues arise—dramatically—for children who are terminally ill. It can be reasonable to provide a child with quality days even though they hasten death. There is a commitment in ECE to childhood as a unique stage in human life, not mere preparation for elementary school and the rest. The joys of accomplishment, friendship, and enlightenment enrich the lives of small children, as they do the lives of adults.

Children who are immunocompromised clearly have important needs in the early childhood setting. There is a concern that they not be exposed to illnesses that, while commonly not serious to healthy children, could well be fatal to them. Accordingly, parents of infected children need to be informed immediately in the event that, for example, chickenpox makes an appearance at the school. While this is what directors are ethically required to do anyway, center staff now have new reasons to take these responsibilities very seriously. Because such communication with all parents should be occurring already, center staff do not need to know, for the infected child's sake, that he or she is immunocompromised and, by implication, HIV-infected. It would be useful to assume that all children are seropositive and that all parents have a life-or-death need to know about outbreaks of infectious illness at the center.

Conversely, parents of all children need to take very seriously the requirement to keep ill children away from schools until the period of infectiousness has passed. Early childhood professionals should take a leadership role in encouraging their communities to meet the need for drop-in sick-child care facilities, especially when parental leave protection is inadequate. Health is not promoted when parents are required to choose between the loss of their livelihoods and the endangerment of other children and their own.

The Argument from Prevention of Harm

Much more common than paternalistic arguments are arguments that appeal to the director's obligations toward the other children. This argument could be set out as follows. The first principle of the Code of Ethical Conduct is ECE's equivalent of the medical profession's norm: above all, to do no harm. Principle 1.1 reads:

> Above all, we shall not harm children. We shall not participate in practices that are disrespectful, degrading, dangerous, exploitative, intimidating, psychologically damaging, or physically harmful to children. *This principle has precedence over all others in this Code.* [Emphasis in original]

If the practice of allowing HIV-seropositive children (or staff members) to participate in a center posed a danger of infection for the other children (and, therefore, a risk of death), then the director would appear to be obligated to refrain from admitting the child to the center, much as children are excluded when they are infected with less serious illnesses like measles and chickenpox. The fact that HIV infection is a mortal illness can justify these standard precautions even though the risk of transmission is substantially lower than that of chickenpox. But the soundness of this argument turns on the truth or falsity of the factual premise that the presence of an HIV-positive individual poses a risk of infection to others at the center. What is known about the magnitude of this danger?

It is well accepted, after years of epidemiological and laboratory research, that *virtually all* transmission of the AIDS virus occurs as a consequence of three types of activity:

1. unprotected vaginal and anal intercourse;

2. direct introduction into the bloodstream of infected blood products (e.g., transfusions, needle sharing among injectable drug users, injection of blood extracts used for hemophilia, accidental clinical needle-stick injuries, and organ transplants); and

3. exposure of a fetus to the blood of an infected mother either before or during birth.

None of these modes of transmission are associated with activities that are even remotely likely to occur in an early childhood center. (Clearly any center where children are at risk because of "vaginal or anal intercourse" or "needle sharing" should be closed down immediately for reasons having nothing to do with HIV infection.)

If, then, we confine ourselves solely to epidemiologically significant modes of transmission, it follows that there is *virtually no risk* of a preschooler's becoming infected by an infected child or staff member. The medical procedures, the perinatal processes, the drug-usage practices, and the sexual activities that are known to be implicated in practically all cases of transmission simply do not take place in early childhood centers. Indeed, children who are infected and whose cases have been examined, appear nearly universally to have contracted the virus perinatally or from the injection of medically prescribed blood products (either transfusions or extracts injected for hemophilia or other blood coagulation disorders).[11] As of this writing, there is not a single reported case in which a child appears to have become infected with the AIDS virus while at an early childhood center.

"Evidence" for Alternative Modes of Transmission

This is not to say that other modes of transmission are impossible or unheard of. Apart from the epidemiological and laboratory evidence for the standard modes, there are arguments for other modes. Three other types of "evidence" are commonly introduced in discussions of alternative risk factors.

Cases in Which the Mode of Transmission Is Unknown Because of Incomplete Investigation
Some commentators note that AIDS was only recently discovered in 1981. They point to data that suggest that, for many who have the virus, how they contracted it is unknown. They take this to be evidence for alternative and unknown modes of transmission and grounds for extreme caution.[12] It is true that, at the beginning of an epidemic, there can be fear associated with a lack of knowledge about modes of transmission. But gradually, as the major modes of infection become known, the nature of our residual ignorance shifts. Although many studies report cases in which the source of infection is listed as "unknown," great care should be taken to distinguish between reports of infected individuals for whom information about the source of their infection (the "risk factor") is unavailable and reports of infected individuals for which investigation has been carefully completed and the "standard" risk factors have been ruled out, leaving open only the possibility of some other mode of infection. Note that this distinction cannot be drawn at the beginning of an epidemic, when none of the standard risk factors are known and so cannot be ruled out. Some discussions of HIV infection and child care suffer for failing to make this distinction.[13]

It is not always easy to confirm that someone has the AIDS virus and that none of the usual modes of transmission is a possibility. Confirmation of both of these is necessary if we are to commence a search for a nonstandard mode of transmission. Among adults, there is an easily understood reticence regarding the details of what may be embarrassing sexual or drug-usage practices. And it can be difficult or impossible to complete investigation in pediatric cases if the family moves and is lost to follow-up or if parents refuse to be interviewed: sexual abuse, a mode of transmission to children, is deeply embarrassing, reportable, and criminal. In many of these cases the mode of transmission is unknown because the data have not been collected.[14] These cases, by themselves, at this advanced stage of our knowledge of the pandemic, do not provide us with evidence for alternative modes of transmission.

Cases in Which the Standard Modes of Infection Have Been Ruled Out

There are, however, anomalous cases in which infection is present, investigation has been carried out, and the standard modes of transmission appear to have been ruled out. We are then left only with evidence that transmission has occurred in some other theoretically possible way. The medical literature contains case reports—what is called "anecdotal evidence"—for other modes of transmission. These have implicated, for example, oral sex, the ingestion of breast milk, nonpercutaneous contact with blood, and biting as possible modes of transmission. (Some of this material is reviewed in the section "Evidence Against Nonstandard Modes of Transmission.") These reports carry weight to the extent that there is evidence that, first, the subject of the case history did not have the virus prior to the exposure; second, the subject of the case history had the virus after the exposure; and third, no other known or theoretically possible mode of transmission could have caused the infection. A single well-documented case of nonstandard but theoretically possible transmission can establish that infection can occur as a consequence of that type of exposure. However, though we would know that there is a risk of infection, we would not know the probability of infection following such an exposure. Although we know that intelligent life can occur on a planet—that is, Earth—we will not know the probability of such an occurrence until we have examined, one supposes, quite a few planets.

Evidence for the "Theoretical" Possibility of Infection

Lastly, there are modes of transmission for where there are no case reports whatsoever—no anecdotal evidence—but that may be "theoretically'' possible. For example, several years ago there was discussion about insect bites (bedbugs, mosquitoes, etc.) as a mode of transmission. While there has never been a case in which infection has been traced to an insect bite, other modes of transmission having been ruled out, some commentators have worried that, given what we know about HIV-infected blood and the transmission of illness through insect bites, it is theoretically possible to become infected with HIV from the bite of an insect that had previously bitten an infected person.

Theoretical possibility calls for laboratory research and epidemiological studies that can provide confirmation or disconfirmation. Laboratory research has been published on the mechanics of disease transmission through insect bites. And, epidemiologically, it has been possible, in high seroprevalence areas with biting insects, to see if unexplained HIV infection shows up among preadolescent children and the elderly. Though these groups are not as much at risk of infection from the standard modes, they would seem to be equally at risk for insect bites. If insect bites were a mode of transmission, the resulting HIV infections would show up in all age groups. It does not, however. Such laboratory and epidemiological research as has been done has largely disconfirmed the theoretical possibility of infection through insect bites.[15]

While the theoretical possibility of a nonstandard mode of infection provides a reason to conduct empirical research, does it provide enough evidence of danger to trigger a professional obligation for teachers to refrain from activities that, theoretically, may be harmful to children? Certainly, where empirical research has disconfirmed the theoretical possibility, we have evidence that there is little or no risk. But even in the absence of disconfirming laboratory and epidemiological evidence, the well-documented case report is of paramount importance. Such a report marks the difference between, on the one hand, not knowing whether or not there is a risk (bare theoretical possibility) and, on the other hand, knowing that there is a risk, but not knowing how great it is. The absence of case reports, especially in an atmosphere where they are zealously sought after and routinely published and read, and especially when virtually all investigated cases of infection are explainable in terms of the standard modes of transmission, suggests that the risk is insufficient to warrant the forbearance called for in Principle 1.1: "Above all, we shall not harm children. We shall not participate in practices that are . . . dangerous . . . or physically harmful to children." Where extensive research, over a period of years, has failed to disclose any risk of infection, it is inappropriate to assert that there is a non-negligible danger of infection. There is no known risk.

I therefore propose that the dangers contemplated by Principle 1.1. must be supported, at the very least, by at least one anecdotal report, that early childhood educators may need to avoid activities in which there is a known risk of harm to children. However, I also propose that early childhood educators may also disregard "negligible" risks, those for which the known risk fails to cross some low threshold level. Sometimes risks are clearly present but at so low a level that they warrant disregard. Consider, for example, the small but very real risks imposed by objects falling from airplanes. If a child is allowed to play outside, there will be a measurably greater risk of being killed by a falling airplane part. But early childhood centers do not keep children indoors on that basis: this risk is negligible. Now if this risk of death is negligible, then any smaller risk is also negligible.

Whether or not a measured risk of HIV infection warrants professional action thus turns, to some degree, on how comparable risks are treated. Appeals to the negligibility of risks is difficult because the parameters for this concept have not been clearly drawn: When is a risk so small that we may disregard it? But fortunately, much of what needs to be said here can be shown without referring to negligible risks. Accordingly, in what follows, only theoretical possibility supported by at least one case report shall be taken as demonstrating danger.

Evidence Against Nonstandard Modes of Transmission

The AIDS virus has been isolated in blood, semen, human breast milk, cervical secretions, cerebrospinal fluid, saliva, urine, and tears. Of these substances, only blood, saliva, urine, and tears are expected to be present in an early childhood center. (The virus is only occasionally to be found in the saliva, urine, and tears of infected persons and, when present, it is much less concentrated than it is in semen and blood.)

Although there have been numerous household and clinical cases in which people have been in regular and extensive contact with the urine of HIV-infected persons (the parents of infected small children, for example) and numerous cases in which there has been regular contact with the tears of HIV-infected patients (among eye doctors, for example), there are no anecdotal reports involving transmission through urine and tears.[16] More broadly, repeated studies have failed to show any risk from "casual contact." Those who live with HIV-infected persons and who do not engage in sexual activities or share needles with them are at no measurably greater risk than those who do not live with such persons. (But note the three reports of household transmission that are discussed below: two involving bites and one involving extensive and repeated contact with blood.)

This suggests that the risks imposed by exposure to tears and urine, while perhaps not zero, are unlikely to be much greater than that. It is important to note that such epidemiological evidence, all alone, could never show that the risk actually was zero. Even if there were one million rigorously documented exposures without a single resulting infection, that would show only that the risk of infection, while perhaps not zero, was unlikely to be much greater than zero. Nonetheless, given the theoretical possibility, it may be a good idea to avoid exposing oneself, extensively and repeatedly, to bodily fluids that might possibly contain the virus. More will be said about such precautions below.

There are, however, two theoretically possible modes of HIV transmission that are associated with anecdotal reports and that are potentially present in early childhood settings. A small number of reports strongly suggest transmission by means of skin contact with the blood of an infected person. And two reports suggest transmission by means of a bite from an infected person. Since contact with blood is not unknown in ECE and since children do bite each other, and since most people are not familiar with epidemiological case reports as a means of scientifically validating risk, these reports will be described fairly completely and examined with care.

What Is Known About the Risk from Nonpercutaneous Exposure to Blood?

In more than 99 percent of the cases in which health-care professionals have been exposed "percutaneously" (i.e., through the skin) to infected blood, they have not seroconverted. These incidents typically involve cuts with contaminated medical instruments or needle-stick injuries in which infected blood (still in the syringe) is injected beneath the skin. Even so, in about 99.6 percent of these "percutaneous" exposures to infected blood, there is no infection.[17] Cases in which blood is introduced beneath the skin are highly unlikely to occur in preschools.

In 1987, however, the Centers for Disease Control (CDC) published three well-documented reports of health-care workers who had seroconverted following "nonpercutaneous" exposure to the blood of infected patients, without any puncturing of the skin. The case reports are of high quality in that (1) there is good evidence that the subject was seronegative at the time of the exposure, (2) there is good evidence that the subject was infected after exposure, and (3) there is good evidence that there were no standard risk factors. All involved health-care workers performing blood-related medical procedures. In each case the skin of the health-care worker was not completely intact: chapping, dermatitis, and acne are mentioned. Here is a typical case:

Case 1: A medical technologist was working with a device used to separate blood components when HIV-infected blood spilled on her hands and arms. She was not wearing gloves and did not recall any open wounds on her hands or any mucous membrane exposure. However, she had dermatitis on one ear and may have touched it. She washed the blood off several minutes after the spill, tested negative five days after the exposure and again six weeks later. Three months after the incident she tested positive by ELISA and Western Blot. She denied sexual contact with anyone except her husband of eight years, who tested seronegative, and denied receiving a transfusion, using intravenous drugs, or having sustained needle-stick injuries in over two years.[18]

A year earlier, the CDC had published details of another case, this one occurring in a home-care setting.

Case 2: The child was diagnosed as having a congenital intestinal abnormality. For more than a year he underwent numerous surgical procedures and transfusions. Following multiple infections, the child's blood was tested for HIV antibody in May of 1985, at about sixteen months of age. ELISA and Western Blot were both positive, as were tests done on the blood of one of the child's twenty-six blood donors. In caring for the child at home (which included drawing his blood, removing intravenous lines, replacing ostomy bags, and changing surgical dressings), the child's thirty-two-year-old mother had had frequent contact with the child's blood and with other bodily fluids, including feces that often contained blood. She did not recall cuts or dermatitis on her hands, but she did not wear gloves and often did not wash her hands immediately after contact with blood. In March, June, and October of 1985, she donated blood, which was screened for HIV antibody. Her blood tested negative in March and June but was positive in October by ELISA and Western Blot. Epidemiological investigations did not reveal any other risk factors. The child's father tested negative.[19]

Cases like these strongly suggest that the risk of contracting the AIDS virus through skin contact with infected blood is marginally greater than zero, especially if the contact is extensive or prolonged and especially if the skin is not intact. The probability of infection through such exposure can be determined only when we have a statistically significant number of infections, documented so as to exclude standard modes of transmission (the numerator), as well as the overall number of nonpercutaneous exposures to infected blood (the denominator). At the present time, the number of cases is too small for the risk to be accurately measured. One study, for example, followed 103 health-care workers who were frequently exposed to HIV-infected blood, either on mucous membranes or on nonintact skin. None seroconverted.[20]

Hospitals and nursing homes have undertaken to reduce and eliminate this small but real risk by instituting what are called "universal precautions." Health-care professionals have learned new techniques to reduce the risk of infection. Dentists and other clinicians wear protective glasses, masks, and gloves. Bleach solutions or other disinfectants are used to clean blood off instruments and surfaces. Since many people who are infected with HIV are not known, even by themselves, to be infected, the only way to reduce risk is to treat all blood as potentially lethal. To confine precaution only to blood from persons known to be infected is to be careless. This means that contact with any blood needs to be taken very seriously. All such mishaps need to be closely investigated with a view toward preventing recurrence.

Incidents like those in Cases 1 and 2 are uncommon in preschools. Early childhood educators do not draw or work with blood. When present, blood is usually the consequence of minor abrasions and cuts; rarely does it flow freely. But early childhood educators, like health-care workers, must learn to approach bodily fluids—especially blood—in new ways. Disposable gloves, towels, and disinfectant should be readily available to all staff at all times, for use in handling and cleaning contaminated objects and surfaces, and hand lotion, to prevent chapping, should be provided. In the age of AIDS (and, while we are on the subject, hepatitis B, which, while less often fatal than AIDS, is about one hundred times as infectious), young children as well as staff need to know about the potential danger.

What Is Known About the Risk from Biting?

While unavoidable and prolonged, extensive, or repeated exposure to the blood of another is probably extremely rare in early childhood centers, biting is common, especially among younger children.[21] There are, however, laboratory studies that suggest that the likelihood of transmission from bites is small at best. Unlike blood, the virus is only rarely capable of being isolated in saliva,[22] and, notably, research exists that shows that saliva kills the AIDS virus.[23] As with nonpercutaneous exposure to blood, it has been impossible to assess epidemiologically the risk levels of biting. One study followed an infected patient who, having sustained brain injuries following an automobile accident, became aggressive and unable to care for himself.[24] He masturbated frequently, was incontinent of urine and feces, and had inflamed and bleeding gums. His aggressiveness made it difficult to cut his nails, which were, at times, soiled with semen, feces, and urine. For more than two years, he inflicted documented bites and scratches on thirty health-care workers. All were scratched on the arm, wrist, or hand, and eight were also bitten. Bites broke the skin in three cases, leaving bleeding puncture wounds. In one of these cases, the wound became infected. Not one of the workers seroconverted.[25]

What about anecdotal evidence of infection by means of a bite? Here there seem to be only two cases.

Case 3: In the course of a fight in early 1985, a 26-year-old health-care worker knocked out some of her sister's teeth, causing bleeding from the mouth. Later in the fight, she was bitten on the leg by her sister, who was infected and whose mouth was still bleeding. The woman had tested negative in August of 1983 but was positive in January of 1987. She claimed never to have injected drugs or had a blood transfusion or needle-stick injury. Of her three sexual contacts since 1983, two tested seronegative and the third was an untraceable one-night stand.[26]

Case 4: This case involved two brothers, one three years older than the other. The younger had had surgery shortly after he was born in 1981, receiving blood from an infected donor. When the child died three and a half years after the transfusion, HIV antibody was confirmed by ELISA and radioimmunoprecipitation. When family members were screened, the older brother tested positive by ELISA, indirect immunofluorescence, and radioimmunoprecipitation. He had significant disturbance of his humoral and cellular immune systems. The mother stated that he had never been given blood or blood products, nor had he been sexually abused. She denied having bedbugs in the house.[27] The mother reported that both children were always under her observation. About six months before the younger child died, he bit his older brother's forearm: the mother observed teeth imprints on the skin but no bleeding.[28]

Case 3 is probably best understood as one involving percutaneous exposure to infected blood (rather than saliva). Assuming that exposure did not occur sexually and that no other modes of transmission were involved, the bite, accompanied by blood in the biter's mouth, could well have introduced HIV-infected blood under the woman's skin, producing seroconversion much as a needle-stick injury could.

Case 4, however, did not involve blood or broken skin. Unfortunately, the report suffers from inadequate documentation. The ELISA test and the others that were mentioned in the case report (in the way they were probably used on the child in 1986) are sensitive but are not specific: they are highly likely to register positive when the antibody is present but also prone to registering positive under other circumstances as well. If the child had had malaria or chickenpox, but not HIV, the ELISA test could have been positive also. That is why, when an ELISA (or some similar test) is positive, it needs to be supplemented by a second test, like the Western Blot test, which is highly specific, that is, highly likely to register negative when the HIV antibody is absent. A positive ELISA followed by a positive Western Blot is the "gold standard" for the presence of the HIV antibody.[29]

The tests done on the child in Case 4 did not meet this standard. Even if other modes of transmission were ruled out, because of the significant likelihood that the child did not contract the virus at all—the tests done were insufficient to have shown this conclusively—it is possible that the child did not contract the AIDS virus at all from the bite. The report also refers to disturbances to the child's immune system. While some—but not all—abnormalities of the child's immune system could be evidence of HIV infection, the report does not describe the abnormalities. Since there is a significant probability that the child never had the AIDS virus, the case does not provide quality evidence for transmission by means of a bite.[30]

Toward a Model Policy for Handling HIV in Early Childhood Centers

Does the danger posed to other children by the presence of infected children or staff warrant exclusion of such persons from participation in the center? If infected children are to remain in the center, what should the parents of other children know?

As of this writing, no cases in which a child has been infected in an early childhood center have been reported. This is not surprising since none of the standard modes of transmission involve activities that are remotely likely to take place in centers. A few case reports suggest two nonstandard modes of transmission that could possibly take place in a center. These cases are so rare and the likelihood of transmission so small that it has not yet been possible for researchers to measure the risk of transmission following such exposure.

Some case reports suggest that it is likely that infection can occur from nonpercutaneous contact with infected blood, especially when the contact is prolonged, extensive, or repeated, and especially when the skin is broken or, possibly, when the exposure is to a mucous membrane. In early childhood centers, the unmeasurably small risk of infection following nonpercutaneous exposure to blood can be reduced or eliminated as it is in other settings, by scrupulous adherence to universal precautions in the treatment of bleeding injuries and the cleaning of blood-contaminated objects and surfaces. Children need to be taught caution. They need to learn how to treat their own nose-bleeds. Where they have open, oozing lesions (impetigo and cold sores are common), children should be sent home until the condition is resolved or until the child's physician assures the director that there is no danger to others.

Two case reports suggest that it is possible that infection can occur from a bite by an infected individual, especially if the biter's mouth is bleeding and if the skin of the bitten person is broken by the bite. The unmeasurably small risk of a child's becoming infected through bit-ing—if indeed there is such a risk—can be reduced or eliminated by excluding all persistent vigorous biters from program activities until the biting behavior stops or until the child's physician assures the director that there is no danger to other children. Children—especially biters—who are bleeding from the mouth because of minor injuries or deciduous tooth loss should be kept from playing with other children until the bleeding stops.

Since the directors of preschools will generally not know whether children or staff are infected, the exclusion of known HIV-positive persons will not have the effect of insuring protection. On the contrary, because parents and staff will often want to avoid exclusion, directors who are known to exclude may be less likely to be told of the serostatus of children and staff. Directors can exclude only if they know, and since they are less likely to know if they exclude, exclusion is not an effective means of insuring safety. Indeed, even daily testing for HIV cannot ensure exclusion of infected people. The best protection is learning to think about and to handle blood and biting behavior in new ways. The responsibility is easier in an early childhood center than in a clinic since there is no need to draw and process blood and since children and staff with open, weeping wounds can be sent home.

Empirical research cannot establish a zero risk of seroconversion. But in light of substantial laboratory and epidemiological investigation, it now appears probable that there is no significant risk in early childhood centers that scrupulously adhere to the precautionary measures set out above. This is not to say that infection is impossible. ("Impossible" does not appear to be a term that is used in epidemiology.) Infection could result from a single accident that somehow simultaneously caused extensive bleeding by a child known to be infected, an abrasion to a seronegative child, and immediate and unavoidable contact between the infected blood and the broken skin. But such accidents may be as rare as injuries caused by falling airplane parts. Since it is highly unlikely that the presence of an infected child could ever pose a significant (i.e., non-negligible) risk to other children, and since it is also unlikely that there are any unknown non-negligible risks, it is not a violation of Principle 1.1 for early childhood centers to admit infected children. Indeed, it would be improper to exclude or refuse admission to an HIV-infected child on the grounds of the danger imposed to the other children. There is no known significant risk, especially if the center is careful about blood and biting behavior.

Given the absence of known danger to other children and the confidentiality provision of the code, parents of healthy children would ordinarily have no legitimate interest in knowing about an infected child in the center. Since contacts of the sort that can be expected to occur at a center are not associated with a known risk of infection, parents of children who have had contact with an infected person need not and should not be informed that such contact has taken place.

Given the widespread misinformation about HIV infection and transmission, it is probably wise for early childhood educators, prophylactically, to educate parents and others regarding what is known about the risks infected children pose to other children, what the school is doing to reduce the risks, and the school's policy, in keeping with the CEC, to allow HIV-positive children to participate in programs. These policies should be circulated and discussed prior to the discovery of the first infected child in the center.

Parents of infected children also need to be informed of the impact of their child's disease on the other children in the center. Consideration needs to be given to how information about the death of their child should be conveyed to the other children. Because the other children will be affected by the illness and death of their classmate, their parents need to be informed appropriately about what the effects on their own children might be and how these can be managed.

Notes

Acknowledgments: Several people have contributed importantly: Donna Marie Anderson, David McEwan, Alan Katz, Joe Elm, Lisa Mendez, Josie Woll, Stephanie Feeney, Eva Moravchic, Annabelle Kaufman, and Michael Davis.

1. The process used to develop the NAEYC code is described in Kenneth Kipnis, "Toward a Code of Ethics for Pre-school Teachers: The Role of the Ethics Consultant," *International Journal of Applied Philosophy* (Summer 1988): 1–11.

2. I helped to found and currently served as an officer of the Hawaii AIDS Task Group, which serves as a channel of communication for people in Hawaii who are involved with the HIV epidemic. Meeting monthly, our two-hour discussions are transcribed and disseminated to about three hundred key individuals statewide.

3. While the Spanish flu epidemic at the end of World War I killed approximately twenty million, it appeared and vanished suddenly. The AIDS epidemic has been evident since 1981 and shows no signs of retreating. The World Health Organization estimates thirty million infections by the year 2000.

4. This language is from the NAEYC Code of Ethical Conduct," prepared by Stephanie Feeney and Kenneth Kipnis. This code was adopted by the NAEYC Governing Board, August 1989, and published in *Young Children* (November 1989): 26–29. The NAEYC is the leading professional association in the field of early childhood education.

5. The fear of contact with HIV-infected children is significantly associated with the belief that a child infected with HIV is likely to infect others. See A. L. Morrow, B. A. Benton, R. R. Reves, and L. K. Pickering, "Knowledge and Attitudes of Day Care Center Parents and Care Providers Regarding Children Infected with Human Immunodeficiency Virus," *Pediatrics* 87 (1991): 876–883. Improved knowledge about the risks of infection may diminish fear.

6. The CEC permits breaching confidentiality only when necessary to protect a child.

7. See L. K. Pickering and A. L. Morrow, "Contagious Diseases of Child Day Care," *Infection* 19 (1991): 61–63.

8. Less has been said on the parallel issues raised by the presence of infected staff. These are treated implicitly in the discussion of infected children.

9. While philosophical discussions of paternalism typically involve decisions made on behalf of competent adults, here decisions are being made on behalf of small children. The issue is whether the director has or ought to have

the authority, as against the child's doctor and parents, over what will best serve the child's interests.

10. Unfortunately, physicians are not uniformly knowledgeable about preschools and the risks these impose on immunocompromised children. Directors should seek advice from well-informed specialists.

11. It is likely that there are several thousand children under the age of 13 in the United States, who are HIV-positive. See M. Gwinn, M. Rogers, R. Berkelman, et al., "Incidence of Pediatric AIDS in the United States: Predictions from Seroprevalance Data: Fifth International Conference on AIDS, Montreal, Canada, June 4–9, 1989 (abstr. Th AO 11). Because of blood-screening practices, infection from blood and blood products is diminishing. As HIV infection spreads among women of childbearing age, however, perinatal transmission to young children should increase.

12. "Caution" is not quite a correct term here, since if we do not know how the virus is transmitted, it cannot be clear what measures we can take to prevent transmission. The history of pandemics is filled with stories of ineffective and counterproductive efforts at prevention; AIDS is no exception. For example, mandatory physician reporting of infected patients, as in Japan, has the effect of discouraging Japanese from going to physicians for diagnosis and treatment. Many Japanese seek anonymous testing abroad.

13. See, for example, C. J. Kasler, "Reading, Writing, but No Biting: Isolating School Children with AIDS," *Cleveland State Law Review* 337 (1989): 337.

14. See, for example, A. R. Lifson, P. Thomas, and G. Scott, "Unrecognized Modes of Transmission of HIV: Acquired Immunodeficiency Syndrome in Children Reported Without Risk Factors," *Pediatric Infectious Disease Journal* 6 (1987): 292–293, for a study of seropositive pediatric patients initially reported to the Centers for Disease Control with "no identified risk." When information is obtained on children with AIDS "initially classified as 'no risk identified,' such children are typically found to have acquired their infection through recognized modes of transmission. Investigation of these cases does not support the existence of new or unrecognized modes of transmission of HIV" (293).

15. A. R. Lifson, "Do Alternate Modes for Transmission of Human Immunodeficiency Virus Exist?" *Journal of the American Medical Association* 259 (1988): 1353–1356.

16. Ibid.

17. Several studies have concluded that the risk of seroconversion from a single percutaneous exposure to infected blood is somewhere between 0.3 and 0.5 percent. See, for example, R. Marcus et al., "Surveillance of Health Care Workers Exposed to Blood from Patients Infected with the Human Immunodeficiency Virus," *New England Journal of Medicine* 319 (1988): 1118–1123. In this fairly typical study, researchers followed 860 health-care workers who had received either a needle-stick injury or a cut with a contaminated sharp instrument. Four (0.47 percent) seroconverted.

18. "Update: Human Immunodeficiency Virus Infections in Health-Care Workers Exposed to Blood of Infected Persons," *Morbidity and Mortality Weekly Report* 36 (1987): 285–289.

19. "Apparent Transmission of Human T-lymphotrophic Virus Type III/ Lymphadenopathy-Associated Virus from a Child to a Mother Providing Health Care," *Morbidity and Mortality Weekly Report* 35 (1986): 76–79.

20. R. Marcus, et al., "Surveillance of Health Care Workers Exposed to Blood from Patients Infected with the Human Immunodeficiency Virus," *New England Journal of Medicine* 319 (1988): 1118–1123.

21. At one large and fairly typical preschool in Honolulu, most bites were inflicted by toddlers. Only rarely—perhaps one incident per year—did these raise a bruise. Puncturing bites were much rarer: none had ever occurred at that center. Bites in which the biter had a bleeding mouth were unheard of. One study reported an incidence of 3.1 episodes of biting per 100 child-days among toddlers (J. Garrard, N. Leland, and D. K. Smith, "Epidemiology of Human Bites to Children in a Day Care Center," *American Journal of Diseases of Children* 142 [1988]: 643–650).

22. In one study, only 1 of 83 seropositive subjects had HIV in the saliva (D. D. Ho, R. E. Byington, R. T. Schooley, et al., "Infrequency of Isolation of HTLV-III Virus from Saliva in AIDS," *New England Journal of Medicine* 313 [1985]: 1606).

23. P. N. Fultz, "Components of Saliva Inactivate Human Immunodeficiency Virus," *Lancet* 2 (1986): 1215.

24. C. Tsoukas, T. Hadjis, et al., "Lack of Transmission of HIV Through Human Bites and Scratches," *Journal of Acquired Immune Deficiency Syndromes* 1 (1988): 505–507.

25. See also J. A. Drummond, "Seronegative 18 Months After Being Bitten by a Patient with AIDS," *Journal of the American Medical Association* 256 (1986): 2342–2343.

26. "Transmission of HIV by Human Bite," *Lancet* (1987): 522.

27. The remark about biting insects reflects the early date of this case report, as well as the concern to rule out all other theoretically possible modes of transmission.

28. V. Wahn, H. Kramer, T. Voit, et al., "Horizontal Transmission of HIV Infection Between Two Siblings," *Lancet* (1986): 694.

29. I am grateful to Joe Elm, M.A., and Alan Katz, M.D., for assisting me with the issues in this paragraph.

30. This defect in the case report has been noted by the Task Force on Pediatric AIDS: "The younger brother bit the older, but the skin of the older boy was unbroken and it is not clear that this act resulted in transmission" ("Pediatric Guidelines for Infection Control of Human Immunodeficiency Virus [Acquired Immunodeficiency Virus] in Hospitals, Medical Offices, Schools, and Other Settings," *Pediatrics* 82 (1988): 803).

5

AIDS in the Workplace: Options and Responsibilities

Al Gini
Michael Davis

Statistics indicate that, while few of us will experience AIDS in private or family life, many will experience AIDS in the workplace. AIDS raises at least three fundamental questions for a manager: How should an employee with AIDS be treated? How should other employees be informed about AIDS and their safety and morale insured? How should the legal, ethical, and human considerations involved be balanced against the needs of business? Such questions will become more pressing as the AIDS epidemic spreads.[1] This chapter considers possible options and strategies for answering them. Let us begin with a case.

Elaine's Cafeteria

Elaine Merkavich operates the cafeteria of Bunyun Hospital under a ten-year agreement, with nine years remaining. As long as she pays the (fixed) rent; maintains the physical plant; satisfies all applicable city, state, and federal laws; and provides full service twenty-four hours a day, she is free to run the cafeteria as if she owned it. Indeed, she insisted on that as a condition for taking over what had been a money loser. The cafeteria's employees, more than ninety of them, are her employees, not the hospital's.

It is one of those employees who concerns her now. Barry, thirty, is a cook she hired only nine months ago. His former wife brought bad news this morning. Barry, she told Elaine ("in confidence" and "out of concern for others"), has AIDS. Barry had been an above-average employee, so hard-working and reliable that Elaine was on the point of promoting him to head cook on the night shift.

Elaine wondered what she should do now. What do you do with such confidential information? How, for example, do you confirm it? The more she thought about that, the more she doubted the information would remain confidential for long. Barry's former wife would probably tell others as well. The news would soon be out. That thought suggested other questions. What effect would news of the disease have on other employees, especially those who work close to Barry or who have become his friends? What effect would the disease have on Barry's ability to manage the night shift, indeed, on his ability to continue to be a hard-working and reliable employee? What effect would news of a cook with AIDS have on customers?

That last question worried Elaine the most. Last year some hospital personnel had refused for a time to take care of patients with HIV. The administration had dealt with that refusal by saying, "Do the job or look for another." Elaine had no such power to get hospital employees to eat in the cafeteria. They were free to bring lunch from home or pay a little extra to go across the street rather than eat food prepared by someone with AIDS. Before Elaine took over the cafeteria, many had done just that because the food and service had been so bad. If many did it again because they feared her cook, the cafeteria would once again be a losing proposition. But this time it would be hers. She would have to do something. But what?

AIDS in Business

A recent study sponsored by Allstate Insurance Company and *Fortune* magazine found that, although a majority of U.S. corporate executives believe that AIDS is one of the major problems facing the country, most companies lack direction in dealing with the problem in the workplace. Only 29 percent of the executives in the 623 companies polled said that their companies have or are planning to formulate a written or unwritten policy on AIDS.[2] The Fourth International Conference on AIDS reported that only 8 percent of U.S. *Fortune* 500 firms and 25 percent of Canadian *Fortune* 500 firms have developed formal policies on AIDS.[3] Seemingly, most companies are unwilling, unable, or unprepared to handle the problem. They teeter between denial and procrastination. Why?

According to Cheryl Russell, editor-in-chief of *American Demographics*, of the 2 million Americans who died in 1987, AIDS victims accounted for only 14,000, less than 1 percent of total deaths. In contrast, heart disease killed 800,000 and cancer another 500,000. Pneumonia, suicide, and cirrhosis of the liver were also far more common causes of death than AIDS. In number of deaths, AIDS ranks with emphysema, kidney failure, and murder. Even if the estimates for

AIDS deaths in 1991 were correct—54,000—this figure would account for less than 3 percent of all deaths that year.[4]

AIDS has killed about 180,000 Americans during its ten years in the United States. During the same period, more than 20 million Americans died. For the nation as a whole, AIDS is an insignificant disease in absolute number of deaths—a mere blip in our mortality statistics.[5] Applied to the workplace, these figures mean that in any given company only a relative handful of employees will have AIDS. For example, in 1983, Control Data Corporation conducted a self-study that predicted that, at most, 104 of its 34,000 employees would die of AIDS between 1983 and 1988—fewer than would die of any other major disease.[6]

So the question remains: Why the hesitance of so many corporations to formulate policies and procedures in regard to AIDS? A large part of the answer at both the human and corporate level is fear, fear fueled by irresponsible headlines and controversies in the press. No other disease in modern times has generated so much fear. In some ways, that is understandable. AIDS touches on many of the basic taboos of human life: sex, homosexuality, illness, suffering, and death. As Reverend Ann Showalter, a Mennonite minister and director of the Chicago-based AIDS Pastoral Care Network, has said, "There are really two epidemics—one of the disease and one of fear. And the fear is much more readily transmitted than the disease."[7] What corporations and individuals alike fear as much as the costs and suffering of the disease are the social stigma associated with it and the unknowns and the intangibles of contagion and cure.

Many social commentators believe that this fear, no matter how exaggerated or misplaced, has immobilized the corporate sector, diminishing its ability to handle a crisis that will not soon go away.

Ethical Issues

The AIDS epidemic raises at least three kinds of ethical issues: First, there are issues of *rights*, both human and civil. Two rights are of special importance here: the right to privacy and the right to work. The right to privacy grants a presumption of confidentiality in regard to health records, financial accounts, and job evaluations or performance records, a presumption operating against both government and private persons until they show a specific need to know. (Does Elaine in fact have a right to know whether Barry has AIDS?) The right to work includes the right not to be discriminated against in matters of hiring, firing, compensation, and terms, conditions, and privileges of employment on the basis of race, color, religion, sex, national origin, or disability. (Can Elaine legally take Barry's disease into account when deciding whether to promote him to head cook on the night shift?)

Second, there are issues of *public health*. Government has an obligation to protect the public from infectious and communicable diseases. This obligation extends to protecting employees in the workplace from disease and unnecessary physical hazards. (What responsibilities does Elaine have to customers and other employees to protect them from Barry?)

Third, there are issues of *social ethics*. What is our commitment to fair treatment and justice for all members of society, in particular political minorities, the young, the aged, and the mentally or physically disabled? (Does Barry's disease even count as a disability?)

Framing these issues, however, are two practical questions. One is factual: Is AIDS readily communicable in the workplace? The other is legal: What legal protections do employees with AIDS have? We must consider these issues first.

How Communicable?

Unlike most transmissible diseases (colds, flu, measles, etc.), AIDS is not transmitted through sneezing, coughing, or eating or drinking from common utensils, or merely through being around an infected person. All scientific evidence so far indicates that transmission is not possible through casual personal contact.

Because of the difficulty of transmission, AIDS is an easily avoidable disease. Risk of contagion is proportional to high-risk behavior. Except for health-care workers engaged in invasive procedures bringing them into contact with blood and other bodily fluids, employees, patients, and customers afflicted with AIDS do not present a health risk under normal working conditions.[8] One has about as much chance of catching AIDS in the workplace as of catching cancer or multiple sclerosis. Although AIDS is a health issue for business, as well as a legal and moral issue, it is not a contagion issue. Businesses should not allow fear and ignorance to disrupt the workplace.[9]

Legal Protection

For employees, the only thing worse than having AIDS is losing one's job because of it. Before 1987, AIDS victims had few legal rights or unambiguous remedies in regard to their status in the workplace.

The doctrine of "employment at will" allowed most employers almost unlimited discretion to fire individuals for any reason or for no reason whatsoever. Only union contracts and specific legislative provisions limited this plenary authority.[10] Employers could solve their AIDS problem simply by firing those with the disease—or even those they feared might have or get the disease. As recently as June 1986, a United States Justice Department memorandum declared that "fear alone" was legitimate grounds for dismissal: "Acting on an irrational fear of contagion is," it reasoned, "not prohibited by law and thus not discriminatory."[11] The memorandum led to a surge of firings, particularly in smaller companies.

Many other employers dismissed employees with AIDS or those simply suspected of having AIDS because the employers feared the threat of reprisals from other workers more than they feared the disease itself. Protests and strikes over health and safety issues have long been sanctioned by the law. Under Section 7 of the National Labor Relations Act, employees have the right to engage in "concerted activity" for their "mutual aid and protection." This means that two or more employees have a right to withhold services to protect their wages or hours or the terms or conditions of their employment. In addition, Section 502 of the Labor Management Relations Act specifically protects the employee's right to stop working because of "a good faith belief" that abnormally dangerous conditions exist in the workplace. Employers had good reason to fear that if, because of health concerns, a group of employees refused to work with a person who had or was suspected of having AIDS, the National Labor Relations Board could view the refusal as a valid protest strike over a health and safety issue.[12]

Since 1987, the legal pendulum has swung to the side of AIDS victims. Employers must now deal with a new legal fact: under the Americans with Disabilities Act of 1991 (ADA), an employee with AIDS is considered disabled and is protected from discrimination just as are other disabled people. The ADA effectively preempts the plenary authority of "employment at will" with respect to AIDS (and HIV), negates the Justice Department's memorandum on fear of contagion, and therefore probably overrides any possible ruling by the National Labor Relations Board in regard to the unwillingness of fellow employees to work with a colleague suffering from AIDS.[13]

This complete turnaround began with the Supreme Court's ruling in *School Board of Nassau County v. Arline*, 480 U.S. 273 (1987). Arline, a Florida schoolteacher, suffered from recurring bouts of tuberculosis but claimed she was not contagious. She argued that her firing by the school district violated Section 504 of the Federal Rehabilitation Act of 1973. Imposing a duty on the federal government, employers with federal contracts, and employers who are recipients of federal assistance not to discriminate against handicapped persons, the act defines "handicap" as "a physical or mental impairment or infirmity which substantially limits one or more of a person's major life activities" but expressly extends coverage to those not only presently disabled, but who have a "record of such impairment" or are "regarded as having such an impairment."

Until *Arline*, appellate courts had applied Section 504 only to conditions such as heart disease, cancer, blindness, epilepsy, multiple sclerosis, diabetes, and dyslexia. The question of whether contagious diseases were covered had never been addressed. When the Supreme Court agreed with Arline and ordered her reinstatement, it effectively extended the act's protection to those with transmissible diseases.[14] Persons suffering from AIDS were (apparently) covered because the ability to fight off infection and preserve health is a "major life function."[15]

The Court did, however, announce in a footnote that it was leaving for another day the question whether persons infected with HIV but free of symptoms qualified for protection as a handicapped person under the 1973 federal act:

> The United States argues that it is possible for a person to be simply a carrier of a disease, that is, to be capable of spreading a disease without having a "physical impairment" or suffering from any other symptoms associated with the disease. The United States contends that this is true in the case of some carriers of the Acquired Immune Deficiency Syndrome (AIDS) virus. From this premise the United States concludes that discrimination solely on the basis of contagiousness is never discrimination on the basis of a handicap. The argument is misplaced in this case, because the handicap here, tuberculosis, gave rise both to a physical impairment *and* to contagiousnss. This case does not present, and we therefore do not reach, the questions whether a carrier of a contagious disease such as AIDS could be considered to have a physical impairment, or whether such a person could be considered, solely on the basis of contagiousness, a handicapped person as defined by the Act.[16]

The Civil Rights Restoration Act of 1987 effectively closed this question. The act states that a person with a contagious disease or infection is disabled if he or she does not "constitute a direct threat to health or safety" and is able to "perform the duties of the job."[17] It was this understanding of disability that the ADA incorporated.

The ADA differs from earlier legislation primarily in extent of coverage. Earlier legislation protected the disabled from discrimination by government or government contractors. The ADA applies to any company with more than fifteen employees.

The legislative history of the ADA is relevant to Elaine's problem. The House of Representatives included an amendment to the (proposed) ADA to exempt "food handlers." This was done out of respect for the interests of the food industry, even though the courts had long ago repudiated the argument that customer preference could excuse otherwise impermissible discrimination. (Many who engaged in racial discrimination in employment had sought to justify their conduct as arising not from their own prejudice but from sound business judgment concerning the prejudices of their customers.)

For that reason, the Senate rejected the House's amendment, while trying to satisfy the legitimate interests of the food industry. The Secretary of Health and Human Services was to maintain a list of infectious and communicable diseases known to be transmitted through food handling (and of methods known to prevent their communication). The ADA permits employers to refuse to assign an employee to a job involving food handling if the employee has one of the diseases on the list and could handle the food in a way capable of transmitting the disease. HIV is *not* on the list.[18]

The ADA classifies all life-disabling, life-threatening, and contagious illnesses under the general heading of "disability" and protects against discrimination all "disabled" employees. The ADA thus closes the door on (legal) summary dismissal of employees with AIDS and provides a framework for dealing with such employees. This framework may be summarized in this way:

1. An employee may not be terminated or otherwise discriminated against solely because of a disability that does not interfere with the performance of the employee's job. An employee with AIDS may be terminated only when his condition substantially interferes with his job performance.

2. While no company is legally obligated to hire workers with AIDS, a business cannot refuse to hire individuals because of their disease. A disability may be a reason to fire, or to refuse to hire, only if it renders the employee either intellectually or physically unable to perform the job (even with reasonable accommodations) or the employee could (even with reasonable accommodations) present a direct threat to the health or safety of herself or others.

3. An employer must make reasonable accommodations for all disabled individuals. The exact accommodations necessary will depend on several factors, such as the nature of the work, the size of the organization, and the costs involved. In general, no radical changes are necessary. Accommodations might include offering flexible hours, part-time work, or transfer to a less taxing position.

4. Given the overwhelming evidence that AIDS is not transmitted from person to person in the ordinary workplace, the ADA implies that employers have *no* demonstrable interest that could justify using blood tests to screen for exposure to the AIDS virus. If the employee or applicant is currently capable of performing the job, the test cannot be used in making employment decisions. Any adverse action premised on the test would be unlawful.[19]

Options for Businesses

Given the ADA, what can businesses do? What should they do? There seem to be three major options: first, guarantee full salary and benefits if the employee agrees *not* to return to work; second, develop no AIDS policy, on the assumption that general policies can handle all possible contingencies; and third, develop a specific AIDS policy, describing both benefits and protections available to an employee with AIDS (or HIV).

The first option, while perhaps within the letter of the law, does not conform to its spirit. The legality of this option remains to be adjudicated. Numerous firms are still unwilling to deal with the personnel problems of an employee with AIDS. They argue that no matter what experts say, retaining an employee known to have AIDS, whether on the shop floor or in the executive offices, creates feelings of anxiety and unrest among a significant portion of their other employees, suppliers, and customers. To resolve the problem while addressing the needs of an afflicted employee, some firms continue to pay the employee's full salary and medical and retirement benefits on condition that the employee not return to work. The employee is, in effect, forced to take paid leave.

One vice-president for personnel management of a *Fortune* 500 firm explained the policy in this way in a private conversation:

> Who are we hurting? For the guy who's got it—we're helping him pay his bills, keep his house, and get first-rate medical attention through our group coverage for as long as he needs it. And from the point of view of the people he worked with, well—I'm sure

they're glad he's taken care of and I know they're relieved by his absence. Look, don't kid yourself, *even* if it isn't contagious, it's just not the same thing as working next to someone who has cancer or a heart condition. As far as I'm concerned, this is just as much of a morale issue as it is a moral one.

When asked about the possibility of civil litigation, the vice-president's answer was equally forthright.

Why would they sue? We haven't fired anyone. We don't even list them as being on leave, and we never put them on disability. They will still be getting full pay without losing any benefits. We'll even give them their annual raise when it comes up. So what could they sue us for—loss of meaningful work? That would be a tough one to win. And even if they did win, it could prove to be a hollow victory if it took longer than forty-eight months to get it through the courts.

I just don't see it happening. It's just not worth the effort and grief involved.

This variation of the first option seems to take advantage of the weak negotiating position of an employee with AIDS. The vice-president does not claim any legal right to force the employee to give up working, merely a practical ability to take (what he obviously considers) "the easy way out." Can an employer justifiably trample on the legal rights of an employee this way? The answer to that question depends both on the *moral* justification of the right and on the alternatives available. Our discussion of the other two options will shed light on both.

The second option seems to be the option of choice for most American businesses. They feel that adopting specific policies that deal solely with AIDS is not advisable for them for at least one of three reasons. First, they don't want to draw attention to the problem and unnecessarily alarm their employees. Second, current company policy on life-threatening illnesses probably covers the situation, and therefore there is no reason to treat AIDS explicitly. Third, a special AIDS policy might prove too restrictive; flexibility is needed because both scientific knowledge and law in this area are changing rapidly.[20]

The key element in this approach is "flexibility." The companies involved believe that each AIDS case is different and must be handled on an individual ad hoc basis. IBM is one of the companies that uses its basic policy on catastrophic illness to deal with "the handful" of AIDS patients among its four hundred thousand employees. If they're fit, they can work. If they want counseling, they can get it. If their coworkers want counseling, IBM offers that, too. The same rules apply to all workers whether they have AIDS or cancer, or have suffered a heart attack.[21]

The third option is to develop, publish, and implement a special policy on AIDS. So far, only a few major companies—including Syntex, Bank America, AT&T, Transamerica, Levi Strauss, Wells Fargo, and Pacific Telesis—have adopted specialized personnel policies to handle the problems that AIDS poses in the workplace.[22]

All such policies are formulated around a commitment to six underlying principles:

1. AIDS is a blood-borne virus that cannot be transmitted through casual social or workplace contact.

2. All human beings gain much of their self-identity and self-esteem from their work. Moreover, good health is often enhanced by working at one's regular job, no matter what the diagnosis. Because of this, all workers should be allowed to determine for themselves, within the limits of safety and physical ability, how long they want to continue to work.[23]

3. All companies have an absolute obligation to provide a safe working environment for all employees and customers. Every precaution must be taken to ensure that an employee does not present a health or safety threat to other employees and customers through loss of physical or mental abilities. As long as medical evidence indicates that persons with life-threatening illnesses do not represent threats to themselves or others, managers should be sensitive to their conditions and ensure that they are treated the same as other employees.

4. The basic posture of every AIDS policy in the workplace must be educational, because while AIDS is a disease that cannot be cured, it can be stopped. Information, training, and counseling should be the cornerstone of any response to AIDS, both for employees with AIDS and for their fellow workers.

5. Special care must be taken with all issues of confidentiality. Management's best course of action is a simple one: except when required by law to do so, never reveal any part of an employee's confidential medical record without that employee's written consent.

6. Any employee refusing to work with an AIDS-afflicted fellow worker is, after appropriate counseling and formal warnings, subject to discharge.

A number of companies have done much to inform themselves and their employees concerning AIDS. Taking the lead in this area is the Business Leadership Task Force, which consists of fifteen major employers based in northern California. These companies have pooled their resources to provide a comprehensive AIDS education program for employees and their families. The basic message of the Task Force is a simple one. They encourage all employers to address the issues of AIDS in the workplace as a means of avoiding hysteria and mistrust. Levi Strauss, for example, a leading member of the Task Force, has developed programs that include lectures for managers by experts on AIDS; resource and support classes for persons with AIDS, as well as for anyone who is related to or knows a person with AIDS; a video presentation that can be checked out for home viewing; and regular updates on AIDS published in the company newsletter. Pacific Bell, another Task Force member, provides AIDS seminars and publishes information on topics not normally covered in a company vehicle, such as sexual activity and sexuality. All of the Task Force members also discuss AIDS in regard to their existing employee benefits programs. This provides them with the opportunity to remind their employees of the protection being provided for them and to reassure them of continued protection.[24]

The real import of a carefully rendered AIDS policy is that it communicates a company's concern to provide a safe, healthful, and efficient work environment. It also demonstrates to workers, suppliers, and customers alike that management cares not only about the continued success of its business but also about the well-being of its employees and the people the company serves. Sadly, however, as BusinessWeek commentator Irene Pave has stated: "Most companies . . . have yet to come to grips with AIDS. But . . . no responsible employer can continue to duck the issue. The peace of mind of future AIDS patients and the stability of a company's work force depend on setting a fair policy without delay."[25]

Conclusion

We have not yet determined what Elaine should do, much less presented an argument for why she should do it. Our purpose here is to sort out issues, to clarify what is at stake, and otherwise to give some structure to what originally might seem overwhelmingly complex. We believe this to be a legitimate service that philosophers can perform for managers. In that spirit, we now make three concluding points:

1. Elaine does not in fact know whether Barry has AIDS. She has only the word of his former wife, who may or may not know what she is talking about. Asking Barry whether he has AIDS, or otherwise

seeking to determine whether he does, has three disadvantages for Elaine. First, she would be inquiring into a disability legally irrelevant to his job. That itself is legally risky. Second, she risks causing Barry a good deal of embarrassment, whether he has AIDS or not. (Imagine how you would feel if your employer asked you whether you have AIDS!) And, third, her seeking such information would suggest that Barry's former wife is justifiably "concerned for others." Elaine would be feeding the very fear she should be trying to kill. She would have been better off if she had just told Barry's wife, "You needn't have told me this. It has nothing to do with me. As long as Barry can do his job, his AIDS is of no concern to me. He can't infect either his fellow employees or my customers. And when he can no longer work, he will go on disability, whether he has AIDS or not."

2. Elaine's competitors across the street are in exactly the same position she is. They too may have employees with AIDS, whether they admit it or not. The problem is to be sure that the hospital's employees understand that.

3. Barry's former wife has done Elaine a service, not by telling her about Barry in particular, but by giving her a push to begin planning for a problem that will be hers sooner or later. She might, for example, want to find out what, if anything, the hospital is doing to inform its employees about AIDS. If the hospital has an educational program, does it include anything about the lack of connection between AIDS and food handlers? Could it? Could her employees take the program?

For Elaine, AIDS in her cafeteria is (among other things) a problem in human relations or employee management. She will probably respond most effectively if she responds to it as she would to any other such problem. While management styles differ, there are certain clear constraints: moral minimums ("Don't lie," "Don't cheat," etc.), the law (e.g., the ADA), and organizational attitudes or traditions that go beyond the moral minimums and the law (e.g., a commitment to treating employees "with respect"). These have a place in every management decision, even one (like this) that may require considerably more sensitivity and inventiveness than most.

Notes

1. Nancy Merritt, "Bank of America's Blueprint for a Policy on AIDS," *Business Week* (March 23, 1987): 127.

2. Allison Kittrell, "Employers Lack AIDS strategy: Study," *Business Insurance* (February 1, 1988): 3.

3. National Public Radio, "All Things Considered," June 15, 1988.

4. Cheryl Russell, "Fear of AIDS May Re-create the Virtuous '50's," In *AIDS*, ed. Lynn Hall and Thomas Modl, p. 199. (St. Paul, Minn.: Greenhaven Press, 1988).

5. Ibid.

6. S. Siwolop et al., "The AIDS Epidemic and Business," *Business Week* (March 23, 1987): 123.

7. "AIDS: Lending a Hand," *Company: A Magazine of the American Jesuits* (Winter 1987): 22–24.

8. Centers for Disease Control, "Recommendations for Prevention of HIV Transmission in Health-Care Settings," *Morbidity and Mortality Weekly Report* 36, no. 2S 35.

9. Merritt, "Bank of America's Blueprint," 127.

10. Patricia Werhane, *Persons, Rights and Corporations* (Englewood Cliffs, N.J.: Prentice Hall, 1985), pp. 80–93.

11. Gary Ward, *What a Manager Should Know About AIDS in the Workplace* (Chicago: Darnell Corporation, 1987), p. 4.

12. Victor Schacter and Susan Seeburg, *AIDS: A Manager's Guide* (New York: Executive Enterprises, 1986), p. 23.

13. Chai R. Feldblum, "Employment Protections," *Milbank Quarterly* 69 (suppl. 1/2 (1991)): 81–110, esp. 86, 102–104.

14. Stephanie Benson Goldberg, "The Meaning of 'Handicapped,' " *American Bar Association Journal* (March 1, 1987): 56–61.

15. Schacter and Seeburg, *AIDS*, pp. 40, 41.

16. *Arline*, 480 U.S. 273, 282 n. 7.

17. Lawrence O. Gostin, "Public Health Powers: The Imminence of Radical Change," *Milbank Quarterly* 69 (suppl. 1/2) (1991): 268–292, esp. 273.

18. Nancy Lee Jones, "Essential Requirements of the Act: A Short History and Overview," *Milbank Quarterly* 69 (suppl. 1/2) (1991): 25–54, esp. 45–46.

19. Jay Waks and Lori Meyers, "An Introduction to AIDS Coverage Under Corporate Policies on Infectious Diseases and Life-Threatening Illnesses," *Business Laws, Inc. (CPS)* (1987): 985–989.

20. Ibid., 986.

21. Irene Pave, "Fear and Loathing in the Workplace: What Managers Can Do About AIDS," *Business Week* (November 25, 1985): 126.

22 Elizabeth Younger and Linda Harris, "AIDS: Employer's Rights, Responsibilities and Opportunities," Washington Business Group on Health, 229½ Pennsylvania Avenue SE, Washington, D.C. 20003, N.p., n.d.

23. A.R. Gini and T. Sullivan, "Work: The Process and the Person," *Journal of Business Ethics* 6 (1987): 249–260.

24. Younger and Harris, "AIDS."

25. Pave, "Fear and Loathing," 126.

6

Leading by Example: AIDS Policy and the University's Social Responsibilities

Howard Cohen

The impact of AIDS on American society is pervasive. It is now generally understood that AIDS represents a health threat that transcends social class, sexual orientation, and other categories with which it was identified in its early history. Moreover, universities and colleges have, for the most part, accepted an educational function with respect to AIDS: campuses typically sponsor programs that inform students about the disease and advocate measures to prevent transmission of the virus. On most campuses, there is widespread recognition that everyone must be prepared to deal at some time or another with someone who has AIDS.

Each individual needs to think about how he or she will respond to persons with AIDS—whether with compassion or fear; with generosity or suspicion; as a supporter, as an uninterested bystander, or as an adversary. But however one resolves personal encounters with persons with AIDS, colleges and universities will inevitably be required to respond at the institutional level as well. Given the current public recognition of the seriousness of AIDS and public acceptance of the importance of AIDS education, policies establishing AIDS education programs are not difficult for a university to adopt. AIDS education, however, is only the first step in a comprehensive institutional policy dealing with the social impact of AIDS. Academic administrators will, sooner or later, be called on to deal with conflicts that cross a range of areas of campus life and that center squarely on intra-institutional responses to persons with AIDS.

One can hope that the development of these policies will be thoughtful, humane, and consistent with the ideals and purposes of institutions of higher education. There is a danger, however, that the policies will be developed in ways that are ad hoc, pragmatic, and aimed at short-term, specific issues. Moreover, given the level of passion that has accompanied public debate about HIV carriers, there is a danger that institutional decisionmakers will have a difficult time sorting out their personal from their institutional perspectives. Indeed, it seems to me that the need to separate personal from institutional responses to AIDS-related issues is neither widely recognized nor uncontested. Feelings about AIDS and about the ramifications of dealing with persons with AIDS are often prominent in discussions about what to do in particular cases. In the interest of a more thoughtful attempt at developing policies to deal with AIDS on campus, I want to consider some of the difficult cases that are likely to prompt policy formulation and then propose a way of thinking through the cases. This decision approach is grounded in an attempt to distinguish the personal desires and inclinations of the campus administrator from the considerations appropriate to the holder of an institutional position. AIDS issues present a kind of acid test for this approach precisely because we are not predisposed to make this separation in these cases.

Difficult Cases

Case 1: An assistant professor in the advanced stages of AIDS wishes to continue teaching as long as possible. Because of intermittent hospitalizations and periods of incapacitation, however, this faculty member misses classes with growing frequency. The faculty member's department chairperson is concerned that the instructor has on numerous occasions come to class unprepared to teach and that this situation can only deteriorate. The assistant professor proposes that the university fund a teaching assistant to provide continuity in the course. The higher-level administration prefers that the instructor go on disability leave. The dean of the college must decide whether to try to force the instructor out of the classroom or to make an effort to support his attempt to teach as long as possible.

Case 2: A private, church-affiliated university has been developing a potential donor who is interested in making a major gift to support the university's writing program. With this support, the university hopes to significantly strengthen its students' basic writing skills and, perhaps, to improve its retention record. The potential donor (an active member of the affiliated church) has expressed strong religious objections to a campus student organization's "safe-sex" condom distribution program. The students have undertaken their program without official university recognition or funds. They do, however, use university space and phones. They also identify themselves as a university student organization. The affiliated church is, itself, in some controversy on the issue of sex outside of marriage in general and on dealing with persons with AIDS in particular. The potential donor is on the conservative side of this debate, and he makes it clear that the elimination of this activity is a condition for the award of the gift. The president of the university must decide whether to suppress the "safe-sex" program so that the university can receive the gift or to inform the potential donor that the condition will not be met.

Case 3: The college cafeteria is run by an independent corporation on a contractual basis. In addition to serving meals, the corporation employs students as kitchen workers. One student, an HIV carrier who has made his condition known publicly, claims to have been denied a job in the kitchen on the grounds that he has AIDS. He wishes to bring a discrimination suit against the Food Services Corporation and requests college assistance in doing so. The vice-president for student affairs must decide whether, and to what extent, to cooperate with the student.

Decision making in these cases is difficult because, whatever the decision, some campus constituencies will feel the decision as a victory and others will feel it as a defeat. Although everyone can be in favor of health education and disease prevention, in many instances, the administrator will be making a decision in a "zero-sum" situation. In each of the examples developed above, whatever decision the administrator makes, some constituents will inevitably feel mistreated. AIDS issues are not, of course, the only zero-sum struggles on campuses. Many issues have this character, and, consequently, what I have to say about decision making in regard to AIDS applies to other decision-making contexts as well. Nevertheless, it is worth focusing on the AIDS cases because they are difficult, because they raise deep personal feelings for many people, and because they still need to be addressed in policy.

In Case 1, the dean has a choice of removing the faculty member from the classroom against the faculty member's wishes or leaving him to teach, providing sufficient support to buffer the students against the consequences of the disease's debilitating effects. No matter how much buffering the dean can arrange, however, there will still be a discernible gap in the perceived quality of instruction, a difficulty that is not likely to be resolved to the satisfaction of all.[1]

A decision to remove the faculty member from the classroom may relieve the department chairperson, who does not want to defend keeping an impaired faculty member in the classroom to students or to their parents. It may also please the president and the university's lawyers, who will not want this case to become a precedent for the future.[2] The dean herself may feel hard-pressed to finance the additional instructional support and may also worry about having to do the same for others in the future.

Nevertheless, a number of others may well be upset or even devastated by the decision to remove the faculty member from the classroom. The faculty member with AIDS for one, may think that the university has turned its back on his suffering and condemned his last days and months to a meaningless wait for death. The faculty members' friends and some of his colleagues in the department may feel the same way. Many would want sympathetic treatment by the university should they find themselves in similar circumstances of deteriorating health. Students who have previously known and admired this instructor might feel hurt and deprived at not being able to take one of his final courses. AIDS activists and supporters of persons with AIDS might see this as a lost opportunity for the university to perform a genuine educational function by demonstrating how persons with AIDS can remain socially integrated and productive, even as they are suffering the effects of the disease.

On the other side, a decision to leave the instructor in the classroom may lead some students, particularly those who have not previously known this teacher, to feel that they have had to suffer through a poor or chaotic learning experience to satisfy the emotional needs of the AIDS patient. They may feel disappointed or bitter about their education in a subject about which they cared very deeply. Their parents, should they learn of the situation, may resent having paid tuition for a course that is held together by a teaching assistant. No doubt some students or their parents will worry about the possibility of transmission of the virus, despite medical wisdom on this point. The department chair may also feel that the dean failed to support her in her effort to maintain a quality program. The dean, too, is likely to worry about complaints from students and parents. Should this situation turn into a more public issue, the dean must also be prepared to defend her stand to higher levels of administration, alumni, and, potentially, a wider community.[3]

In Case 2, there is probably no way to both permit the safe-sex condom distribution activity and have the more developed writing program. One might hope that the president could convince the donor to drop the condition, but given the religious basis of the objection and the orientation of the church toward issues of sexuality, that is quite unlikely. The president might, alternatively, try to support the writing program from another source, but the pool of donors is not limitless. In any event, this very substantial gift will be lost. There will be some price to pay for permitting the safe-sex program to continue.

A decision to eliminate the safe-sex program would likely be extremely upsetting to the morale of the students who are committed to it. These people have undertaken progressive and socially important work on a voluntary basis with little or no institutional support. Now they would be asked to stop doing it for reasons that have nothing to do with the cost, value, or effectiveness of the program. Some student groups, faculty, and other employees on campus are also sure to see this as, at best, bad health policy and, at worst, callous disregard for purely monetary reasons of a potential risk to student lives. Many others are likely to see the suppression of this activity as an attack on freedom of inquiry. Others may see the acceptance of the gift as a signal that the university wishes to be more closely associated with the conservative wing of its church. This has the potential to provoke divisiveness among members of the university community and alumni. Should the university try to deny that signal and distance itself from that church faction, the decision to accept the gift is likely to appear to be simply cynical. There is also the possibility that the university's action will be seen as a sanctimonious public posturing on the sexual morality of its students or as a pretext to undermine a valuable AIDS prevention effort.

On the other side, a decision to refuse the gift may cause faculty in the writing program to feel that a significant program at the core of the university's mission has been sacrificed. Students who realize that they have been admitted with inadequate skills may also resent the fact that the university passed up the opportunity to help them succeed. There will also surely be those on the faculty who feel that the academic mission of the university is primary and must always take precedence over nonacademic student activities, such as athletics, student clubs and organizations, and health services. It is not that these faculty members would argue that such services are unimportant in life; rather, they would claim that the university is not responsible for supporting them. To this constituency, for the university to forgo a chance to improve its writing program to permit a safe-sex program is to misunderstand its responsibilities and its mission. In their view, each individual should take responsibility for his or her own health care. They would have the students learn about safe sex entirely off campus so that they may learn to write better on campus. The cynics on this side of the fence might also think that the president feared the students and did not wish to risk a confrontation with them.

In Case 3, the vice-president is being called on not to make a judgment of whether discrimination has occurred but rather to aid in the investigatory process. Thus, it may appear that the vice-president need not "take sides" in this dispute. Nevertheless, what is at stake here is whether or not the university will undertake to support the investigation. On this matter, it is not possible for the university to be neutral. The student and his supporters will surely regard neutrality as a covert support for the Food Services Corporation. Indeed, the corporation may read neutrality in the same way. From the corporation's perspective, having the university as a party in the investigation would probably make its defense a more formidable task; it would have to overcome the presumption that the university thought that the charge was justifiable by its entrance into the investigation. Whether the vice-president likes it or not, the student has made the university's participation into an issue of confidence in the disputing parties. There is really no way for the vice-president to express confidence in both sides.

A decision to support the student in the investigation of possible discrimination by the Food Services Corporation will likely be seen by the corporation as a sign that the university suspects it engaged in discrimination. At best, it will feel that the university is trying to "micromanage" an independent contractor. It may feel that the university is pressuring the corporation to hire the student as a way to bury an issue that can only hurt the university if it becomes highly publicized. The corporation might also feel that the university was trying to score moral points with its students at the expense of an independent contractor. It might wonder whether the university would be so quick to support the student if it ran its own food services. Others on campus who did not like the student or who were put off by AIDS activists might feel that the university had allowed itself to be taken advantage of for political purposes.

The decision to support the student would, however, be warmly greeted by the student and by those who feel that persons with AIDS are badly treated in our society. Given the widespread discrimination against persons with AIDS that has been well documented in many contexts, there is at least an initially warranted presumption that discrimination may have occured here. Even if there has been no discrimination in this case, the willingness of the university to investigate the possibility would serve notice on others who might consider discriminating against such persons in the future. Those on campus who favor the vigorous defense of civil liberties would be pleased by the vice-president's decision to support the inquiry.

On the other side, a decision to stay out of the dispute between the student and the corporation is likely to be perceived by some as institutional insensitivity to possible discrimination. Refusal to permit a student to work in food services because that person is an HIV carrier is discriminatory, and the university would be implicated if it permitted a contractor on its premises to engage in such a practice. Even though the Food Services Corporation is an independent contractor, virtually everyone but the university administration (and lawyers) would identify it as part of the university. To most of the world, a decision to remain netural would be perceived as a decision by the university to avoid investigating itself. The university may technically be a third party, but it will be perceived as being a participant rather than a neutral party.

Decision-Making Roles

In each of these cases, no "creative" solution will permit all parties to feel that their concerns have been satisfied. While that may not be true in all instances, a theoretical approach to decision making must address the most difficult cases. Moreover, as we have just observed in working out the possible reception of the decisionmaker's choices, there will be hard feelings in every case. Whatever the outcome, someone is likely to take it personally—and take it badly. Still, the fact that an administrative decision will satisfy some, but not all, of the campus constituency should not be news. This is true of many decisions that administrators make. It is simply not always possible to solve a disputed issue in a way that will satisfy all parties. The job of the administrator, however, is not to satisfy all parties—or even to satisfy as many parties as possible. The job of the administrator is to make the decision that is in the best interest of the institution, whether that decision happens to be agreeable to many, some, or few of the people who are associated with that institution.[4] In the best circumstances, all of the parties will feel that their concerns have been taken into account and that the decision was made on unbiased grounds.

These cases are especially difficult for administrators because it is not always clear what the administrator is supposed to take into account when deciding what is in the best interest of the institution (or when determining what, in fact, the best interest of the institution is). In the cases describe above, many interested parties are bringing multiple concerns to the issue at hand. Some of these concerns may have seemed more relevant than others as we began the initial diagnosis of the disputed ground. In the course of trying to gauge the relevance of these multiple concerns, the administrator must also be aware of his or her personal reaction to persons with AIDS, their supporters, and their detractors. It would be a misuse of institutional authority to let those reactions drive the policy decisions that must be made. What is needed, then, is a framework from which we can evaluate the relevance of the various concerns and considerations.

The problems that arise in decision making around the AIDS-related cases we have been exploring are characteristic of the more general problems of making legitimate decisions that are binding on a group of individuals with conflicting interests. These problems are complicated in the first place because groups can have many members with a wide range of interests, some of which clash, and some of which do not. The more heterogeneous the group, the more difficult to determine the extent of clashes and conflicts. The problem of reconciling conflicting interests among members of a group is, however, further complicated by the fact that each individual has not one interest, but several, depending on the various roles and offices the individual occupies in society. Jean Jacques Rousseau was particularly attuned to this dimension of decision making.[5] Indeed, Rousseau saw in the reconciliation of conflicting interests *within* individuals the solution to the problem of reconciling conflicting interests *among* individuals.

In the arena of politics, Rousseau attributed to each person a "double capacity" of private individual and public citizen. Rather than attempting to reconcile all of a person's differing private individual interests, he argued that each individual possesses a "general will," or an interest sufficiently generalized that, at that most abstract level, the interest of any one citizen is identical with the interest of all of the others. Thus, one need only determine one's own general will to determine what is in the best interest of the group.[6] Rousseau illustrates this point by describing this overlaying of interests as a multiplicity of "wills" within the magistrate or legislator:

> In the person of the magistrate we can distinguish three essentially different wills: first, the private will of the individual, tending only to his personal advantage; secondly, the common will of magistrates, which is relative solely to the advantage of the prince, and may be called corporate will, being general in relation to the government, and particular in relation to the State, of which the government forms a part; and in the third place, the will of the people or the sovereign will, which is general both in relation to

the State regarded as the whole, and to the government regarded as part of the whole.[7]

If we can sidestep the very difficult problem of trying to determine what Rousseau meant by "will," the thrust of his point about individual interests, or (as he says) "advantages," is quite helpful here.[8]

An individual, in our case a university administrator, who occupies a complex social position will have overlapping (and sometimes conflicting) interests. These interests can range from the purely personal (individual), to the familial (spouse, parent, sibling), to the professional (dean), to the political (Democrat), and so on. These interests can be differentiated and identified in terms of the *perspective* from which the interest is assessed, the *benefit* of the outcome to the individual, and the *scope of information* that may be taken into account in coming to determine one's advantage. To illustrate, a dean of a college may have a personal interest in the resolution of an issue: for example, she may benefit personally from a decision to raise administrative salaries. That interest is distinguishable from, but compatible with, her interest in keeping the university competitive in attracting competent, high-quality personnel. At another level, that same dean may also have decanal interest that is sometimes different from her personal interest. For example, it may be in the dean's (professional) interest that all promotion recommendations arise from the faculty even though this dean (a member of the sociology department) will be personally thwarted by colleagues who refuse to initiate a recommendation in her case. As an administrator of the university, the dean may have yet another level of interest that differs from her interest as dean. The university, for example, might benefit from the creation of an additional college. As a member of the university community, the dean, as administrator, will share in the advantage that comes to the university as a result of this expansion—even if the growth results in the decrease in the number of faculty in the dean's own college (to the disadvantage of the dean as dean). At an even more rarefied level of generality, the person/dean/administrator is also what Rousseau calls a "citizen," That is, a member of society with the most general interests of society at heart. The dean as citizen may have an interest in the expansion of educational opportunities to the broadest segments of society even while the dean as administrator/dean/sociologist/person has grave concerns about the institutional capacity to prepare that wider class of students who are admitted to her college.

What is clear from all this is that our multiple interests (or advantages) may be compatible or in conflict in a variety of combinations. In the best of situations, my interest as dean will be the same as my interest as citizen, as administrator, as person, and so on. More commonly, however, will be cases in which one or more of these interests is out of sync with the others. What remains unclear is how we are to recognize conflicts within our own set of interests and resolve them. Rousseau observed that our wills are hierarchical from the most particular to the most general. The best social decisions—the only decisions he recognized as having legitimacy—are those that are guided by the general or sovereign will. Despite this, Rousseau thought that the decisions people most commonly make are those guided by the most particular level of personal interest. In short, people tend to decide and to act "in an order exactly the reverse of what the social system requires."[9]

The challenge of approaching administrative decision making along these lines is that the administrator must find ways to sort through and prioritize the multiple interests he or she brings to the work. This is particularly important in dealing with AIDS-related matters, since personal feelings tend to be strong and institutional policies tend to be inadequate to cover the difficult cases. If we are to begin identifying and prioritizing our interests, we need to find ways to more carefully differentiate them according to our various roles. As I noted earlier, we can characterize these interests in terms of the perspective from which we view our situation, in terms of the benefits that accrue to us in our respective roles, and in terms of the scope of information we are entitled to take into account when acting in a role capacity. Let me amplify each of these points.

For each role or position that one occupies, one has a somewhat different vantage point from which to view one's circumstances. For example, at the personal level, I see the world from the vantage point of the totality of my undifferentiated interests. That is, in developing my intentions, I make no effort to see the world through the restricted eyes of my work, my family responsibilities, my social associations, or any other segmented part of my life. I do not try to put myself into one of my roles or into another's position. I treat myself as a whole person, standing in my own shoes. This is, in a sense, the baseline of who I am. It is arguably my "authentic" self. To the extent that I take what may happen to others into account, it is because what happens to them may affect me. To the extent that I take my role positions into account, it is because what happens to me as, say, a father affects me as a person. My perspective as a person is unrestricted and unfiltered, and is not externally structured. When I move to the level of considering my interests as the occupier of a role, I view the world from a narrower perspective, for example, that of the office of the dean. As a dean, one views policies and decisions for their impact on the dean's office and the ability of the dean to carry out his or her responsibilities and plans. Presumably, whoever is dean should be able to adopt the dean's perspective—no matter how different that perspective might be from one's personal perspective.[10]

One might also approach one's interests from a more general perspective. The dean is also a university administrator, and she may view a problem or issue from a perspective that takes the university's advantage into account without specifically considering the advantage to the dean (or dean's office). From the most general perspective, that of human being or citizen of the world, one would presumably see an issue from the point of view of humanity—without qualification. At this level, if Rousseau's perception is correct, the advantage of each is identical to the advantage of every other.

Benefit, the second dimension of interest, assesses and evaluates the outcome of a decision. In the context of our current discussion, we are looking at the benefits of a decision or action for a single individual. Benefit, like perspective, may be calculated in relation to a role, and the benefits of a decision to an individual may differ when considered from the perspective of the individual's differing roles. Thus, even for a single individual, multiple benefits must be taken into account. At the personal level, taking everything into account, we may say that in the end, or "on balance," an action or decision benefits an individual (or not). Once we differentiate roles, however, we face the issue of conflicting benefit within a single individual. As we noted earlier, the dean (as member of the sociology department) might benefit from a decision to leave promotion decisions in departmental hands, even though the dean (personally) may fail to be promoted.

Finally, to fully differentiate levels of advantage or interest, it is useful to characterize them by what they may take into account in their calculation of benefit. With regard to one's personal interest, all of one's knowledge is relevant to the determination of one's action or decision in a given situation. When I am trying to decide what to do as a person, I can, and should, take into account my beliefs, values, wants, interests, feelings, and so on. I may (and should) also take into account any general knowledge I have about how others are likely to react should my decision be put into effect. All of the general knowledge I have about the impact of possible policies and decisions on others, on society, on nature and the environment, and on future generations is also relevant, with the understanding that this knowledge is to be filtered through my perspective and viewed in terms of my own advantage.

To arrive at a decision from a more general role perspective, I must sort out my personal beliefs, values, wants, interests, feelings, and so on, from those beliefs and that knowledge that are particularly associated with the role in question. That is, I may take into account only my detailed knowledge of my office, its duties and responsibilities, and its organizational purpose. The process here is like what John Rawls describes as putting oneself behind a "veil of ignorance."[11] The veil is selective—permitting one to have sufficient general knowledge to make a decision without having the personal knowledge that would risk a self-interested decision. In making a decision as dean, I may take into account knowledge of my job, how best to do it, and how to further the effectiveness of the office within the organization, all of which are relevant to determining my advantage (as dean). In this exercise, I need to know how individuals participate in the organization, but I should not take into account the personal (nonorganizational) circumstances of their lives. Again, any general knowledge I have about how people will react to organizational decisions and policies is relevant, as is any general knowledge I have about the impact of decisions on the human and natural world.

To arrive at the most general institutional perspective, I must take into account the goals, purposes, and mission of the organization in which I play a role. I must (again) set aside my personal beliefs, values, and so on; the personal beliefs and values of others in the organization; and the interests of the various organizational offices. I must also set aside the information that would help me determine my advantage from my perspective as dean. At this more general level, my more differentiated role interest, like my personal interest, should be subservient. I must treat the organization as if it were an undifferentiated whole. I should know, and take into account, the organization's goals and purposes. I should set aside any particular knowledge I have of the personal circumstances of the membership. My general knowledge about the way in which organizations function in the world and have an impact on it remains relevant.

At the most general level, which Rousseau set at the level of citizenship, or which we might take to the even more abstract level of humanity, only the most general information about people and the world may be taken into account. At this level, akin to Rawls's original position, the interest of the individual and the interests of all other individuals are presumably congruent.[12] At the most general level, none of us has a perspective that differs from any other, has a special or differentiated advantage, or is permitted to take into consideration knowledge of the special circumstances of oneself or others. This most general level need not be driven to the level of humanity in all cases. For the purposes of decision making, it need be only the most abstract level at which all members of a group share a common purpose. In the case of a university, that may be the institutional level for some issues. For other issues, the members of the university share a common purpose with a wider society, and the necessary level of generality must go beyond the university walls.

Through the mechanism of articulating the perspective, benefit, and relevant information for each of my roles, I can differentiate my interests and determine which are compatible and which are not. This differentiation of interests, however, is only half the battle. The issue that looms behind it is the prioritizing of interests. When an individual's several interests are in conflict, which is to take precedence? Rousseau's answer to this question is that the most general interest should take precedence, despite his belief that this would rarely be the case. I suggest that the answer to this question is slightly more complex. When one is trying to make a decision or take action, it is important to first identify one's personal interest, the interest that is represented by the perspective of the role to which the decision is assigned, and the most general interest one has in common with the others who are affected by the decision. The perspective of the "decision-making role" becomes the starting point for decision making. If one's interest from that perspective is in conflict with one's interest at a more general level, the decision should accommodate the more general perspective if one wishes to maintain group cohesion. If one's interest from that perspective is in conflict with one's personal interest, one's personal interest must accommodate that interest for the same reason. In short, *one must act from one's role*, unless that role conflicts with more general institutional or societal goals. Furthermore, acting from one's role may encompass acting from one's personal interest if there is no conflict. If there is, either a compatible soluton must be found, one's personal interest must give way, or one should resign from the decision-making position.

Resolving Issues from the Decision-Making Role

Let us now return to the three AIDS-related cases that require campus policy. How would an administrator approach these cases from the method of decision making I have just outlined?

In Case 1, the dean must identify, then set aside, her own personal feelings about persons with AIDS—whether those feelings are grounded in compassion, loathing, or something in between. She must also identify, then set aside, considerations of personal convenience—the matter of whether one or another decision will create fewer distasteful ramifications. These matters may be reconsidered only after the dean has determined her interest strictly from the perspective of the dean. If a decision from that perspective can be crafted to avoid personally distasteful ramifications, so much the better. If not, the dean must "bite the bullet." The question of her future effectiveness as an administrator, an issue for her standing in her role, is relevant but, as Rousseau notes, must also play a subordinate role. That is, as long as the dean's future effectiveness is in the interest of the university (the next relevant higher level of generality of perspective), the dean may take it into account as a priority. Another element of this situation, the chairperson's personal discomfort, if any, about having to deal with this situation should not be taken into account directly. It is of indirect relevance to the extent that general information about any chair's comfort in attending to certain tasks may be taken into account at the dean's or university's level of interest. The chairperson's effectiveness in implementing the departmental curriculum is, likewise, important to take into account in a subordinate way (as above). With respect to each administrator who has a role to play in this case, the dean must be concerned with the ability of that administrator to do his or her job. The dean's decision must be clear, must be an acceptable precedent for the future, and must not run afoul of broad institutional constraints such as federal or state regulations.[13]

What of the faculty member with AIDS? His courage and persistence are admirable, even heroic, but should the dean take this into account? The issue for the dean must be: Are heroic efforts on the part of health-impaired faculty sufficiently educational to overcome the educational burdens that faculty member is imposing on the students? Because this is a question of institutional policy, the answer to this question cannot consider the character or personality of this particular person with AIDS, other than the general information that the person wishes to continue teaching as long as possible, and it must not presume that this will be an isolated case. The dean must, however, be satisfied that the faculty member is capable of actually teaching (and not merely attending) the class.

With respect to the students and their parents, the dean must, similarly, set aside consideration of their feelings of loyalty, disappointment, admiration, or fear. The question to answer must be the dean's-level question: Can students learn effectively in this context?

This is, I would emphasize, a question about what is possible, not about how well particular students will or will not succeed. What the students are to learn in this setting must also be part of the decision. There is, of course, the necessity that they be able to learn the content of the curriculum that is to be taught in the instructor's courses. The dean should also take into account the value of learning from impaired persons and of learning that teaching can take diverse forms. This must all be balanced against the presumed reduced effectiveness of a disrupted and discontinuous learning context.

Once the dean has considered this issue from the perspective of the dean's role, taking into account and determining compatibility with what is to the advantage of the institution and considering only general information, she should be ready to articulate a finding in this case and, by implication, a policy for the university. One hopes that the finding would be indisputable. In theory, anyone who reasoned this case from a perspective compatible with the interest of the institution would see the compatibility with the dean's decision. Unfortunately, as any student of Rousseau knows, divining the common interest is subject to human interpretation and, consequently, human error. Our knowledge of learning theory and human psychology are, after all, far less than perfect. Nevertheless, I would hazard the judgment that the dean should permit the faculty member to continue teaching, suitably supported with assistants. This judgment is grounded in my general belief that students have much to learn from the commitment of their instructors to their discipline and from their instructors' love of teaching and learning—as they are manifest in the extraordinary effort of a person with AIDS to continue to teach.

How is the president to approach Case 2? In the first instance, the president will need to identify, then set aside, his personal feelings about the potential donor, whether they be affection and friendship, admiration of or contempt for the donor's religious convictions, anger about the condition for the gift, or whatever. The president should also try to identify, then set aside, his own speculations about the personal consequences of his decision, whichever decision he finally makes. It is worth engaging in this speculation to clarify his individual interest and the magnitude of its importance to him, but once contemplated this information should be isolated and not taken into account. The personal feelings of others who will be affected by this decision are also not relevant in the process of discerning the presidential and the institutional interests he must promote in this case. Thus, the feelings of the donor, of the students engaged in the condom distribution program, of the writing program faculty, and of others in the campus community should also be acknowledged but set aside.

The president does need to be mindful of the consequences of his decision on the office of the president. The president's "corporate will" should attend to the costs and benefits of accepting or refusing the gifts for the presidency. Will turning down this gift make it more difficult to raise money from donors in the future? Will accepting the gift mark the presidency as corrupted? Will a public battle with the student organization over this issue harm the credibility of the president's office? These considerations are, to Rousseauu's mind, important but subordinate to a more general level of consideration even though they do achieve a higher level of generality than do personal considerations.

To determine the interest of the institution, the president needs to think about the research, teaching, and service functions of the university, and also of its church affiliation. There is some case to be made that accepting the gift would improve the university's teaching function. It would certainly improve teaching in the writing program. However, an overall assessment of improvement needs to take place in the context of evaluating the damage that would be wrought by the same act. Suppressing the safe-sex condom distribution program would have a cost in terms of health education and AIDS prevention. But more to the point, the act of censoring health education for financial gain is a deep and serious assault on the university's teaching and service missions. My point here is not that universities ought to sponsor or foster safe-sex programs—these programs may, in fact, be of lower priority than writing programs. Moreover, such programs, once created, may be eliminated for a variety of reasons. For example, they may be ineffective or less important to the university's purposes than other programs competing for the same resources. The problem here is that the university would be compromising the integrity of its societal function by participating in a kind of intellectual dishonesty that can only cast doubt on its willingness to promote and defend the advancement and dissemination of knowledge.

The church affiliation of the university complicates the president's decision considerably. The president may personally agree with the views of the potential donor, but he would have already set this consideration aside. At the institutional level, however, the presidency may be an office that speaks for the values of the church as well as for the values of education. It may be the president's duty, as president, to take a stand on condom distribution as an approach to AIDS prevention. At any rate, this may be so if the church took a firm position in accord with that of the potential donor and tolerated no deviance from that view. However, that is not true in this case; the issue is a matter of contentious discussion within the church. As long as that is true, the president remains on the hook. Indeed, given the church's need for resolution on its orientation toward persons with AIDS, it is probably the responsibility of church-affiliated universities (as curators, discoverers, and disseminators of knowledge) to promote consideration of the issue.

It is the suppression of what the university accepted as a responsible program that casts doubt on its ability to pursue its mission at a high intellectual standard should the president accept the gift and suppress the student organization's program. It is the role of the university to be fearless and incorruptible in the pursuit and transmission of knowledge. The president must hold up this highest institutional value, despite the cost of the donation.

In Case 3, similar patterns of reasoning should prevail. The vice-president should ignore her personal distaste for (or, alternately, admiration of) the student who is pressing for support. Similarly, cordiality with the head of the Food Services Corporation should be set to one side. Likewise, the preponderance of opinion on campus should not figure into the vice-president's decision. As before, the vice-president must acknowledge the interest she has to protect and develop her office, but this interest must also be subordinate. What is relevant here is discrimination law, federal and state policy, and the university's legal obligations as a contractor of services. Within that framework, the university must not take a position that would hinder a just outcome in the investigation that will follow. The institutional role of the vice-president is to keep the procedure moving along so that a determination of discrimination is not lost for delay or despondency on the student's part. The university must rise above tactics to become a partisan of inquiry. The vice-president must help the student keep the investigation on course without joining the student in bringing a charge.

Setting the Person Aside

I readily acknowledge that it would be possible for others to arrive at different decisions or policies in these cases while professing to follow the process of identifying and subordinating lower levels of interest. This is partly because the general knowledge that we bring to bear on these cases is imperfect and incomplete. It is partly because the missions of universities are not entirely precise and are certainly not uniform. It is also partly because setting aside our personal and role interests is not a simple matter. Nevertheless, we have, I think, improved our clarity about what should, and what should not, be relevant in making a decision about each of these cases. There may be more to be said in each of these cases, but the field of the dispute is circumscribed.

This approach to administrative decision making, particularly with respect to AIDS-related issues, runs counter to many people's perceptions that more sympathy, not less, is required of administrators. If we could rely on closer individual relationships between persons with AIDS and administrators to produce concern and understanding, this might be so. Unfortunately, there is no particular reason to believe that those who react negatively to persons with AIDS will not continue to do so on closer proximity. Even if some administrators should become more sympathetic to those with AIDS, surely others will not. It is those administrators particularly who need another way to sort out their personal from their official reactions to the kinds of cases I have sketched here.

Those administrators who are strongly sympathetic toward persons with AIDS must also be watchful that the use of their offices to benefit those persons does not engender resentment in others. With virtually every decision they make, university administrators direct resources toward some individuals and away from others. Because others perceive the stakes to be significant, the administrator's actions are generally carefully scrutinized for fairness. Thus, however much an administrator may wish to act from personal feeling, the need for accountability will ultimately require defensible reasons for administrative action.

None of this is to say that the administrator should be unfeeling about persons with AIDS. As I have noted, the requirement is that one's personal interest be subordinate to one's "decision role" and institutional interests. If they are compatible, so much the better. If not, the administrator may wish to identify that fact for others. There is nothing wrong with the president in Case 2 saying to the potential donor: "If it were my personal decision, I would go along with your request, but the university does not belong to me, and its needs conflict with our desires. You should know that I find my own decision personally unsettling." To the extent that administrators can educate their constituents on this distinction, they will pave the way for better acceptance of their difficult decisions in the long run.

Finally, one may feel that this approach to dealing with issues raised by AIDS on campus has, in the end, a much broader application than specifically with AIDS. I am content with this consequence of my analysis. Part of the difficulty, in my view, associated with developing AIDS-related policy is that reaction to persons with AIDS is overly visceral. We would do well to abstract somewhat and see persons with AIDS in terms of broader categories of health impairment and disability. This is not to deny their particular agony or to slight the pressing nature of their plight. Rather, it is to say that we must show our personal affection and sympathy at a personal level and accept AIDS sufferers as social equals—with general wills of their own—at the institutional level.

Notes

1. I am not saying that it is impossible or inconceivable that the buffering strategy will work, but only that it is likely to be regarded as second best to a solution that puts a fully capable instructor in the classroom. In any event, the dean cannot be sure that the buffering solution will provide a comparable educational experience for the students and should make her decision on the assumption that things will not work out perfectly.

2. The lawyers, of course, will not be entirely pleased. They will be concerned that the faculty member might bring a discrimination charge against the university. In that case, the burden of proof would be on the university to demonstrate that for any classroom teacher with any debilitating illness known in advance to the employer, the university would require the instructor to take a disability leave.

3. The dean will probably have these worries about making either decision. In a situation in which not all can be satisfied, some party is likely to complain or protest. Therefore, the dean's worries on this score should balance out.

4. The point here is that administrators are not poll takers. There are, of course, moral and social constraints on the decisions administrators may make. I am not arguing that the administrator is merely an institutional "good soldier" who may act without consideration of the moral or social value of the university's interests.

5. Jean Jacques Rousseau, *The Social Contract* (Buffalo, N.Y.: Prometheus Books, 1988).

6. While this citizen self-knowledge might be acquired through solitary exploration, it is, perhaps, more effectively accomplished through debate and discussion with other citizens.

7. Rousseau, *Social Contract*, p. 65.

8. My intention here is to develop a model of administrative decision making based on Rousseau's insights. It is not my intention to defend this model as historically correct interpretation of Rousseau.

9. Rousseau, *Social Contract*, p. 65. If Rousseau is correct about the relative dominance of the personal interests of individuals over their role interests, an institution would do well to hire individuals whose personal beliefs, values, and interests are as similar as possible to the institution's mission. Then, even when the administrator was acting from his or her personal advantage, the interests of the institution would more likely be served. This would be a kind of backup system to ensure against the prospective failure of administrators to act from their role responsibilities.

10. See Joseph Martin, *To Rise Above Principle: The Memoirs of an Unreconstructed Dean* (Urbana, Ill.: University of Illinois Press, 1988), esp. p. 81. The dean's capacity to adopt the dean's perspective when it differs radically from the dean's individual perspective is a good measure of his or her insight into the requirements of the job. In practice, it is all too likely, in such cases, that the dean will follow his or her individual advantage.

11. John Rawls, *A Theory of Justice* (Cambridge, Mass.: Harvard University Press, 1971), pp. 136–142. The process of determining the general will is like the process of determining the principles of justice from the original position in *A Theory of Justice*. The common point is that both processes ask the decision maker to arrive at a principle or policy taking account only of information available from behind a "veil of ignorance" of one's and the other's personal circumstances.

12. Rawls imposes a more severe veil of ignorance than I have imagined here. He is asking us to think about fundamental principles at the most basic level and, therefore, requires that only the most general knowledge be taken into account.

13. AIDS is classified as a disability and is protected by federal laws and executive orders regarding disabled persons.

7

What Would a Virtuous Counselor Do? Ethical Problems in Counseling Clients with HIV

Elliot D. Cohen

As the AIDS pandemic continues to escalate, counselors are increasingly confronting ethically hard cases involving clients who have HIV.[1] This chapter addresses some of these cases.

First, three paradigmatic cases involving HIV-seropositive clients are presented. Second, a conceptual analysis of a virtuous counselor is developed, to be used as a basis for addressing these cases. The analysis proceeds first by examining "fiduciary" and "autonomy" models of counseling ethics. These models are, in turn, used as bases for developing a final model, a "human welfare" model. This last model is then applied to the cases at hand for purposes of answering the practical question of how a virtuous counselor would respond to the specific ethical exigencies raised by each of the three cases.

Case 1: Peter, age thirty-two, was in therapy with Dr. T. for purposes of working through a depression. Peter's profile included a history of depression and an attempted suicide. After three months of therapy, Peter, who was very resistant to the therapeutic process, reluctantly revealed to Dr. T. that he was HIV-positive (which he said was probably the result of having had intercourse with prostitutes). He told Dr. T. that he had attempted suicide after finding out about his positive HIV status. Moreover, Dr. T. was aware that Peter was regularly having (vaginal) sexual intercourse with his fiancee, Donna, without using any means of protection. When Dr. T. asked if Donna knew about his HIV status, Peter responded that he could not bring himself to tell her because she would then surely leave him.

Case 2: Jason, age twenty-five, was in therapy with Dr. C. due to problems of coping stemming from the fact that he was in the early stages of AIDS. Among other problems, Jason was experiencing rejection by close relatives and friends, who disassociated themselves from him when they found out that he had AIDS. In the course of therapy, however, Jason revealed to Dr. C. that he was engaging in sexual activities with multiple, anonymous sex partners—routinely "picking up" women at singles bars and having unprotected oral, anal, and genital sex with many of them. When Dr. C. advised Jason to cease his promiscuous, high-risk sexual activities and to wear a condom, Jason agreed to do so. Two months later, however, he admitted that his sexual practices had not changed and that he still did not wear a condom.

Case 3: John and Sue, husband and wife of one year, were seeing Dr. B. for marital problems, which seemed to be getting progressively worse as time went on. In the course of therapy, in an individual session in which Sue was not present, John revealed to Dr. B. that he was regularly having oral and anal sex with other men (John usually being the recipient in both kinds of sex) without using any means of protection. Unbeknown to Sue, several evenings each week he would "pick up" other men at gay bars and have sex with them. John also told Dr. B. that he found these sexual encounters much more gratifying than any heterosexual experience he had ever had. However, Dr. B. was aware that John was also having (vaginal) sexual intercourse with Sue, and that the two did not use any means of protection. Nevertheless, when Dr. B. advised John to get tested for HIV, John refused, saying that he was "better off not knowing." Moreover, he was unwilling to inform Sue of his sexual activities for fear that she would leave him "just as his first wife did when she found out."

Each of these cases raises a problem of professional ethics for the counselor in question. The ethical problem in each case concerns the obligations of the counselor, *as* counselor, to the client or clients and to the respective third party or parties, given certain information acquired in the course of therapy—such as the client's HIV status, sexual activities, sex partners, and so on.

From a practical, moral standpoint, the question is what the counselors in each case should do. One approach to answering this practical moral question, the approach taken here, is to ask what a (morally) *virtuous* counselor would do in each case.

The Concept of Virtue

In defining "virtue" I am, generally speaking, following Aristotle, who recognized three components to virtue: "In the first place, he [the virtuous person] must have knowledge, secondly, he must choose the acts, and choose them for their own sake, and thirdly his actions must proceed from a firm and unchangeable character."[2] Since virtue involves knowledge and choice, the virtuous person is not to be viewed as a mere robot who exhibits certain conditioned responses to particular stimuli. Rather, the virtuous person is a rational agent. To say this, however, is not to say that the virtuous person lacks emotion. Indeed, according to Aristotle, the virtuous person is one whose passions are rationally in order—feeling anger, compassion, and the other emotions in the appropriate situations and in the correct proportions.[3]

Moreover, the virtuous person, in the Aristotelian sense, does not simply occasionally do morally correct things but rather is disposed to do so—his or her actions "[proceeding] from a firm and unchangeable character." On this understanding, such dispositions of character are not inborn traits but rather "come about as a result of habit," that is, by repeatedly doing virtuous deeds.[4]

Finally, the virtuous person acts according to principles of ethics that he or she has internalized. For example, honest people think that they ought to be honest and choose to do so for its own sake.

According to Aristotle, "the function of man is an activity of soul which follows or implies a rational principle," and a state of character is a virtue insofar as it is a fulfillment of this rational human nature.[5] For example, courage can be counted as a virtue since it involves a rational response to fear.

However, Aristotle's "rational teleology," which includes his view of human nature, will not be utilized in this discussion. For purposes of articulating a counseling ethics, more specialized "teleologies" (standards of virtues selection) are needed, that is, ones that concern the function of a counselor. Three such models of virtues selection are examined: (1) the fiduciary model (the counselor as a professional who is worthy of clients' trust); (2) the autonomy model (the counselor as a facilitator of clients' autonomy); and (3) the human welfare model (the counselor as a helping professional). The third model incorporates the first two and offers a more comprehensive and credible model of counseling ethics.

The Fiduciary Model of Virtues Selection

According to the fiduciary model, a state of character (disposition to act, think, and feel in certain ways under certain conditions) is a virtue in a counseling ethic when a counselor must have that state of character to be worthy of her clients' trust (that is, so that the counselor can be reasonably relied on to use her professional knowledge and abilities in a manner promotive of her clients' interests).

A general version of the fiduciary model has been discussed by Michael Bayles.[6] While Bayles did not intend this model to apply exclusively to counseling ethics—but to professional ethics in general—what he says can be applied, *mutatis mutandis*, to counseling ethics.

According to Bayles, the fiduciary model itself is justified insofar as "the weaker party [the client] depends upon the stronger [the professional] in ways in which the other does not and so must *trust* the stronger party."[7] In the case of counseling, clients may be especially vulnerable to the unethical counselor. Frequently, clients come to counselors because they have dependency issues to work through. Unethical counselors can use their position of power to exploit this dependency for self-serving purposes.[8] Therefore, a counseling ethic that takes trustworthiness as its central criterion of virtues selection will include those virtues likely to militate against exploitation of such client weakness.

Bayles maintains that at least six virtues can be justified on the standard of trustworthiness. They are honesty, candor, competence, diligence, loyalty, and discretion.[9] A professional—in particular, a counselor—who did not exemplify each of these virtues would, therefore, on the Baylesian analysis, not be worthy of clients' trust.[10] Each of these virtues is briefly discussed here in the context of counseling ethics.

Honesty

The connection between honesty and trustworthiness is an analytic one since "by definition, a dishonest professional is not worthy of a client's trust."[11] An example of professional dishonesty in counseling would be extending the duration of therapy beyond what the therapist knows would be beneficial to the client, for the purpose of continuing to receive payment for the unneeded services. A virtuous counselor, on the Baylesian understanding, would be disposed against such a practice since it would require modes of thinking and acting that are inconsistent with honesty and, therefore, with the professional–client trust.

In addressing honesty, however, Bayles notes that the sense of honesty he is considering amounts to "an obligation to the client" and "does not directly require honesty towards others." He notes that "professionals can be honest with their clients, and in acting in their behalf be dishonest with others."[12] While Bayles does suggest that professionals who act dishonestly toward others are more likely to do the same to their clients,[13] the standard of client trust that undergirds Bayles's professional virtues does not *require* a professional's honest treatment of nonclients. Therefore, on Bayles's standard, there can be virtuous counselors who are dishonest in their treatment of nonclients.

While it has been argued that professional virtue is consistent with the disregard for the welfare of nonclients (for example, Charles Curtis has claimed that good lawyers must learn to treat everybody but their clients as "barbarians and enemies"),[14] the moral position taken in this chapter is that persons who are not clients can also have legitimate (moral) claims on professionals. As will be argued, in cases such as those outlined above, consideration for the interests of third parties may sometimes provide instances of such claims. If a counseling ethic is to clearly recognize these third-party claims, then a further criterion of virtues selection, in addition to promoting clients' trust in their counselors, must be introduced.[15]

Candor

According to Bayles, the virtue of candor requires "full disclosure" and not merely truthfulness, whch may be consistent with the withholding of relevant information.[16] What constitutes full disclosure will, however, be a function of what a client would *reasonably* want to know.[17]

There is also an important conceptual link between the concepts of professional candor and clients' informed consent, since a professional who withholds relevant information from a client (perhaps to influence the client's judgment) thereby deprives the client of the opportunity to give informed consent.[18] For example, in counseling, a client would be entitled to information about the modality of therapy being used, since this information could reasonably be expected to influence the decision of the client to remain in therapy. A virtuous counselor, on the Baylesian analysis, would thus be disposed to provide to clients information consistent with their informed consent. Otherwise, the counselor would not be worthy of the client's trust.

There are, however, some situations under which a virtuous counselor would, arguably, be justified in at least temporarily withholding relevant information from a client. For example, if a client with a history of attempted suicide is experiencing suicidal ideation at a given juncture, the counselor might reasonably decide, out of consideration for the client's welfare, to withhold certain material information from the client—for instance, the results of a psychological evaluation that the counselor believes would adversely affect the client's psychological state.

It is questionable, however, that exceptions to candor like this one are essential to preserving clients' trust in their counselors, since counselors who do not make such exceptions but instead maintain an unconditional policy of candor might arguably merit greater client trust. But a policy of unconditional candor would inevitably run into conflicts with other morally relevant considerations, for instance, the welfare of the client (as in the above case).

The disclosure of the results of a psychological evaluation to a suicidal client, who is likely to be further disturbed by those test results, might serve the client's *interest*—in knowing what the diagnosis is—without also serving the client's *welfare*. Since the fiduciary relationship is one in which clients can trust counselors to further client interests, this relationship does not, ipso facto, safeguard client welfare. A further standard outside the fiduciary model of counseling ethics, one that addresses client welfare (such as that to be developed later in this chapter, under "The Human Welfare Model of Virtues Selection"), would therefore be required to do this job.

Competence

Since an incompetent counselor is not trustworthy, this attribute must be included within the fiduciary counseling ethic. According to Bayles, however, competence is "not a moral virtue."[19]

In any event, the notion of competence in counseling is logically tied to a further state of character, which *is* a moral virtue, namely, benevolence. By the latter is meant a state of being "disposed to do good for others when reasonably situated, and to do no harm," this concern for the well-being of others being "for its own sake." Moreover, benevolent persons are "disposed toward *feeling* certain ways under certain conditions," such as experiencing sorrow at another's misfortune or pleasure in helping another.[20]

To benefit another, one must first have the requisite knowledge and understanding. For instance, a benevolent counselor must know what type of therapy is likely to fit the specific needs of individual clients, for instance, that one client, a very yound child, is a good candidate for play therapy while another, older, client would be more likely to benefit form cognitive-behavior therapy. Moreover, because benevolent counselors want to benefit their clients not harm them, they will tend to carefully look for the relevant facts, grounding their probability assessments of alternative hypotheses on these facts, before choosing their modus operandi.

Accordingly, since the disposition to help another assumes the knowledge and ability to do so, a benevolent counselor would also need to be a competent counselor. Conversely, on at least one theory of counselor competence (the Rogerian approach, to be discussed in the next section of this chapter), a competent counselor would also need to be a benevolent one. This is because counselors' own feelings and motives may themselves figure as major causal factors in helping clients get better.

If competence *does* require benevolence, then, since trustworthiness requires competence, it follows that trustworthiness requires benevolence. In other words, it follows that benevolence must be included within the fiduciary counseling ethic. In that case, however, according to the fiduciary model the benevolence in question need only extend to clients—since it is clients' trust and not that of others that is relevant on that model. A broader concept of benevolence, which includes the benefit of third parties within its scope, would therefore need to be justified on further grounds.

Diligence

Since nondiligent counselors would not be worthy of clients' trust, diligence must also be included within the fiduciary counseling ethic.[21] Diligent counselors are ones who maintain adequate records, return client calls on a timely basis, maintain an answering service or at least an answering machine, keep appointments, do not cut short clients' session time to accommodate other clients, do not make clients wait excessive amounts of time to get appointments, and so on. Counselors who are not disposed to handle such matters expeditiously would, indeed, fall short of being worthy of their clients' trust.

Loyalty

Loyal counselors are ones who are disposed to respect, and work to advance, the interests of their clients. According to Bayles, such loyalty requires the professional to exercise "independence of judgment," that is, unbiased judgment on the client's behalf.[22]

One way in which a counselor can lose independence of judgment is when she allows her personal dislike for the client, or her disapproval of something the client is doing (or has done), to adversely affect the quality of therapy. For example, a counselor may find it hard to counsel a child molester due to her own negative feelings toward the offender.

Another manner in which a counselor can lose independence of judgment is when she gets personally or emotionally involved with the client to the extent that she becomes incapable of making objective discernments. One example of this is the counselor who develops a "dual-role relation" with a client, for instance, becomes a sex partner.[23] Another is the counselor who engages in countertransference with the client, thereby using therapy to work through her own problems.[24]

A loyal counselor is one who is disposed to avoid such breaches of loyalty. Indeed, a counselor who was not so disposed would not be worthy of clients' trust. Moreover, a virtuous counselor who, on a particular occasion, knew that she could not maintain independence of judgment would so inform her client and, if in the interest of the client, would make a referral to another (virtuous) counselor. Indeed, such remedial action is what one would expect from a candid and loyal counselor.

Discretion

The discrete professional respects the privacy of the client through nondisclosure of information about the client. Bayles uses the term "discretion" to include information that is a matter of public record as well as that which is, strictly speaking, confidential (learned from the client in the course of therapy).[25] Thus, on this broad use, the discrete counselor would be disposed not to speak openly to others about what has transpired in a court proceeding in which one of his clients was a litigant, even though such information was a matter of public record. In this chapter, the term "discretion" will be employed in a manner compatible with this broad sense, although the central issues will focus on information that a counselor learns from a client in the course of therapy.

This chapter is also concerned with the *ethical* status of confidentiality in counseling and not with its current legal status. Thus, in some states, communications between counselor and client are protected by statute as "privileged communication." The concern here is not with whether a counselor would be guity of violating such a statute through disclosure of confidential information but rather with the ethics of doing so. It is worth noting, however, that a satisfactory understanding of the ethical questions surrounding confidentiality can lead to a more enlightened treatment of the legal questions.

Since counselors who are not discrete (in the explained sense) are not worthy of their clients' trust, discretion must be included among the virtues of a counselor under the fiduciary criterion of virtues selection.

Nevertheless, there are situations in which even discrete, virtuous counselors may, arguably, be disposed to breach such confidentiality, for example, to save the life of a third party.[26] Since, however, such a (nonconsensual) breach of confidentiality is not essential to making the counselor worthy of the client's trust, the disclosure could not be warranted under the fiduciary conception. Again, a further selection criterion would be needed to do this job.

According to Standard B.4 of the American Counseling Association's (formerly, American Association for Counseling and Development) Ethical Standards (1988), "when the client's condition indicates that there is clear and imminent danger to the client or others, the member must take reasonable personal action or inform responsible authorities." Assuming that such exception to confidentiality is warranted and will be exercised, the fiduciary standard would then require counselors to inform clients of this exception to confidentiality at an early juncture in the course of therapy. Otherwise the counselor would not have afforded the client informed consent to the material conditions of therapy and would therefore not have been candid with the client.

The Autonomy Model of Virtues Selection

While the fiduciary model is justified because counselors must be trusted not to exploit client dependency, a more positive ethical mission of counseling is to help foster greater independence and autonomy in clients.[27] The latter mission, however, is not included within the purview of the fiduciary model. A further autonomy model of virtues selection, which takes this autonomy- and independence-enhancing mission of counseling as a primary standard, would therefore remedy a significant shortcoming of the fiduciary model.

According to the autonomy model, a state of character is a virtue in a counseling ethic when a counselor must have that state of character to effectively facilitate (that is, serve as a catalyst for) the self-actualization of clients as independent, autonomous persons.

A version of this standard of virtues selection is implicit in the "person-centered" approach to psychotherapy, which has been developed by Carl Rogers.[28] (The term "implicit" is used here because Rogers was primarily concerned with constructing a therapy, not a counseling ethic, although the two appear to coalesce in the emerging theory.)

According to Rogers, "therapy is not a matter of doing something *to* the individual, or inducing him to do something about himself. It is instead a matter of freeing him for normal growth and development, of removing obstacles so that he can again move forward."[29] On this view, those in need of therapy have been in some manner deprived of certain requisite conditions of normal psychological growth and have consequently had their natural growth potential thwarted. The job of therapy is thus to introduce, or reintroduce, those conditions into the client's life and thereby "to free the client to become an independent, self-directing person."[30]

Furthermore, Rogers holds that "the individual has within himself vast resources for self-understanding, for altering his self-concept, his attitudes, and his self-directed behavior—and that these resources can be tapped if only a definable climate of facilitative psychological attitudes can be provided."[31] From the Rogerian standpoint, this "definable climate of facilitative psychological attitudes" is completely definable in terms of three counselor attitudes: (1) congruence, (2) unconditional positive regard, and (3) empathetic understanding. According to Rogers, these conditions are both necessary and sufficient for client growth and development. Moreover, they apply to constructive change within all personal relations, not just client–counselor ones—for instance, parent and child, leader and group, teacher and student.[32]

What follows is a brief discussion of each of the three Rogerian attitudes as they are viewed as counselor virtues within an autonomy-driven ethic of counseling.

Congruence

According to Rogers, the more congruent the therapist is—that is, the more genuine she is, permitting herself to be "herself in the relationship, putting up no professional front or personal facade"[33]—the more likely it is that the client will also realize a similar freedom. Such openness or transparency about oneself means that the congruent counselor will be disposed to express her beliefs, feelings, and attitudes rather than to hide them from the client. She is thus prepared to "own" her own thoughts and feelings, to take responsibility for them. Consequently, she provides an impetus for clients to take similar responsibility for theirs.

This does not mean, however, that counselors must be congruent in an absolute sense. "Congruence exists on a continuum rather than on an all-or-nothing basis."[34] For example, counselors do not have to disclose *everything* about themselves to clients, for not all self-disclosures are even relevant to clients' situations. Similarly, some information may be confidential and therefore should not be disclosed. In the latter case, it may be enough simply to say that the information in question is confidential. There are therefore some rational limits to the extent of counselors' congruence.

Given that counselors' congruence, in the sense just discussed, is a necessary condition for facilitating patients' autonomy, it must be included within an autonomy-driven counseling ethic. The virtuous counselor must then be congruent. Moreover, this virtue would appear to go beyond a client-restricted sort of genuineness. The virtuous counselor, on this model, would need to have acquired a disposition toward genuineness with others if she is to be genuine with clients. Otherwise, such client-restricted genuineness would be itself a sort of professional posture that is not congruent with the counselor's private self. The congruent counselor must therefore be disposed to present herself as the person she is, both inside and outside of therapy.

Unconditional Positive Regard

On the Rogerian model, a second condition of constructive client change (toward greater independence and autonomy) is satisfied when counselors are disposed toward having unconditional positive regard for their clients as persons. This is an attitude of deep, genuine caring for the client, which does not depend on what the client thinks, feels, or does. "It is not an attitude of 'I'll accept you when . . .'; rather, it is one of "I'll accept you as you are.'"[35] It is an attitude that "resembles the love that a parent sometimes feels toward an infant."[36] This does not mean that counselors must always share their clients' perspectives or that counselors must always approve of what their clients say or do. It does mean that counselors will continue to care deeply for their clients regardless of what their clients think, feel, or do, and it means that counselors will communicate the same to their clients. Thereby, clients encounter a therapeutic environment in which they are free to be whatever they are without thereby jeopardizing their counselors' regard for them as persons.

Although counselors who have an attitude of unconditional positive regard for their clients may evaluate their clients' behavior, these counselors will be disposed against evaluating their clients as persons. Thus, such counselors may sometimes communicate negative moral evaluations of clients' behavior to clients—for instance, "What you are doing is, in my estimation, morally wrong because you are, through your conduct, destroying the life of another human being." However, counselors who have unconditional positive regard for their clients will be disposed against condemning *them*—for instance, "Because you have harmed another, *you* are a bad person." The former sort of evaluation (that which sticks to an assessment of client behavior) is consistent with a caring attitude toward clients; the latter sort (that which degrades clients as persons) is not.[37]

Empathy

According to Rogers, the third facilitative condition of constructive client change is satisfied when counselors are disposed toward experiencing empathetic understanding of clients' subjective worlds. Such a counselor "senses accurately the feelings and personal meanings that are being experienced by the client and communciates this understanding to the client." In so doing, the empathetic counselor "assists the client in gaining a clearer understanding of, and hence a greater control over, her own world and her own behavior."[38]

While empathy involves a sense of personal identification with the client's subjective world, counselors must be careful not to overidentify with the client's feelings; that is, they must not lose a sense of their own identity and separateness. Otherwise, counselors may be unable to help clients clarify and understand their own subjectivity— for example, as when a counselor allows his own negative feelings toward his wife to interfere with the client's working through of similar feelings. Since, according to Rogers, clients' self-understanding promotes greater control over their own world and behavior, counselors who overidentify with clients' subjective worlds (thereby failing to facilitate clients' self-understanding) are apt to thwart client autonomy. If so, then an autonomy-driven counseling ethic would justify the cultivation of a type of empathy that does not absorb counselor identity but instead enables the counselor to "sense the client's private world as if it were [the counselor's] own, but without ever losing the 'as if' quality."[39]

The Human Welfare Model of Virtues Selection

According to the human welfare standard, a state of character is a virtue in a counseling ethic when counselors, as such, must possess that state of character for them to maximize human welfare.

The Concept of Human Welfare

Human welfare is here interpreted to include (but is not necessarily restricted to) the human goods of survival, pleasure, and the absence of pain and frustration. This hedonistic interpretation makes sense in the context of therapy since the usual reasons that clients are in therapy (for instance, the alleviation of anxiety, depression, stress, guilt, inability to cope, dysfunctional relations, etc.) involve relief from pain and frustration and the establishment of more pleasurable modes of living and relating.

On the model in question, counselor trustworthiness and the promotion of clients' autonomy are to be valued, not for their own sake, but because they are instrumental to the promotion of client welfare in the described sense. First, when counselors are trustworthy, clients are more likely to disclose information of a personal nature. When such disclosure occurs, the likelihood that clients will work through their problems is significantly increased. Therefore, counselor trustworthiness is justified on grounds of client welfare, and the virtues that are justified on a fiduciary model—namely, honesty, candor, competence, benevolence, diligence, loyalty, and discretion—are also, *ceteris paribus*, justified on a human welfare model.

Second, clients who become more independent and autonomous are more likely to experience greater pleasure and less frustration than those who lack self-direction. Therefore, the virtues that are justified on an autonomy model—namely, congruence, unconditional positive regard, and empathy—are also justified, *certeris paribus*, on a human welfare model.

Some Comparative Advantages of a Human Welfare Model

As suggested in the discussion of the fiduciary model, while the fiduciary standard is of considerable value as a criterion of virtues selection in counseling ethics, it does not provide a sufficient standard. In particular, this standard does not, per se, warrant counselors' intrinsic regard for the welfare (not just the interests) of both clients and nonclients. A human welfare model of counseling ethics, which takes the production of human welfare to be the primary standard of virtues selection, remedies this shortcoming.

This does not mean that the human welfare model dissolves the special responsibilities that the counselor has to the client. It does, however, avoid the naive assumption that the term "client" can be adequately defined and understood apart from a broad social and professional context. Thus, Gerald Corey states:

> In recent years there has been an increased interest in developing ethical standards and an increased awareness of the responsibility of counselors and psychologists to alleviate human suffering. . . .
> The therapist has a responsibility primarily to the client. But, because the client does not live in a vacuum and is affected by other relationships, the therapist has a responsibility also to the client's family members, to the therapist's own agency, to a referring agency, to society, and to the profession.[40]

While recognizing important counseling virtues, the autonomy model also has significant shortcomings. First, it does not offer any method for resolving conflicts between competing virtues. For instance, how should a counselor proceed when congruence requires disclosure of confidential information, or when congruence, unconditional positive regard, and empathy are not sufficient to prevent harm to the client or others? There are morally justified limits and exceptions to these autonomy-driven virtues, but the autonomy model does not itself provide any way of determining them. A standard of human welfare, however, addresses this shortcoming.

Second, although a proper understanding of the virtues countenanced by the autonomy model would require that these virtues be "universalized" to nonclients (for instance, proper congruence would demand being congruent both inside and outside of therapy), the autonomy model does not explicitly recognize that. The practical danger of this is that the therapist who subscribes to the autonomy model may nevertheless fail to recognize the ethical imperative for considering the welfare of nonclients. It is one thing to act morally and another to understand just why one's act is moral. A human welfare standard as a basis of counseling ethics provides such an explicit standard of recognition.

Third, a human welfare standard provides a sort of "common denominator" from which both fiduciary and autonomy virtues can be derived. In so doing, it systematizes the ethics of counseling and offers a much more comprehensive model of ethics.

Finally, and relatedly, the autonomy model does not include all virtues relevant to the ethical practice of psychotherapy. For example, it does not clearly address the importance of being diligent or of being discrete. On the other hand, a welfare standard does clearly sanction such morally significant dispositions.

Respect for Human Worth and Dignity

The human welfare model requires counselors' respect for human worth and dignity. Indeed, the virtuous counselor must be disposed to treat clients as well as nonclients as "ends in themselves," not as "mere means." That is, counselors must be disposed against manipulation and deceit if they are to maximize human welfare. Counselors who do not respect the dignity of clients cannot facilitate the development of client autonomy, nor can they be worthy of their clients' trust. Consequently, they cannot promote their clients' welfare.[41]

Moreover, counselors who are disposed toward treating nonclients as mere means, say, to advancing clients' interests, cannot promote the welfare of nonclients either. Nor can such manipulative treatment of nonclients appear to be compatible with such essentially universalizable virtues as congruence. (It would not be possible to be congruent *only* with clients since such client-restricted genuineness would render counselors' private selves incongruent with their professional selves.)

Resolving Ethical Conflicts

On the present model, virtuous counselors may sometimes be pulled in opposite directions at once. For instance, on the one hand, they are disposed toward being discrete with client information. On the other, they are disposed toward honest and kind dealings with nonclients. In situations where honesty with a third party demands disclosure of confidential information, a virtuous counselor may be disposed to move in two opposing directions. While no formula is offered here for the resolution of such dilemmas, a virtuous counselor will attempt to go as far as possible in *both* opposing directions with as little sacrifice of the integrity of each as is possible under the circumstances. For example, this may mean taking care not to release any more information than is necessary and to make such disclosure only to appropriate third parties. Here there is no wholesale departure from virtue. The goal is to stay on course, to reconcile as much as can be reconciled, with the understanding, however, that a "perfect" solution is not an option. Without exercise of such discretion, the probability of causing unnecessary pain or injury is increased.

On the human welfare model, a virtuous counselor must therefore be morally autonomous. This means that she must be disposed toward making her own moral decisions, that is, "to come to her own decisions about moral issues on the basis of her own moral principles [and understanding of the situational facts]; and then in turn to *act* upon her considered judgment."[42] A counselor who simply follows the rules of her agency or institution without wrestling with the moral issues, or who takes the legal route just because the law enjoins it is not morally autonomous in the described sense. Such a counselor cannot therefore be morally virtuous because such a counselor is a mere cog, not a moral agent.

This does not mean that morally autonomous counselors will act without regard for institutional rules, codes of ethics, or law; however, they will not mechanically pursue these rules, without appreciating the rationales for applying them, nor will they pursue them without holding open the possibility for exercising discretion when the rules do not clearly apply or are judged to be overridden by further morally relevant considerations such as human welfare.

Concern for the Welfare of Third Parties

It is assumed, on the present model, that counselors will ordinarily maximize human welfare when they strive to promote client welfare. This assumption is in concert with Standard B.1 of the American Counseling Association's Ethical Standards, which states, "The member's primary obligation is to respect the integrity and promote the welfare of the client(s)."

Since the human welfare model is concerned with the welfare of nonclients as well as clients, however, the virtues justified on a fiduciary model must be broadened on the present model to include concern for nonclients. Thus, a virtuous counselor must not only be honest with clients, she must also be honest with others who may never themselves be clients.

Similarly, the benevolence of virtuous counselors will extend to the welfare of nonclients as well as clients. That is, virtuous counselors will be disposed toward having intrinsic concern for the welfare of other human beings, whether or not they are clients. Virtuous counselors will normally be motivated by such concern to try, within reason, to prevent foreseeable, substantial harm to third parties and will feel remorse when such harm does occur.

The human welfare standard does not, however, justify a general disposition of counselors to base their ethical decisions on what will create the greatest happiness. This standard necessarily operates at the meta-level of justifying virtues but does not *necessarily* operate at the level of counselors' ethical decision making. This is because it would be self-defeating, from a human welfare perspective, to recognize such a general disposition. If counselors generally based their ethical decisions on what is conducive to the greatest happiness, they would cease to be worthy of their clients' trust, clients would accordingly be less apt to place such trust in their counselors, and, consequently, the therapeutic process would not effectively promote client welfare.

When keeping the confidences of clients poses a clear and imminent danger to the lives of certain third parties, however, the welfare of those third parties must also figure in the ethical reasoning of a virtuous counselor. Hence, in such a case, there *is* recourse to the primary standard of maximization of human welfare, not merely the welfare of the client.

Yet even here, the virtuous counselor will be disposed toward exercising discretion in the *amount* of information disclosed and *to whom*.[43] It is one thing to disclose only relevant, necessary information to the affected third party and quite another to make wholesale disclosures—to disclose information that need not be disclosed for the purpose of alerting third parties to the danger. It is also one thing to inform a relevant third party and quite another to publicize the information. If counselors are not disposed toward being discrete about the scope of disclosures, even when danger to the welfare of a third party hangs in the balance, clients' welfare will be unnecessarily compromised and, therefore, human welfare will not be maximized.

It has been arugued that, if exceptions to confidentiality are made for the purpose of warning third parties of impending danger, then potentially dangerous individuals who would otherwise seek therapy will be deterred from doing so, or if they do seek therapy, they will not place in their counselors the trust that is requisite for their successful therapy. Consequently, human welfare will be compromised rather than served by making such exceptions to confidentiality.[44]

First, however, such exceptions to confidentiality are, in fact, now generally permitted (by state statutes, legal precedent, and professional codes), and there is still no proof that this allowance has had an overall negative effect on human welfare. In the case of clients who are HIV-seropositive and who are engaging in high-risk sexual activities with uninformed third parties, the claim that many of these individuals will be deterred from seeking or from cooperatively participating in therapy unless they are guaranteed unconditional confidentiality is speculative and requires empirical evidence.[45]

Second, a genuinely warm, caring attitude toward clients, which is a condition of successful therapy, seems to be psychologically incompatible with the willingness to allow third parties to come to harm. Indeed, it may be asking too much of counselors to expect them, on the one hand, to be genuinely warm and caring to their clients while, on the other, to simultaneously intentionally permit serious harm to others.

Third, even if some counselors are capable of so dichotomizing their benevolent dispositions, these counselors would not be congruent role models for their clients.

Finally, counselors who unconditionally keep confidences without ever attempting to rationally balance client welfare against third-party welfare would not function as autonomous moral agents but instead would be more like programmed automatons. This again would not project an adequate role model for clients who themselves lack self-determination.

On the human welfare model, the virtuous counselor would also recognize certain exceptions to the general rule of candor, in particular cases in which making a material disclosure to the client would jeopardize the client's welfare. In addition, while counselors should not lie or misrepresent the truth to third parties (since this is what is entailed by being honest with them), a counselors' disposition toward candor (in the sense of full disclosure) to third parties (who are not also clients) does not appear to be warranted on the human welfare standard. First, virtuous counselors must usually (although not without exception) keep clients' confidences even if the information in question is material to the decision of some third party. Otherwise, clients would be disinclined to make disclosures of personal information to their counselors, which would impair the therapeutic process.

Moreover, it is impractical to expect counselors to regularly seek out third parties, with whom they are not familiar or closely related, to convey *any* information that they believe is in some way relevant to the lives of these individuals. Indeed, this would take valuable time away from counselors' case loads, and it would seem unlikely that such unsolicited information would typically be received with open arms by nonclients.

The Virtuous Counselor and the HIV-Positive Client: Applying the Human Welfare Model to the Cases

In what follows, the human welfare model will be used as a basis for providing ethical analyses of each of the AIDS cases presented in the first part of this chapter. These analyses are not intended to yield absolute answers to the practical problems posed by these cases. Within the ethical framework provided by the human welfare model, however, they will provide reasonable responses to the question of how a virtuous counselor would proceed in addressing those problems.

An Ethical Analysis of Case 1

Assuming that Dr. T. is a virtuous counselor, at an early juncture of therapy (preferably the first session), she will inform Peter of the confidential nature of the client–counselor relationship. Since Peter, like many clients, is resistant to the therapeutic process, such assurance can facilitate Peter's disclosure of very personal information, which in turn may be instrumental to Peter's successfully working through his depression. In the interest of honesty, however, Dr. T. will not misrepresent the bond of confidentiality as being unconditional. Since clear and imminent danger to the client or others is just grounds to breach confidentiality, Dr. T. must *inform* Peter of the same. This can be done by providing him with some *clear* illustrations of when such breaches are justified, for instance, to prevent the client from committing suicide or to prevent the client from killing another human being. (These illustrations *might* include the example of preventing a client from transmitting AIDS to a sexual partner, although, as will be discussed, the ethical warrant for disclosure in such cases is very provisional; consequently, clearer, less contingent examples may be preferable.)

Since Peter has had and continues to have unprotected sexual intercourse with Donna, there are strong probabilities of Donna's contracting HIV in the future, or of her having already contracted it, from Peter. If Donna has not yet contracted the disease, then informing her about the potential danger could encourage her to take adequate precautions, for instance, discontinuing sexual intercourse entirely or using protection such as condoms. If Donna has already contracted the disease, then, by virtue of being informed of such, she will be allowed the option of early detection, monitoring of the disease through periodic medical examinations, medication to prevent AIDS-related complications, increased longevity, and generally greater control over her life. So it is in her best interest to be informed, whether or not she has contracted the disease.

As a virtuous and hence benevolent counselor, Dr. T. will *care* about the plights of Peter and Donna and will try to promote the welfare of both. Dr. T. is aware that, whether or not Donna has contracted the disease at this juncture, it is in her best interest to be informed about Peter's positive HIV status. He is also aware, however, that Peter is presently unwilling to do the informing. Moreover, given Peter's history of depression and attempted suicide, Dr. T. has reason to believe that, if she does the informing herself, and Donna subsequently leaves Peter, then there are the prospects of the client's withdrawal into worse depression, the loss of future rapport with the client, and the possibility of another suicide attempt. Thus, while Dr. T.'s informing Donna of Peter's positive HIV status is likely to promote Donna's welfare, it might also adversely affect Peter's.

While there is no formula for predicting dangerousness, Dr. T., as a competent counselor, can make a reasonable assessment of the prospects of Peter's attempting suicide if Donna leaves him. If these prospects appear to be great, then involuntary commitment may be indicated. Although providing the benefit of possibly saving the client's life, this paternalistic option is likely to run contrary to the interest of the client in not being hospitalized. Moreover, the client is manipulated and treated as a means, albeit to his own survival. For Dr. T., who cares about the autonomy and dignity of her client, this option will be avoided if there are less degrading and restrictive ones available.

Under the circumstances of this case, Dr. T. will be more inclined to try at first to work within the therapeutic process to get Peter to disclose on his own. This option has the advantage of maintaining confidentiality and, therefore, the client's trust. It also places the responsibility in the client's own hands, thereby facilitating client self-determination and independence.

Although Dr. T. does not approve of Peter's initial refusal to inform Donna, she does not attempt to coerce or intimidate him into changing his mind. She abstains from telling him that he is bad; although she *will* openly express her own ethical position that Peter should inform Donna. Despite Dr. T.'s disagreement with what Peter is doing, Dr. T. continues to convey to him an attitude of deep, genuine caring, thereby encouraging him to freely explore his own thoughts and feelings and to be himself. Moreover, Dr. T. attempts to get inside Peter's subjective world, understanding what he must be going through in these difficult times, reflecting back this subjectivity with even greater lucidity than Peter has expressed it, thereby helping this client to reach greater depths of understanding of what and how he is feeling—his fear of dying, of being out of control, of abandonment, his anxiety, his anger. Dr. T. is no phony. She deeply cares and Peter knows it. She is there for him and she understands him. While not necessarily a cure-all, such are some *ethical* conditions that may help to facilitate change toward greater self-directiveness and independence. And such is the hope that Peter will, through the therapeutic process, which includes these conditions, take up on his own the ethical responsibility of informing Donna.

Of course, Dr. T. knows that the risks of Donna's contracting the disease increase as time goes on. Since she is diligent, she will realize the urgency of the matter and will take recourse in a timely fashion. While Dr. T. will try at first to facilitate Peter's self-disclosure, she may reasonably conclude that the only timely disclosure Donna is likely to receive is one from Dr. T. herself. If so, then Dr. T. will let Peter know that she will be informing Donna, for to act without Peter's knowledge would be to act with less than candor, and this would be almost sure to destroy the bond of trust that has been formed in the therapeutic venture. Nor will Dr. T. impart this information to Peter with the implication that herein marks the end of Dr. T.'s genuine concern for Peter's welfare. On the contrary, she will continue to convey unconditional positive regard for Peter, empathizing with him, still being there for him.

In the event that Dr. T. herself informs Donna, she will not then simply turn her back on Donna. Realizing that the bomb that she has dropped is likely to be traumatic, she will offer Donna her counseling services, and if they are declined, she will make a suitable referral. Such would be the actions of a benevolent, virtuous counselor.

An Ethical Analysis of Case 2

In this case, Jason knows that he is subjecting others to a deadly disease. Yet despite this knowledge he continues to do so. Viewed in this light, it is easy to understand how one might feel a sense of moral outrage at this sort of conduct. However, Dr. C., as a virtuous counselor, will not allow her personal disapproval of Jason's conduct to taint the quality of her therapy. She will still be there for Jason, deeply caring for him and putting on no facade, empathizing with him. Jason is experiencing a deep sense of alienation, abandoned by those whom he thought really cared about him, and this at a time when he desperately wants their companionship and support. His subjective world is a painful one to be in. Dr. C. will put herself in these subjective shoes, feeling what he is feeling and understanding his behavior. While uncovering no moral justification in the depths of this subjectivity, Dr. C. will at least appreciate "where Jason is coming from."

However, Dr. C. is also a human being, and her own personal disdain may get in the way of such a display, destroying her authenticity, clouding her independence of judgment, compromising her loyalty to this client. If that happens, then Dr. C. will recognize it, and she will refer Jason to another counselor, one whose loyalty, she has reason to believe, will not similarly falter.

The case of Jason is significantly different from that of Peter. Unlike those in Peter's case, the third-party "victims" in Jason's case are nameless, and Dr. C. does not have a phone number or an address where they can be reached.

It might also be argued, at least by some, that Jason's victims are not victims after all, since they have also accepted the risks of promiscuity. But death for sexual indiscretion is too high of a price to pay, and Dr. C., who cares about other human beings, none of whom are perfect, will feel regret and a sense of tragedy, which she will not rationalize away with the simple brushstroke of a "they deserve it anyway." She will want to do whatever she can reasonably do about this exigency instead of allowing it to persist. But what can she do about it?

As a virtuous counselor, Dr. C. will work diligently to provide Jason with competent, loyal counseling services. First, she will desire to help Jason work through his problems because she has intrinsic regard for Jason's own welfare, but second, she will be aware that her success with Jason can be instrumental in helping Jason relinquish his dangerous sexual activities. In other words, the most efficacious way Dr. C. will have for harmonizing her intrinsic regard for Jason's welfare and for the welfare of those who may be harmed by him is to provide Jason with her best possible counseling services.

Obviously, there is no guarantee that Jason will relinquish his dangerous sexual activities, even with the help of very competent counseling. Jason can continue to pay lip service to the idea of giving up these activities, or he may prematurely discontinue counseling, without accepting a referral.

In cases such as these, Dr. C. may have done all that she can reasonably do. One further possibility, however, would be for Dr. C. to apprise the police of the situation. This would involve a breach of confidentiality that would make *public* information out of very personal, private features of Jason's life, including the fact that he has AIDS. This, in turn, would probably subject Jason to further painful discrimination. Moreover, it would be likely to mark the end of any trusting relationship that Jason would have with a counselor and, therewith, of the likelihood of working through his problems in therapy.

Of course, Dr. C. could merely *threaten* to go to the police if Jason does not cease his dangerous sexual activities. Under these conditions, however, he could cease to be honest with Dr. C. about his sexual activities, thereby also destroying her chances of getting him to alter his sexual conduct.

Reporting Jason to the police assumes that the proper legal machinery is in place to make such an apprisal feasible. First, this option supposes that the state in which Dr. C. practices would regard Jason's alleged sexual misconduct as a criminal offense. Second, since there are no complainants, the police would be required to engage in covert activities to "catch" the alleged perpetrator in the act of fornication. Third, the police would need to have legal grounds for subjecting Jason to an AIDS test or for gaining access to the results of his previous tests.

Virtuous counselors will be disposed against subjecting clients to these privacy intrusions, even if lawful, insofar as they violate human dignity, treating clients as means rather than as ends in themselves. However, virtuous counselors will also be disposed against knowingly permitting harm to third parties when such harm can be avoided.

Dr. C., as a virtuous counselor, will thus be pulled in two opposing directions. In the end, she will assert her own moral autonomy, weighing client welfare against third-party welfare. If after a careful evaluation of the relevant facts and probabilities she believes that human welfare will be maximized through apprising the police of the situation, then that will be the route she will choose.

On the other hand, if she believes that harm to the client resulting from such a disclosure, which is bound to be considerable, would override any likely positive results for third parties, then she will opt for nondisclosure. Either way she decides, however, the decision will be a hard one because there will be a sacrifice of human welfare, and while recognizing that a "perfect" solution cannot realistically be found, she will nevertheless deeply regret any harm to her client or to others that may result from her decision.

An Ethical Analysis of Case 3

One salient difference between the present case and the case of Peter (Case 1) is that the endangered third party in this case (namely, Sue) is also one of the counselor's clients. As a virtuous counselor, Dr. B. will therefore be disposed to treat Sue in the same equitable fashion as he would treat any other client. Thus, not only will Dr. B. be disposed toward making full disclosure of material fact to John; he will also be disposed toward making full disclosure of material fact to Sue. Since Sue's husband's sexual activities are materially relevant to the course of Sue's own therapy, disclosure of such fact to her would seem to be part of her informed consent.

Still, John has trusted and confided in Dr. B., and it is only because of this bond of trust that Dr. B. has learned about John's promiscuous sexual activities with other men. If Dr. B. discloses this information to Sue, then John would probably view the disclosure as a betrayal of his trust, which would probably mean the end of their counseling relationship and, perhaps, the last time John would ever accept any counseling. Since Dr. B. cares about John, he will not want to lose him as a client.

On the other hand, he also cares about Sue, whom he believes is presently being placed at high risk of contracting AIDS.[46] Moreover, if Dr. B. is to be honest with Sue, then he cannot allow her to remain in a state of ignorance about such an urgent matter, at least for very long.

Because Dr. B. is concerned about the welfare of both clients, he will choose the course of action that is most likely to promote the welfare of each as much as is possible under the present circumstances. However, the welfare of each seems best served where Dr. B. helps to facilitate, through the process of therapy, John's self-disclosure of the pertinent facts to Sue.

First, Sue will receive the information she needs to exert significant control over her own life; and therapy will proceed, if she so deems it, with a more realistic picture of her marriage and the warrants for "saving" it. Second, from the perspective of John's own welfare, it is important that John himself accept responsibility for the disclosure. John is a homosexual in a primarily heterosexual society, in which admitting to be a homosexual is typically greeted with discrimination. It is therefore understandable if John tries to hide behind a heterosexual facade. John's marriage is such a facade, but this is surely not congruence, nor is it personal autonomy, that is, the exercise of control over his own life.

The process of therapy can serve John's welfare by facilitating change toward increased powers of self-determination. By exhibiting the quality of congruence in relating to John, Dr. B. will himself be setting up an example for John to emulate, thereby helping John to surrender his own phoniness and to move toward greater personal autonomy. Through Dr. B.'s own experience of unconditional positive regard for John, John will have a model of self-acceptance from which to draw his own positive self-concept. A fuller therapeutic message conveyed will be that "my value as a person exists and does not depend on my sexual preference or on what others might say or think of my homosexuality." The success of therapy will, in this instance, depend on whether or not the client internalizes this message. If he does so internalize it, then the task of confronting Sue will be much easier for John to perform and more likely to occur.[47]

Dr. B. will also place himself in the subjective shoes of John, however, without losing a sense of his own separateness. If Dr. B. is himself a homosexual, he will have worked through any "unfinished business" of his own that might lead him to overidentify with the feelings of anger, alienation, and frustration that can come from trying to cope with one's homosexuality in a society that treats homosexuals as outcasts. If Dr. B. is a heterosexual, he will have worked through any "unfinished business" regarding his own sexuality so that he will not be blocked from empathizing with his homosexual client. Dr. B. will therefore maintain independence of judgment throughout the therapeutic process, unfaltering in his loyalty to John and Sue alike.

Nevertheless, Dr. B. may reasonably conclude that therapy is not serving—and is not likely to serve—to facilitate John's self-disclosure to Sue. Dr. B. will then wrestle with the ethical question of whether or not *he* should make the disclosure or remain silent. On the one hand, there is the possibility that such a disclosure will foreclose any future help that John might reap through therapy—although, unfortunately, the possibility that John will be benefited by therapy may have already grown quite dim. On the other hand, Sue's welfare may be jeopardized if she is not informed. Dr. B. will take account of these harms, along with their respective probabilities, and he will make a decision consistent with what he thinks will create maximum human welfare under these particular circumstances.

If Dr. B. decides to disclose, he will inform John of his intention to do so, thereby also giving John a final opportunity to do it on his own. He will also convey willingness to make the disclosure in John's presence, for instance, in a session in which both clients are present. Moreover, Dr. B. will inform John of exactly what he intends to tell Sue. Therefore, Dr. B. will remain candid with John throughout the process of disclosure.

Dr. B. will also exercise discretion in *what* he discloses. He will restrict the disclosure only to information that is needed to inform Sue of the potential danger. For example, he may say, "John is in a high-risk category for contracting HIV, and it would be in your best interest to discuss this matter further with him." He may not say, "John is a homosexual who has had affairs with other men behind your back and now may well have contracted, and infected you with, HIV." While the former statement respects confidentiality as far as is consistent with the purpose of making the disclosure, the latter statement contains unnecessary breaches of confidentiality. Hence, making no wholesale surrender of either virtue, Dr. B. will try his best to harmonize candor and discretion, being "discretely candid" and "candidly discrete," conceding to each whenever feasible.

Conclusion

While the foregoing case analyses have not been intended to address all of the permutations of counseling exigencies surrounding the counseling of clients who have HIV, they do point to some important ways a virtuous counselor, as defined by a human welfare model (as that model has itself been understood), would respond to some of these exigencies.

One virtue of a virtues perspective of counseling such as the one taken here—as opposed to a rule-based one in which certain rules of ethics for counselors are constructed and defended—is that, while counseling ethics involves rule-governed activities, it also involves emotional and attitudinal elements that go beyond simple adherence to rules. For example, being empathetic, benevolent, and congruent, and experiencing unconditional positive regard are not activities that are done simply by following the rules. Yet as argued here, they are important dimensions of counseling ethics.[48]

A rule-governed treatment of counseling ethics would fail to address this "gut level" of counseling and would therefore risk presenting an oversimplified and artificial view of counseling ethics. In cases involving clients who have HIV, such an externalized perspective is bound to be of lesser value to ethically concerned counselors who must themselves wrestle with these problems from inside the trenches.[49]

Notes

1. In this chapter, the term "counselor" includes a wide variety of mental-health professionals such as mental-health counselors, marriage and family counselors, addictions counselors, psychiatric nurses, clinical social workers, psychologists, and psychotherapists.

2. Aristotle, *Nichomachean Ethics*, bk. 2, ch. 4, 1105a32.

3. Ibid., bk. 2, ch. 6, 1107a1.

4. Ibid., bk. 2, ch. 1, 1103a15.

5. Ibid., bk. 1, ch. 7, 1098a6.

6. Michael D. Bayles, *Professional Ethics*, 2d ed. (Belmont, Calif.: Wadsworth, 1989), chap. 4.

7. Ibid., p. 78.

8. Gerald Corey, Marianne Schneider Corey, and Patrick Callahan, *Issues and Ethics in the Helping Professions*, 3d ed. (Pacific Grove, Calif.: Brooks/Cole, 1988); William H. Van Hoose and Jeffrey A. Kottler, *Ethical and Legal Issues in Counseling and Psychotherapy*, 2d ed. (San Francisco, Calif.: Jossey-Bass, 1987).

9. Bayles also includes the virtue of fairness, by which he primarily intends impartiality. Bayles states, however, that "if a professional provides diligent and loyal service to each client, then each is treated fairly" (*Professional Ethics*, p. 95). Moreover, the issues raised in Bayles's treatment of fairness that are relevant to this chapter are also raised in his treatment of loyalty. Accordingly, a separate discussion of fairness has been omitted from this discussion.

10. Ibid., p. 80.

11. Ibid.

12. Ibid.

13. Ibid.

14. Charles Curtis, "The Ethics of Advocacy," *Stanford Law Review* 4 (1951): 3–23.

15. Bayles himself later recognizes the need for such a development of the fiduciary model. According to Bayles, the later model "states that a professional is not completely directed by the client but offers independent advice

and service. To the extent professionals are free moral agents, they are responsible for effects on third parties and subject to obligations to them" (*Professional Ethics*, p. 112).

16. Ibid., p. 81.

17. See the opinion in *Canterbury v. Spence*, U.S. Court of Appeals, District of Columbia Circuit, May 19, 1972, 464 *Federal Reporter*, 2d Series, 772.

18. Bayles, *Professional Ethics*, p. 81.

19. Ibid., p. 84.

20. Elliot D. Cohen, "Pure Legal Advocates and Moral Agents: Two Concepts of a Lawyer in an Adversary System," *Criminal Justice Ethics* (Winter/ Spring 1985): 40.

21. Bayles, *Professional Ethics*, p. 86.

22. Ibid., p. 90.

23. Karen Strohm Kitchener, "Dual Role Relationships: What Makes Them So Problematic?" *Journal of Counseling and Development* 67 (1988): 217–221.

24. Corey, Corey, and Callahan, *Issues and Ethics*, p. 49.

25. Bayles, *Professional Ethics*, p. 96.

26. See, for instance, the Tarasoff case, in which a client confidentially informed his therapist that he intended to kill a young woman and subsequently carried out his intention. *Tarasoff v. Regents of the University of California*, 131 *California Reporter* 14 (1976).

27. Van Hoose and Kottler, *Ethical and Legal Issues*, p. 7.

28. Carl Rogers, *On Personal Power* (New York: Delacorte Press, 1977).

29. Ibid., p. 6.

30. Ibid., p. 7

31. Ibid.

32. Gerald Corey, *Theory and Practice of Counseling and Psychotherapy*, 3d ed. (Pacific Grove, Calif: Brooks/Cole, 1986), pp. 106–107. The autonomy model of virtues assumes that Rogers's three psychological attitudes are at least *necessary*, even if not sufficient, conditions of helping clients become more independent and self-directing. This view appears to be accepted in some form by many counseling theories. See, for example, ibid., p. 181; Susan Whalen, Joseph DiGiuseppe, and Richard Wessler, *A Practitioner's Guide to Rational-Emotive Therapy* (New York: Oxford University Press, 1980), chap. 2.

33. Rogers, *On Personal Power*, p. 9.

34. Corey, *Theory and Practice*, p. 108.

35. Ibid.

36. Rogers, *On Personal Power*, p. 10.

37. The distinction between evaluating behavior as opposed to evaluating persons or selves is an important aspect of cognitive approaches such as rational-emotive therapy. See, for example, Albert Ellis, "The Philosophical Basis of Rational-Emotive Therapy (RET)," *International Journal of Applied Philosophy* 5, no. 2 (Fall 1990): 37.

38. Rogers, *On Personal Power*, p. 11.

39. Carl Rogers, *On Becoming a Person* (Boston: Houghton Mifflin, 1961), p. 284.

40. Corey, *Theory and Practice* p. 325. See also the Preamble to the National Association of Social Workers Code of Ethics (1980).

41. The human welfare model derives Kantian standards from a utilitarian one. It is not assumed, however, that Kantian standards *require* a utilitarian justification. Moreover, a mixed deontological model of counseling ethics, in which Kantian and utilitarian standards are used jointly as criteria of virtues selection, would also be possible. For a general discussion of Kantian and utilitarian ethics, see the section "AIDS and Professional Ethics" in the Introduction to this book.

42. Cohen, "Pure Legal Advocates," 41.

43. See Elliot D. Cohen, "Confidentiality, Counseling, and Clients Who Have AIDS: Ethical Foundations of a Model Rule," *Journal of Counseling and Development* 68 (January/February 1990): 285.

44. See, for example, the dissenting opinion in *Tarasoff*.

45. Craig D. Kain, "To Breach or Not to Breach: Is That the Question? A Response to Gray and Harding," *Journal of Counseling and Development* 66 (January 1988): 224–225.

46. Dr. B.'s evidence for thinking that Sue is at high risk of contracting AIDS from John does not include a test for HIV. Admittedly, Dr. B. would rationally need to take this fact into account when assessing the probability of harm to Sue. Given John's present high-risk sexual activities, however, Dr. B.'s belief that Sue is at high risk of contracting AIDS from John still appears to be a reasonable one.

47. It is not assumed here that Rogers's person-centered therapy is a sufficient therapeutic basis for such positive change. Here, therapists who do not accept Rogers's approach as a sufficient basis of therapy would also employ other therapeutic techniques, for example, cognitive-behavioral ones.

48. For a rule-based analysis of ethical problems of counseling clients who have AIDS, see Cohen, "Confidentiality, Counseling, and Clients Who Have AIDS."

49. I wish to thank Gale S. Cohen, Licensed Mental Health Counselor, for her helpful comments on earlier drafts of this paper.

8

The Attorney, the Client with HIV, and the Duty to Warn

Martin Gunderson

Attorneys can be of great help to those with HIV infection. They can help with such complicated matters as estate planning and securing medical benefits. They can also help to protect the rights of HIV-infected persons who encounter various forms of discrimination. In states that have made intentionally exposing another person to HIV infection a criminal offense, attorneys may even be called on to defend persons with HIV against criminal prosecution.

Within the context of a discussion of the impact of HIV on the professions, it is worthwhile devoting time to the legal profession because of the way it differs from other professions. As we shall see, the legal profession is unique among professions because it is based on an adversarial relationship between the client and others. While this is most obvious within the context of courtroom litigation, it is also relevant for other forms of legal counseling. A lawyer working out an estate plan for a client, for example, must do so with an eye to those who might want to challenge the plan in the future. Within the context of a discussion of confidentiality in the legal profession, it is worthwhile discussing clients with HIV infection. Clients with HIV infection differ from other clients because of their vulnerability to discrimination and because whether they are subjected to this discrimination depends in part on the lawyer's willingness to preserve attorney–client confidentiality.

Much light can be shed on these features of the relationship between the attorney and the HIV-infected client by looking at the ethical considerations involved in those unusual cases in which the attorney learns that his or her client intends to engage in activities that pose a risk of exposing another person to HIV. When, if ever, should the attorney in such cases warn the person at risk or inform others so as to stop the client from exposing another person to HIV infection? It is worthwhile looking at this issue because it places in sharp focus the conflict between the demands of the adversary system coupled with the vulnerability of the client, on the one hand, and the protection of third parties, on the other hand.

Those who have written on this question have typically argued that attorneys should be permitted to warn third parties of potential exposure and that attorneys should in fact sometimes warn third parties.[1] The literature does not, however, discuss the specific moral reasons that should influence the attorney's decision in a particular case. Nor does the literature discuss how the various competing reasons should be weighed. In particular, the current literature on this question does not take into account the vulnerability of the HIV-infected client. In this chapter I examine these moral factors. I proceed by discussing the role of the attorney within the adversary system and legal considerations regarding the duty to preserve confidentiality and the duty to warn. This background is then applied to a consideration of the factors that ought to inform the decisions made by individual attorneys. As we shall see, it is not possible to formulate a general moral rule regarding confidentiality for HIV-infected clients and the duty to warn because the weight of the various determining factors depends on circumstances that differ in different cases.

The Attorney's Role

Both the law governing attorney–client confidentiality and the moral factors that influence decisions by individual attorneys are responsive to the role attorneys play in our society. This can be made clear by contrasting the role of the attorney with the roles of the physician and psychotherapist.

A major area of difference between attorneys and other professionals such as medical professionals is, of course, their area of expertise. Physicians, in particular, can be expected to have a knowledge of HIV and AIDS that is not shared by the average attorney. In this respect the physician is typically in a better position than the attorney to judge whether a particular behavior is likely to pose a risk of HIV infection to other persons. Determining the extent to which an HIV-infected person poses a threat to others depends on two primary factors: (1) determining the likelihood that a person will behave in a certain way and (2) determining whether that behavior poses a significant risk for others. The attorney may be in as good a position as the physician to determine whether the first factor is met, although a psychotherapist may be in a better position to predict behavior than either the attorney or the physician. The physician, however, is likely to be in a better position than the attorney and possibly the psychotherapist to determine whether the second factor is in play. In short, both the physician and psychotherapist are likely to have knowledge not shared by the attorney, which produces for them a stronger reason to warn third parties at potential risk.

Another factor needs to be taken into account in considering the roles of the attorney and physician. Physicians are subject to mandatory reporting laws that require them to report various communicable diseases and various other conditions such as gunshot wounds.[2] For sexually transmitted diseases, including AIDS and HIV infection, these reports are often followed up by health officials, who attempt to warn others who may have been infected and in turn to discover their contacts. This is relevant because it determines the extent to which the client or patient is likely to rely on the professional to preserve confidences. Since the physician, unlike the attorney, is subject to reporting laws that often result in contact tracing, the patient is much less likely to rely on the physician to keep his or her confidences regarding communicable diseases than is the client of the attorney, who is not subject to such laws.

Perhaps the most obvious difference is that the attorney, unlike the physician or psychotherapist, functions within an adversarial system. The attorney's client is often involved in an adversarial relationship with others, and the attorney has the duty of advocating the client's interests within the adversarial relationship.[3] As a result of this, the attorney, in advocating the interests of the client, will often be involved in situations in which he or she engages in activities that harm others.[4] For example, an attorney may help a client collect a debt, an action that may have the effect of seriously harming the debtor. In treating the medical problem of a patient, physicians and psychotherapists are rarely thereby involved in directly harming the interests of another. Even when an adversarial relationship is not directly present, the lawyer must still work with an eye to adversarial proceedings. The lawyer working out a tax plan or a trust agreement, or drafting a contract remains cognizant of the possibility of a future challenge by an adversary.

As a result of the attorney's role in the adversary system, disclosure of a client's confidence often "frustrates the very objectives of the specific legal consultation."[5] To tell an opposing party the plans of one's client may make it impossible for the client to carry out those plans. Of course, the doctor who warns a third person that he or she may be exposed to a disease from the physician's patient may frustrate the plans of the patient, but the doctor was not hired specifically to help with those plans.

There is also a way in which the advocacy role of the attorney indirectly influences the extent to which the attorney has a duty to warn third parties. Because of this role, people not represented by an attorney do not rely on the attorney to keep them safe from harm. To the contrary, the assumption is that the attorney works solely for the client and is willing to harm others on behalf of the client, though not, of course, to engage in unlawful activity on behalf of the client. In the case of physicians and psychotherapists, however, people close to the patient may rely on the medical professional to help the patient in such a way that they themselves will not be endangered by the patient. Because of this reliance on the part of third parties close to the patient, physicians and psychotherapists may have a reason not shared by the attorney to warn third parties.

As many writers dealing with legal ethics have noted, such an adversarial system cannot function adequately without a rule creating at least a prima facie duty to preserve the confidences and secrets of the client. Attorneys cannot effectively represent their clients if they do not know all of the relevant facts about the matter regarding which they are representing the clients, and clients often do not have the legal knowledge to sort out what is and what is not relevant. Therefore, clients have to be able to trust their attorneys enough to tell them everything conceivably related to the matter at hand without restricting themselves to what they believe is legally relevant. Clients will be willing to do this only if they believe that their secrets will be kept by the attorney.[6] Clients must also be willing to tell attorneys things that would be of use to their adversaries. Clients will be willing to do this only if they know that attorneys will maintain their secrets. If there are good moral reasons for the adversary system, then the attorney has a moral reason to keep the secrets of his or her client.

Legal Considerations

The law governing the attorney–client relationship must be responsive to the needs of the client within an adversary system. This responsiveness is gained by several legal considerations that constrain attorneys from divulging a client's secrets and hence from disclosing a client's HIV status. The various codes of professional conduct adopted by the states are an obvious source of constraint. Most states have adopted a version of the American Bar Association's Model Rules of Professional Conduct. Attorneys who violate the mandatory provisions of these rules may be disciplined. Rule 1.6 states that with two exceptions a lawyer may not reveal information related to the representation of a client.[7] The exception that is relevant here is that a lawyer may reveal information that the lawyer reasonably believes is necessary to prevent a client from committing a criminal act likely to result in imminent death or substantial bodily harm.[8] It is quite clear, on this rule, that a lawyer may not warn persons who have been previously exposed to HIV infection by his or her client even if those exposed are unaware that they have been exposed. For it to be permissible under Rule 1.6 for an attorney to warn a person who may have been exposed by his or her client, two conditions must be met. First, the client must be about to commit an illegal act. In states that have made intentionally exposing another person to HIV a criminal offense, this condition will be met.[9] Even where intentionally exposing another to HIV is not itself a criminal offense, it may constitute a different offense such as reckless endangerment.[10] In most states some such statute exists under which knowingly exposing another person to HIV can be considered a criminal act even if it is not explicitly made illegal. Second, the exposure must be likely to result in imminent death or substantial bodily harm. Exposing another to HIV infection does not cause imminent death. Even in those cases in which it does cause death, the death typically occurs years after the exposure.[11] Exposing a person to HIV may or may not be likely to result in substantial bodily harm, depending on how likely it is that the exposure will result in the transmission of HIV. A single act of oral sex may expose someone to HIV, but it is unlikely that transmission will occur.[12] Even a single act of vaginal intercourse is unlikely to result in transmission.[13] Repeated acts of unprotected sexual intercourse, however, are likely to result in transmission of HIV.[14] In short, an attorney wishing to comply with Rule 1.6 must make a calculation of likelihood of harm on the basis of a variety of factors. In particular, the attorney must know in some detail precisely what sort of behavior the client is likely to engage in and how frequent the behavior will be.

Another constraint on attorneys involves the possibility of a suit under tort law for violation of privacy. Most states allow recovery in tort law for damages that result from the public disclosure of private facts. To establish a claim under this tort the plaintiff must show that the defendant made a public disclosure of private facts and that such a disclosure would be offensive to a reasonable person of ordinary sensibilities.[15] The information must not be part of a public record, and the plaintiff must not have consented to publication by the defendant.[16] Cases split on whether the information must be made public to a large number of people.[17] Certainly the public disclosure that a person has HIV would be the disclosure of a private fact that would be offensive to a reasonable person of ordinary sensibilities. In those jurisdictions that do not require that the information be shared with a large number of people, this tort acts as a constraint on an attorney's sharing his or her client's HIV status with others even for purpose of warning.

Apart from general legal considerations protecting attorney–client confidentiality, some states have laws that specifically protect the confidentiality of persons infected with HIV. These states make it illegal for anyone except a physician or public health authorities to disclose the HIV status of a person without that person's consent.[18] In such states attorneys are simply forbidden from disclosing the HIV status of a client.

The adversary system is not the only value that informs the law, of course. There are also legal considerations that have the effect of encouraging an attorney to warn others he or she believes may be exposed to HIV infection by a client. The most important of these is legal liability under tort law for failure to warn another who may be endangered by one's client. The duty to warn has been most fully developed in medical and psychiatric contexts. Physicians who fail to warn others that they have been exposed to a disease carried by a patient may be liable for damages under negligence law.[19] Psychother-apists also have a duty to warn those who may be endangered by the violent acts of a patient. The classic case is *Tarasoff v. Regents of the University of California*.[20]

There are fewer cases dealing with an attorney's duty to warn those who may be hurt by a client, but cases in some jurisdictions have indicated that attorneys who fail to warn potential victims of crimes their clients intend to commit may be liable to the victims of those crimes. A relatively clear case is *Hawkins v. King County Department of Rehabilitation Services*.[21] *Hawkins* held in part that an attorney has a duty to warn anyone endangered by a crime of the client when (1) the potential victim is unaware that he or she is threatened by the client, (2) the attorney has personal knowledge of the client's intent to commit the crime, and (3) the attorney knows that a specific person is likely to be the victim, not merely that the client is dangerous in general.[22]

In summary the Rules of Professional Conduct provide a narrow area within which the attorney has discretion to warn a person who may be exposed to HIV by his or her client. Within this area, however, the attorney must weigh his or her exposure to liability from suits by the client for violation of privacy against suits by those who may be harmed by the client. Legally, the duty to warn would take precedence, but only if the factors set out in *Hawkins* are clearly met. From a practical point of view the attorney must also calculate the likelihood (usually remote) of a suit by a third party harmed by the client against the likelihood (possibly high) of a suit by the client whose confidentiality was breached.

Weighing Moral Reasons in Particular Cases

Most writers on the duty of attorneys to warn third parties note that the adversary system provides a reason for keeping the confidences of clients. On the other hand, the fact that the third party may be threatened with severe harm by a client provides a reason to warn the person at risk. How these conflicting reasons are to be weighed depends on a variety of subsidiary factors. Consider first the reason for maintaining confidentiality based on the role of the attorney in an adversary system.

Needs of the Adversary System

Whether or not the adversary system is the best possible system, it is the system we have. Thus, from the point of view of an individual attorney involved in the practice of law there is good reason to act so as to enable his or her client to act effectively within the adversary system. Doing so enhances the client's autonomy and the client's ability to seek an advantageous position. Since, as we have seen, the adversary system has as one of its corollaries the principle that confidences ought generally to be kept, the attorney will have a baseline reason for keeping the confidence of all clients, including, of course, HIV-infected clients.

It could be argued that this general rationale applies with less force in the case of HIV-infected persons who intend to expose another to HIV infection in violation of the criminal law. As Bruce Landesman points out, the force of the argument for confidentiality based on the adversary system is considerably weakened regarding the expression of an intention to commit future crimes. The intent to commit future crimes is seldom relevant to anything the attorney needs to know to defend the client regarding legal matters having to do with past and present activities.[23] There are two ways in which one might argue that the intent to commit future crimes may be irrelevant to what the attorney needs to know about a current case so that the attorney can represent a client. First, it might be argued that it is not relevant for the gathering of evidence that the attorney needs to know to represent the client. In the case of the HIV-infected client, however, facts about sexual relations may actually be relevant to the representation of the client. This would be true of an attorney representing an HIV-infected client in the area of family law (e.g., divorce) or estate planning (e.g., drafting a trust with a sexual partner as beneficiary). The problem is that in some states this may amount to disclosure of criminal activity. Hence, the disclosure of the intent to commit future criminal acts may be relevant to the attorney's representation of the HIV-infected client.

Second, it might be argued that the intent to commit future crimes is not relevant because warning the person at risk will typically not interfere with the specific matter in which the attorney is representing the client. This may or may not be true when the client is a person with HIV. An attorney who is helping a client draw up an estate plan may, of course, have to worry about adversarial relationships with those who may oppose the estate plan (e.g., those who are not beneficiaries of the will and government officials who may challenge interpretations of the tax code), but the attorney may have no worry about the disclosure influencing these particular adversarial relationships. In this respect, the attorney is in the same position as the physician. Disclosure may harm the professional relationship by undermining trust, but it does not directly undermine the function the professional is performing. Drawing up an estate plan is the moral equivalent of mending a broken wrist, in spite of the potential for adversarial proceeding regarding a challenge to the estate plan. This is also true for the attorney who is hired by the HIV-infected person to help secure Medicaid or to help with other financial matters.

This is not always true, however. There are situations in which disclosure of a client's HIV status to a third party would directly undermine the nature of the attorney–client relationship. For example, if an attorney is representing a man in a divorce, warning the wife that she may be exposed to HIV by her husband may adversely affect the very interests of the client for which he is seeking representation. This may also be true of the attorney representing an HIV-infected client accused of violating a state law by intentionally exposing another person to HIV. In such cases, whether the attorney can warn the third party without directly undermining his or her representation of the client depends on whether the third party can be warned in a manner that cannot be traced back to the attorney's client.

In general, the role of the attorney in the adversary system gives the attorney a baseline moral reason for not breaching the client's confidentiality. This moral reason is often weak in the case of a client who expresses an intent to commit future crimes. In the case of the

HIV-infected client, however, who expresses the intent to expose another to HIV infection, this general moral reason may or may not be weakened depending on the facts of the particular case.

Promises Made to the Client

The extent to which the attorney is morally obligated to keep the client's secrets also depends in part on whether the attorney promised to keep the client's secrets.[24] If an attorney specifically tells the client that he or she will preserve all of the secrets of the client, then the attorney has at the outset a very strong moral reason for keeping the client's secrets. If, however, the attorney tells the client that he or she will not keep the client's secrets when it is necessary to keep the client from violating a criminal law and posing a significant risk to others, then the attorney does not have this strong reason for preserving the client's secrets, although, as we shall see, there may be other reasons for not divulging the client's secrets.

What if the attorney says nothing, however? Then what matters is whether an implicit promise has been made. If the attorney knows that the client is familiar with the law regarding attorney–client confidentiality, then the attorney can correctly reason that the client is not relying on confidentiality insofar as the Rules of Professional Conduct give the attorney discretion over whether or not to warn a third party. On the other hand, if the attorney does not have reason to believe this, the attorney can reason that the client is probably relying on the attorney to keep his or her secrets. This is because in our culture generally, attorneys are thought to be bound by a strict code of confidentiality. If the attorney knows that the client is relying on his or her confidentiality and the attorney does nothing to dispel that reliance, then in light of the general mores regarding attorney–client confidentiality, the attorney has made an implicit promise to keep the client's confidences.

Unlike the explicit promise that gives the client a clear reason to rely on the attorney, the implicit promise may give the client more or less reason to rely on the attorney depending on how clear the attorney's behavior is and on what the client knows about the law governing attorney–client relations. Because this is a matter of degree, the reason for not divulging the client's confidence can be stronger or weaker depending on the extent of the client's reasonable reliance on the attorney.

In short, the attorney's role in the adversary system and promises made by the attorney typically provide reasons for preserving the confidences of clients and therefore for not warning third parties.

These reasons may be stronger or weaker, however, depending on such things as the degree to which the atttorney's representation of the client will be adversely affected by warning the third party and the extent to which the attorney has implicitly promised the client not to divulge information necessary for warning the third party. There are, however, countervailing reasons to warn those placed at risk by the client. We turn now to reasons for warning a third party placed at risk by an HIV-infected client.

The General Duty to Warn

In general, there is a strong moral reason to warn those who are at risk of serious harm. For those who base their ethics on a form of consequentialism, the duty to warn is a way in which harm can be minimized, since the warning enables the person warned to take steps to avoid the harm. Those who base their ethics on individual autonomy also have a moral reason to warn others. Warning another of harm enables the person warned to decide autonomously what steps to take in light of the danger warned against. It gives the person warned more control over his or her life. The Kantian would argue that we cannot universalize the maxim that one not warn those who are in serious danger when it is inconvenient to do so, because it would involve us in an inconsistency in willing. After all, we ourselves would want to be warned of serious risks that we face. While there is clearly a general moral reason for warning others who are at risk, the reason may be stronger or weaker, and whether it is compelling in an individual case depends on the circumstances of that particular case. This in turn requires balancing a number of factors.

Significance of the Risk to Third Parties

Perhaps the most obvious factor is the significance of the harm risked.[25] Since the whole purpose of warning is to avoid harm, the more significant the harm risked, the stronger the reason to warn. To determine the significance of the harm risked, the person considering warning needs to take into account both the degree of harm risked and the likelihood of the harm occurring. Hence, the greater the harm risked and the more likely the harm is to occur, the greater the moral strength of the reason for warning.

In the case of HIV infection, the degree of harm risked is great—possible death. On the other hand, the degree of risk can vary considerably depending on the type and frequency of behavior. For example, suppose that an attorney has a client who is an HIV-infected physician and that the attorney finds out that her client plans to perform a surgical operation on a patient without informing the patient of his HIV infection. The chances of a physician transmitting HIV infection to a patient from an operation is exceedingly small. There is no reported case of this happening. The only known case of a health-care worker transmitting HIV to a patient through medical treatment is the case of a Florida dentist who probably infected six patients.[26] What risk there is depends on such factors as the physician's overall infection control procedures, the number of times the physician cuts him- or herself in such operations, and the physician's experience in conducting the operation. Also, some surgical operations are more prone to risk than others.[27] On the other hand, if the physician states that he will not tell his wife and plans to continue having unprotected sex, the wife may be in considerable danger.[28] Even then the precise degree of risk depends on the type of sex they have and such physical factors as whether they have genital ulcers or infections.[29]

Knowledge of Risk

In deciding whether to warn someone, the warner also needs to take into account both the degree to which he is certain that there is a risk and the extent to which the person warned is likely to already be aware of the risk.[30] The need to warn persons grows in proportion to knowledge of the risk. As we have seen, the degree of risk depends in part on the physical conditions of the partners in cases of sexual relations, and the attorney is not in a good position to determine the precise degree of risk. This is sometimes true of other behavior as well. As noted, the degree of risk posed by a physician to his patients depends on a variety of factors concerning the physician's technique, factors not likely to be known by the attorney.

The extent to which the person about to be warned is aware of the risk may also vary depending on the situation. A woman in what she thinks is a monogamous marriage may have no idea that she is at risk of HIV infection. On the other hand, a man who picks up a stranger in a gay bar has reason to believe that there is a fair risk that his new partner will be HIV-infected.

The attorney also needs to consider whether the third party is likely to be warned from other sources and hence be aware of the risk. If the attorney's client is seeing a physician, the attorney may be able to rely, depending on the state in which he or she practices, on reporting laws and contact tracing to alert partners such as spouses and long-term lovers. In addition, the physician who does the reporting is likely to be in a far better position to assess the exact risks undergone by various partners of her patient and therefore in a better position to assess whether to warn them.

Likelihood of Success

If one knows that one's warning is not likely to be heeded by the person warned, then there may be little reason to make the warning.[31] The extent to which a warning is likely to be effective depends, in part, on how it is made. If the attorney sends a note saying that the addressee is at risk but does not divulge the client's name, the warning is less likely to be effective than if the attorney states who the client is. The problem is that the most effective forms of warning are likely to be the forms that pose the greatest risk to the attorney and to his or her client.

Responsibility for Risk

If someone is partially responsible for the risk, that person may have a stronger reason to warn than if that person is not responsible for the risk. Typically, the attorney will not be even partially responsible for the risk created by the person with HIV. There are exceptions, however. An attorney who helps a client apply for insurance may be enabling a fraud if the client fails to divulge that he or she has HIV infection.

In sum, the reason for an attorney to warn a third party placed at risk by a client may be stronger or weaker depending on the significance of the risk to the third party, how certain the attorney is of the risk, whether the person at risk is likely to know of the risk, and whether the attorney is in any way responsible for the risk. As has already been noted, these reasons must be balanced against reasons for not warning based on the attorney's role in the adversary system and promises, implicit or explicit, made by the attorney. The reasons for warning the third party must also be balanced, however, against reasons for not warning based on risks to the client and the attorney.

Significance of Risk to Client

In general, as we have seen, when someone poses a risk to another, there is a reason to warn. If, however, the risk to the third party is small and the risk to the person who poses the threat extremely great (e.g., the third party will react by killing the person who threatens her), then the reason in favor of warning the third person may be overridden. Such factors also need to be considered in the case of HIV-infected clients. The risks associated with divulging the client's confidence by warning a third person may be extreme. If the person warned decides to tell others, then the client may be subject to all the discrimination to which HIV-infected persons have too frequently been subjected.

It might be objected that the client forfeits his right to confidentiality when he exposes another to the danger of HIV infection. As we have seen, however, merely exposing another to HIV can create more or less of a risk depending on the type of exposure and the frequency of exposure. There is another factor as well. The third party may or may not have assumed the risk of exposure to HIV infection. Whether the client forfeits his right to confidentiality depends on whether the third party is subjected to an unreasonable risk. Whether the risk is reasonable depends on factors such as those mentioned above.

This risk can be minimized in several ways. First, the attorney should tell the client that she will warn the third person unless the client agrees not to endanger the person. Second, if the attorney does warn the third party, the attorney can withhold the name of the client. Depending on who the others are, however, the third person may be able to infer the identity of the client. Third, the attorney needs to make absolutely certain that the client really does pose a significant danger to an unsuspecting person.

Significance of Risk to Attorney

Any potential risk to the person who warns also needs to be considered. If warning someone places the warner at risk, then the overall reason to warn is weaker. In the case of an attorney, there are several potential dangers in warning others of a client's HIV infection. First, the client may have a potential suit against the attorney for violation of privacy or a malpractice suit for breach of confidentiality. Second, for attorneys who have a practice in which they work with a large number of gay or HIV-infected clients, breaching confidentiality may result in the destruction of the attorney's practice. Third, in those states in which statutes forbid divulging a person's HIV status, the attorney may run the risk of prosecution, fine, and disbarment.

Sometimes there are risks to be run for a failure to warn. The attorney must weigh the risk of whether the third party is likely to bring an action for negligence or malpractice for a failure to warn. How these risks are weighed is a matter of degree. Attorneys may be more or less at risk of being sued depending on the circumstances of the case.

Weighing the Factors

It should be obvious from all of this that there is no obvious or mechanical way in which all of the factors can be weighed against one another. It is not clear, for example, just when the amount of harm to a third party is great enough to merit breaking a promise to a client. Nor is it clear just how much harm to the client should be discounted when it is balanced against harm with which the client threatens others. In addition, the situation is complicated by the fact that most of the factors to be weighed are a matter of degree and are therefore more or less present depending on the individual case. The situation is far from hopeless, however. By considering the sorts of factors noted above, it may become clear that the reasons for warning (and for not warning) are far stronger or weaker than they appeared at first glance. In a particular case, then, it might be quite clear which reasons carry more weight.

Dealing with Clients

From the above discussion, several questions arise concerning how attorneys should deal with particular clients. Some questions concern how active the attorney should be in determining whether the client poses a risk to others. Should the attorney actively attempt to find out whether his or her HIV-infected client poses a risk to others? Several reasons militate against this. Quizzing HIV-infected clients to determine if they pose a risk to others threatens the attorney–client relationship at the outset by exhibiting a lack of trust and respect on the part of the attorney. The HIV-infected client who seeks an attorney's advice in estate planning and is then questioned about whether he or she is endangering others is right to feel insulted and has good reason to be suspicious of the attorney.

It might also be asked whether the attorney should tell the client what the limits of attorney–client confidentiality are at the outset. An advantage of this is that it respects the client's autonomy by telling the client how information he or she provides may be used. A disadvantage is that the attorney may not find out about threats to others. Another disadvantage is that it informs the HIV-infected client that the attorney suspects that there may be reason to suppose that the client does in fact pose a danger to others. These problems can best be avoided by simply making sure that the client is seeing a physician and by not spelling out the limits of confidentiality. On the whole, however, it is better to inform clients generally of the limits to confidentiality in the attorney–client relationship. Given the stress on confidentiality generally within the legal profession and the history of preserving client confidences, not to spell out the limits of confidentiality is to make an implicit promise to the client that all confidences will be kept, or at least to induce reliance on the part of the client. This, as we have seen, creates an additional reason for not divulging confidences even when the client poses a serious threat to others. In addition, it could be argued that informing the client of the ground rules under which he or she is speaking shows respect for the client's autonomy. It allows the client to keep control over information he or she does not want divulged.

The limits of confidentiality should be spelled out as part of a standard procedure that is given to all clients whether or not they are HIV-infected. This is necessary so as to avoid implying that the attorney suspects that his or her HIV-infected clients are especially dangerous. In those cases in which the attorney believes that the client will not freely discuss her legal problems unless the attorney promises unconditional confidentiality, the attorney can modify the original statement and promise greater confidentiality depending on his overall assessment of the risks and benefits.

Once it is decided that someone should be warned, what procedure should be used to warn that person? In some states the attorney may be able to inform the state health department, which will then engage in contact tracing. The attorney might also attempt to anonymously warn someone at risk. The attorney could also reveal his identity but not the identity of the client. Finally, the attorney could reveal the identity of the client. Based on the moral considerations given above, the most plausible answer is that the attorney should warn the person at risk in the manner that is most likely to keep information regarding the identity of the client confidential while still making the warning effective.

Conclusion

The law regarding attorney–client confidentiality leaves an area of discretion in which the attorney is permitted to warn others of a client's intentions if the client intends to violate a criminal law and poses a risk of substantial bodily harm. The literature regarding the HIV-infected client typically argues that there is moral reason to preserve attorney–client confidentiality but that this moral reason may be overridden in the case of an HIV-infected client who poses a risk of exposing others to HIV infection. This chapter deals with the various factors that the attorney should use in determining whether the attorney ought morally to warn another in a specific case. We have seen that the attorney must weigh not only considerations based on her role in the adversary system but also such considerations as promises made to the client, the likelihood of third parties being harmed, the likelihood and degree of harm to the client and the attorney, the degree to which the third party and attorney are aware of the risk, and the likely effectiveness of the warning. There is, then, no simple rule for determining how the attorney ought to act in all cases.

A consideration of these factors is important in determining what overall ethical theory one adopts to account for attorney–client confidentiality. It is clear that if one wishes to adopt a consequentialist approach one must explain how these various factors can all be understood in terms of harms and benefits and how all of these can be weighed against one another. The consequentialist, for example, needs to come up with a way of balancing the weight of an explicit promise to keep confidentiality against the severity of risk to a third person. The deontologist must also account for these factors. He or she must find ways of explaining, for example, how the principle that attorneys ought to keep their client's confidences is to be limited by a principle regarding the prevention of harm. It is still an open question whether any such theory can succeed in finding a principle that can be used to weigh all of these factors against one another. In any case, by looking first at the individual factors that an attorney must consider in dealing with client confidentiality and the risk of harm to others, we are in a better position to begin a consideration of the background ethical theory that accounts for attorney–client confidentiality.

Notes

1. See, for example, the following law review articles: W. James Ellison, "Legal Ethics Condones AIDS Transfer: A Disclosure Dilemma," *Whittier Law Review* 12 (1991): 327–348; Anne L. McBride, "Deadly Confidentiality: AIDS and Rule 1.6(b)," *Georgetown Journal of Legal Ethics* 4 (Fall 1990): 435–458; Nancy J. Moore, "Limits to Attorney–Client Confidentiality: A Philosophically Informed and Comparative Approach to Legal and Medical Ethics," *Case Western Reserve Law Review* 36 (Winter 1986): 177–247; David P. T. Price, "Between Scylla and Charybdis: Charting a Course to Reconcile the Duty of Confidentiality and the Duty to Warn in the AIDs Context," *Dickinson Law Review* 94 (Winter 1990): 435–487.

2. As of April 1992, twenty-four states required confidential reporting by name of HIV-infected persons to local or state health officials. Another eleven states required reporting without a name (Centers for Disease Control, "Public Health Uses of HIV-infection Reports—South Carolina, 1986–1991," *Morbidity and Mortality Weekly Report* 41 [April 17, 1992]): 246.

3. Moore, "Limits to Attorney–Client Confidentiality," 208–209. Moore notes that one of the chief ways in which the role of the attorney differs from the role of the physician or psychotherapist is that the attorney's client is often involved in an adversarial relationship.

4. Ibid., 208 n. 145.

5. Ibid., 108.

6. For a version of this argument, see Monroe Freedman, *Lawyer's Ethics in an Adversary System* (Indianapolis, Ind.: Bobbs-Merrill, 1975), esp. p. 4. See also Michael D. Bayles, *Professional Ethics* (Belmont, Calif.: Wadsworth, 1981), pp. 83–84.

7. American Bar Association, Model Rules of Professional Conduct (Chicago, Ill.: American Bar Association, 1983).

8. Ibid., Rule 1.6(b)(1). This is somewhat more restrictive than the American Bar Association's previous Model Code of Professional Responsibility, which stated that a lawyer may reveal "the intention of his client to commit a crime and the information necessary to prevent the crime" and which made no mention of likelihood of death or substantial bodily harm (Idem, Model Code of Professional Responsibility [American Bar Association, 1981], DR 4-101[C][3]).

9. Idaho and Georgia, for example, have both made it a criminal offense to knowingly expose another person to HIV, although Georgia allows a person who is HIV-infected to have sexual relations with an uninfected partner provided the infected person discloses his or her HIV status. See Idaho Code, sec. 39-601 and Code of Georgia Annotated, sec. 16-5-60.

10. See the Model Penal Code, sec. 211.2, which states in part that "a person commits a misdemeanor if he recklessly engages in conduct which places or may place another person in danger of death or serious bodily injury." For a discussion of how reckless endangerment can be applied to transmission of HIV infection, see Ellison, "Legal Ethics," 335–346.

11. James W. Curran, Harold W. Jaffe, Ann M. Hardy, et al., "Epidemiology of HIV Infection and AIDs in the United States," *Science* 239 (1988): 610–616.

12. Lawrence A. Kinsley, Roger Detels, Richard Kaslow, et al., "Risk Factors for Seroconversion to Human Immunodeficiency Virus Among Male Homosexuals," *Lancet* (February 14, 1987): 345–348; Warren Winkelstein, Jr., David. M. Lyman, Nancy Padian, et al., "Sexual Practice, and Risk of Infection by the Human Immunodeficiency Virus: The San Francisco Men's Health Study," *Journal of the American Medical Association* 257 (January 16, 1987): 321–325.

13. While it is not known precisely what the risk of transmission from a single act of heterosexual vaginal intercourse is, one medical writer estimates the risk of an infected woman transmitting the virus to an uninfected man to be 1 in 2,000, while the risk of an infected man transmitting the virus to an uninfected woman is between 1 in 500 and 1 in 1,000 (George J. Pazin, "HIV Transmission Among Heterosexuals," *Pennsylvania Medicine* 92 [December 1989]: 48–49).

14. If one person in a heterosexual couple is infected with HIV, the chance of the other person becoming infected through sexual intercourse is between 10 and 70 percent (William L. Heyward and James W. Curran, "The Epidemiology of AIDS in the U.S.," *Scientific American* 259 [October 1988], 79). Another study indicated that for women who had over 100 sexual contacts with an HIV-infected male the chance of transmission of HIV was 31 percent (Nancy Padian, Linda Marquis, Donald Francis, et al., "Male-to-Female Transmission of Human Immunodeficiency Virus," *Journal of the American Medical Association* 258 [August 14, 1987]: 788–790).

15. W. Page Keeton, Dan B. Dobbs, Robert E. Keeton, and David G. Owen, *Keeton and Prosser on Torst* (St. Paul, Minn.: West, 1984), pp. 856–857. See also idem, *Restatement of the Law 2d Torts* St. Paul, Minn.: American Law Institute, 1977), sec. 652D.

16. *Cox Broadcasting Corp. v. Cohn*, 420 U.S. 469, 494–495 (1975).

17. Keeton, Dobbs, Keeton, and Owen, *Keeton and Prosser on Torts*, p. 856.

18. California is an example of such a state. See California Health and Safety Code, secs. 199.21 and 199.25.

19. For early cases establishing that physicians have a duty to warn third persons of threats from their patients, see *Skillings v. Swenson*, 143 Minn. 323, 173 N.W. 663 (1919); *Davis v. Rodman*, 147 Ark. 385, 227 S.W. 612 (1921); *Jones v. Stanko*, 118 Ohio St. 147, 160 N.E. 456 (1928).

20. *Tarasoff v. Regents of the University of California*, 17 Cal. 3d 425, 551 P.2d 334, 131 Cal. Rptr. 14 (1976).

21. *Hawkins v. King County Department of Rehabilitation Services*, 24 Wash. App. 338, 602 P.2d 361 (1979).

22. *Hawkins*, 602 P.2d at 365.

23. Bruce M. Landesman, "Confidentiality and the Lawyer–Client Relationship," in *Ethics and the Legal Profession*, ed. Michael Davis and Frederick A. Elliston (Buffalo, N.Y.: Prometheus Books, 1986), pp. 377–379.

24. Landesman claims that in general the prima facie obligation to keep the confidences of others depends in part on the promise (whether explicit or implicit) to keep the information secret and in part on the speaker's need to divulge the information while keeping control of it ("Confidentiality," 372).

25. For a general discussion of the role of harm risked in the duty to warn, see Martin Gunderson, David J. Mayo, and Frank S. Rhame, *AIDS: Testing and Privacy* (Salt Lake City: University of Utah Press, 1989), chap. 7, esp. p. 124.

26. J. J. Witte, "Update: Investigations of Persons Treated by HIV-Infected Health-Care Workers—United States," *Morbidity and Mortality Weekly Report* 42 (May 7, 1993): 329–330.

27. Centers for Disease Control, "Recommendations for Preventing Transmission of Human Immunodeficiency Virus and Hepatitis B Virus to Patients During Exposure-Prone Invasive Procedures," *Morbidity and Mortality Weekly Report* 40, no. RR-8 (July 12, 1991): 3.

28. McBride, "Deadly Confidentiality," 438–439; Padian et al., "Male-to-Female Transmission," 788–790.

29. See Kinsley et al., "Risk Factors," 345–348; D. William Cameron, J. Neil Simonsen, Lourdes J. D'Costa et al., "Female to Male Transmission of Human Immunodeficiency Virus Type 1: Risk Factors for Seroconversion in Men," *Lancet* (August 19, 1989): 405–406.

30. Gunderson, Mayo and Rhame, AIDS, p. 124.

31. Ibid., p. 125.

9

AIDS: A Transformative Challenge for Clergy

Joseph A. Edelheit

> For a true Christian and Jewish ecumenism, . . . we must
> never again do theology in such a way that its construction
> remains unaffected, or could remain unaffected, by Ausch-
> witz.—Johann Baptist Metz[1]

For the last thirty years, significant Christian and Jewish thinkers have
all argued that the unthinkable event of the holocaust has been transformative in shaping the way theology has been done. An event of
unspeakable evil has required religious thinkers to find a new vocabu-
lary and take risks in dialogue that were inconceivable before Auschwitz. It is my contention that just as the challenge presented by Metz,
a noted European Christian theologian, demands a response for those
who profess fundamentalist and systematic theology, a similar challenge now emerges for those who expound practical or pastoral theology because of the HIV/AIDS pandemic. Let me state, without equivo-
cation, that by no means am I equating the realities of the holocaust's
radical evil and mass human extermination with the currently incurable
disease and worldwide pandemic of HIV/AIDS. Rather, for the purpose
of this reflection, I draw attention to the transformative shift the events
of Auschwitz caused for religious thinkers, and in like manner, though
the causal event is fundamentally different, the changes caused by HIV/
AIDS in the way clergy confront several essential issues of pastoral and
practical theology. It is the transformative change that HIV/AIDS demands in the way we think as clergy that corresponds to Metz's
challenge.

As of this writing (the statistics will change dramatically by the
time this is published), more than 180,000 persons in America have
died because of HIV/AIDS, and another 1.5 million persons are infected
with the HIV/AIDS virus. Millions of people worldwide are infected,
and epidemiological projections by the year 2000 stagger the imagina-
tion. But it is not the statistical reality that transforms the clergy;

rather, it is the single human life confronted with HIV/AIDS. In less than a decade clergy have been forced, often against their desire and will, to deal with these lives, and the unyielding demand will continue into the foreseeable future. It is unlikely that any active congregational clergyperson, or hospital clergyperson, will be able to remain disconnected from HIV/AIDS. HIV/AIDS requires immediate changes in the clergyperson's knowledge and behavior, attitude and commitment. All of these components are primarily practical. The overwhelming majority of these active clergy were ordained long before seminaries began to teach courses about HIV/AIDS ministries; courses dealing with this issue have been introduced only within the last five years. Therefore, the transformative nature of the pandemic has taken place among persons who were basically unprepared and lacked any institutional and traditional guidelines or denominational philosophies. It may well be another twenty-five years before we have enough perspective about HIV/AIDS to fully measure the complete impact of this transformative shift among clergy.

With these historical caveats in mind, I hope to sketch the basic characteristics of the change and the future challenge that will lead to further reevaluations in the way clergy deal with HIV/AIDS. Fundamental to this transformation is the conflict between tradition and the complex human realities of HIV/AIDS. The conflict centers on issues of sexuality, drug abuse, homosexuality, and dying and death. Still other conflicts illuminate the clergy's social responsibility, a responsibility extending beyond individual pastoral obligations. Are clergy and their religious institutions responsible for participating in the prevention of HIV/AIDS transmission. Even asking the question creates a conflict for some who do not see their religious calling to be a prophetic response to social justice and social gospel. HIV/AIDS forces clergy to deal with issues of confidentiality in a way unlike anything they may encounter in their careers. It is my position that every significant counseling/pastoral role in which a clergyperson attempts to transmit religious values requires a new sense of purpose or a greater degree of nonjudgmental pastoral support. Helping a person who just found out he or she is HIV-positive may mean doing suicide intervention work or crisis intervention to help the person cope with rejection by a lover or parents, as well as requiring social-service networking to facilitate the full array of backup services now needed to deal with an HIV infection. Just one case, even a relatively simple case, can consume the time and tax the skills of a clergyperson who does not know his or her community's networking regarding HIV/AIDS service providers. Even more dangerous is the clergyperson whose ignorance of HIV/AIDS terms, concepts, and facts can be a source of potential harm or even moral liability. For all these reasons a clergyperson cannot refuse to accept responsibility for knowledge and sensitivity.

Transformations in Clerical Thinking

William E. Amos, Jr., writes about his experience with AIDS and his middle-class white ministry in Florida in his book *When AIDS Comes to the Church.* He stresses the complete lack of preparation clergy have in dealing with the complexities of HIV/AIDS. This awareness of ignorance is the initial step necessary in accepting responsibility, which people in need place on the clergy, especially in an emergency. This ignorance and our inability to recognize it often represent the denial with which we are dealing with HIV/AIDS. If the denial could be limited to our own human frailty, fear, or anger, or even to a phobia, it wouldn't be worth mentioning. But ignorance that is fostered by denial and in turn helps rationalize the denial can endanger a person in grave need who comes to a clergyperson. Such a person might have realized that he or she has been involved in a high-risk behavior and after some episode of "illness" is considering the value of an HIV-antibody blood test. An ignorant clergyperson might refer to the antibody test as an "AIDS test," confusing HIV seropositivity with the diagnosis of AIDS. Most people are aware of the fatal and incurable nature of AIDS. Such a mistake is dangerously irresponsible and might lead to either a refusal to be tested or even an attempted suicide. The very first transformative challenge for clergy, therefore, is facing their own ignorance regarding HIV/AIDS. This pandemic demands literacy because of the danger that can be caused by anything other than complete and confident knowledge. I participated in a series of clerical seminars during the sixteen months in which Illinois required an HIV-antibody premarital blood test.[2] My experience of the reality of the clergy's ignorance and the importance of knowledge has been confirmed again and again in various questions asked by other clergy. Given the contexts in which clergy intersect with events and lives, no one can claim, ten years into the pandemic, "I don't know anything about it." If the discomfort or judgmental religious posture of a clergyperson helps to support his or her ignorance, then minimally such a person must be able to refer someone in need to a known expert who is nonjudgmental.

The second most significant shift comes from the resolution of the conflict between religious traditions' view of sexuality and the reality of lives facing HIV/AIDS. Western biblical tradition is unequivocal in its position on male homosexuality (as stated in Lev. 18:22) as well as on any sexual relations outside of marriage. Hence, clergy must answer for themselves, their own faith-communities, and the person with HIV/AIDS, How will I cope with a scriptural tradition that judges as "sin" one of the primary modes of HIV transmission? If we respond that anyone who is sick requires our pastoral care, sinner or not,[3] then has the stigma of HIV/AIDS biased the clergy's compassion and acceptance of the person with HIV/AIDS? This is not a mere homiletical emphasis; it is more an affirmation of God's wrathful punishment of homosexual behavior. To be truly accepting of a person, regardless of their sexual orientation, the clergy must confront the text, not ignore it. HIV/AIDS is not a gay disease, but a predominant number of persons with HIV/AIDS who want pastoral care are gay; therefore, we cannot ignore the scriptural biases.

Often a family member comes to the clergyperson after a death to attempt a reconciliation that was not realized during life. The historical rejection of gays and lesbians by institutional religion often translates into the presumption that a clergyperson would have been judgmental, even if that clergyperson had been neutral on the topic. The historical position of Judaism and Christianity on homosexuality has created a serious credibility gap in the minds of most persons. Someone who is only casually acquainted with tradition will assume that a clergyperson is forced by doctrine to consider the mode of transmission as a "sin." This presumption prevents many persons with HIV/AIDS and their family and friends from asking for pastoral care.

Rather than risk rejection or judgment, people who both need and want a clergyperson's care will suffer alone and become more embittered about religion's failure to care about them. Several social thinkers have noted that HIV/AIDS has shattered many different kinds of traditional presumptions.[4] Clergy are forced to reread traditional texts in an attempt to find a more inclusive, less harsh interpretation; a reading in which the predisposition of sinner is removed. Persons with HIV/AIDS, their family, and friends must give clergy a chance to change. There is a risk taken by both parties, one that transforms both clergy and persons in need of religious/pastoral care alike.

The key to a clergyperson's change is *people* with HIV/AIDS. This is not the same as the *idea* of people with HIV/AIDS. Charles Gerkin, professor of pastoral theology at Emory University, offers us compelling arguments that we as clergy have a prophetic context for our pastoral theology when we think of human lives as documents. Gerkin offers us a hermeneutical mode for doing pastoral/practical theology and counseling. This model is especially helpful in dealing with HIV/

AIDS. When I wrote about the first person I met with AIDS, it was *his* story, *his* life, that became the goad to my own transformation. Gerkin states, "Each individual living document has an integrity of his or her own that calls for understanding and interpretation, not categorization and stereotyping."[5] Furthermore, Gerkin notes correctly, "Persons coming for pastoral counseling are usually aware of the suffering that comes from their embeddedness and their own history."[6]

Gerkin helps refine the issue. The clergyperson must deal with his or her own prejudgment of sexuality and then accept the fully alive and complex reality, not merely the idea, of the person with HIV/AIDS. Finally, and most important, the clergyperson must accept the suffering with which the person comes asking for help. This suffering means that any additional suffering caused by the clergy through ignorance or judgment is counterproductive and cruel. The second transformation then is the resolution of conflict that stems from the transmission of HIV/AIDS by sexual acts.

The third area of transformation is the systemic integration of HIV/AIDS awareness through a clergyperson's various duties. Once sensitized to the issue of HIV/AIDS through the life of a person having the virus, the clergyperson is changed. He or she must then decide how to share this change with his or her congregation and community, whether through teaching, preaching, or community effort. HIV/AIDS is not a private topic. When a clergyperson is thrust outside into the full scope of needs in the AIDS community, this becomes even more clear. For instance, a person whose grandchild has AIDS comes to a clergyperson and needs help because the landlord has denied the grandchild a new lease—can the clergyperson get housing? Consider the HIV-positive woman who needs help finding health care or a dentist because she has been denied such help at her health maintenance organization. There may be an AIDS sufferer who has no family in the area and requires home-delivered meals or a lawyer who can provide advice about a will. A single mother comes to ask for help because she needs a respite from care. She cannot afford to pay for a babysitter to care for her child with AIDS, and yet she needs the time away to attend a support group for parents and caretakers of persons with AIDS.

These are all examples of real-life requests that come to the clergy. They go far beyond counseling, requiring the clergyperson to get involved in the always-widening circles of social-service needs within the HIV/AIDS community. The reality of these needs within the lives of real people transforms the issues from political and social to fundamental and non-negotiable. The text *AIDS and the Religious Community*, edited by the Reverend Scott Alexander, is an anthology of local projects to provide a religious response to the basic human needs of persons with AIDS. Common to many different kinds of programs is the realization that people come to their churches and synagogues expecting the kind of help that cannot be found elsewhere. For example, "in 1987 it became clear to many concerned citizens in the Baton Rouge area that there was a desperate need for safe and affordable housing for persons living with HIV/AIDS. A vacant house was donated to Our Lady of the Lake."[7] "The Yom Rishon AIDS Food Drive, a project of the Washington Committee of the National Jewish AIDS Project, coordinates the collection of non-perishable food items from synagogues."[8] "Rev. Katrina of Finley realized that the spiritual needs of people with AIDS were unmet once they left the hospital. In 1987 she founded the Interfaith AIDS Ministry of Boston."[9]

These and other examples of public responses to HIV/AIDS are transformative shifts for clergy. The pandemic demands a significant social-service network that public, government, and even private institutions cannot provide entirely; surely they cannot provide the spiritual and pastoral components. Hence, once a clergyperson pierces the veil of initial awareness, he or she must decide where that ministry will lead publicly. Often the church is willing to follow the lead of the clergyperson; still other clergy find like-minded persons in their denomination or movements, regionally or nationally. Those unable to get significant support within their congregations have turned to a regional or even national AIDS committee. A congregation uncomfortable with a sermon on AIDS or even an adult education program on HIV/AIDS because their clergyperson represents *them* may be able to listen to a visiting clergyperson or send people to participate in their denomination's or movement's program on AIDS. All of this affirms the necessary shift to public and communal networking.

Clergy who want people in their congregations to volunteer for multiple events and needs, from office help to youth group chaperons, must realize the extent to which people volunteer because they want to help those with AIDS. "Many AIDS volunteers unexpectedly found themselves able to do the things beyond the realm of prior experience or expertise." The response to AIDS (by volunteers) suggests an increasing trend of citizens taking issues of governance into their own hands through voluntary associations if not direct participation in electoral process."[10] Clergy must confront their own understanding of Robert Bellah's communitarian values as more than a topic for preaching. Every book that gives testimony of how AIDS changes church and synagogue lives underscores the community involvement in the complex needs of persons living with HIV/AIDS. A clergyperson, however, cannot merely raise up those who are supportive. There is also an essential context of prophetic response to discrimination, because the majority of persons with HIV/AIDS—gays, drug abusers, African-Americans, Hispanics (most of whom are poor)—are very vulnerable to various forms of discrimination. Mary Katherine Bateson raises the question of whether AIDS will even change the basic character of human life, triggering religious and social scapegoating, paranoia, and the failure of hope and compassion the way society is actually organized as a social unit. Several volumes raise the issues of ethics and confidentiality, housing, and health-care insurance, to say nothing of the fundamental loss of privacy. Clergy who are true to their calling of caring for those most spurned by society must stand up for people with HIV/AIDS. This is a religious issue that is as essential as any other question of human rights. There is a desperate need for the unequivocal translation of scripture and later religious tradition into the meaning of our society's response to AIDS. We still risk the social rejection of persons, the forced testing of whole communities, and even government isolation of infected persons; thus, clergy must become even more aware of their role as the prophetic conscience of society.

Other Transformations in Clerical Practice

In two very practical areas clergy must deal with radically different issues because of HIV/AIDS. Marital counseling is forever changed because of the sexual means of HIV/AIDS transmission. Whether or not a state requires an HIV premarital blood test (as of this writing none are required anymore), every clergyperson who does premarital counseling cannot ignore HIV/AIDS as a topic. Since we know that exposure to the virus has a possible ten-year period of incubation, and that only one exposure is necessary, any premarital or extramarital sexual act is now a high-risk act. Promiscuity is no longer an issue of quantity. Surely, the statistical possibility of exposure increases exponentially if a person has multiple partners and multiple experiences, but even one experience with one person has the possibility of being high risk. Regardless of the journalistic revisionists who want us to think that heterosexuals are at lower risk than gays and drug abusers, there is still a possibility of exposure, no matter how small, that could result in the transmission of an incurable and fatal disease.

How one raises the issue requires knowledge and a clergyperson's own self-awareness about human sexuality. Should a clergyperson suggest HIV-antibody testing prior to the wedding service if the groom admits in private that his fraternity all "had a prostitute" one night?

Should a clergyperson counsel a recently divorced woman who wants to date for the first time in twenty-five years that she should use a condom if she is not going to be chaste? If clergy require or recommend various blood tests prior to conception for such diseases as Tay–Sachs or sickle cell anemia, then should a couple be tested for HIV antibodies prior to conception? What was once better left unsaid and in the past may now have a critical impact on another person's life. Therefore, should a clergyperson pry into the issues of drug abuse as a context for high-risk exposure? If a clergyperson who has been told in marital counseling that a bisexual husband is having extramarital gay affairs, should the wife be informed? Since HIV/AIDS is so lethal, clergy cannot afford the luxury of ignoring this virus as a critical component in every marital counseling context.

Another area in which very practical changes must occur is funerals. Often the need to maintain secrecy, even "denial," forces the clergyperson into a eulogy of euphemism. The state may require embalming for the deceased, and the family may want cremation, both of which are prohibited in certain traditions. Still other complexities involve the inclusion of the lover or life partner of the person with AIDS and the person's family. Since most religious communities do not recognize the formal life partnership of gays, where does a person's lover of twenty-five years fit into the traditional funeral ritual? Does a person's family have the "religious right" to exclude a lover because of their own denial?

Still another problem is the need for spirituality for those who are grieving, many of whom have previously been rejected by the church or synagogue. I have found it particularly poignant that Jews who have considered themselves "outside" the institutional community crave Jewish tradition, especially during a funeral. Their grief is a mixture of mourning over the dead and their rage and sense of loss over the years of alienation by the religious community. We clergy who officiate at AIDS memorials must be aware that we are ministering to the living, many of whom *we* have rejected and still might. How do we serve people we neither know nor understand and whose lives do not intersect with our congregation? This is a serious problem in the African-American community, where black churches have little influence on the lives of those who are either gay or drug abusers. Yet their families often desperately need the church so that they can face death and grieving. Clergy who deal with the deaths of persons with AIDS and the needs of those who grieve for them know after just one AIDS funeral that change is inevitable.

Finally, the clergy's most important role, that of teacher, is also confronted with a transformative set of conflicts and resolutions. Are clergy responsible for the prevention of HIV/AIDS transmission? Should we expect religious leaders to share the challenge of preventing deaths by changing people's behavior vis-à-vis sex and drugs? If public high schools pass out condoms to prevent high-risk exposure among sexually active adolescents, should clergy be supportive? The prevention of HIV/AIDS transmission will save lives. Is this a religious challenge that requires clergy to overcome other traditional conflicts like condoms as birth control? Should all religious spokespersons preach and teach only the assumed religious message of abstinence? These and other questions plague clergy, seminaries, and denominational leaders. These are not theological or political issues; these are questions about life and death, especially among the young.

Clergy can have a significant role in the prevention of new transmission, since the only known mode of prevention is behavioral change, and the likelihood of a cure or vaccine is remote. Can there be any argument about the moral imperative of saving lives by changing behavior? But clergy face a significant conflict personally, theologically, and institutionally, because changed behavior as it relates to the transmission of the HIV virus directly relates to the exchange of bodily fluids. Once clergy have reiterated the sacred axiom of chastity, abstinence, and "say no to drugs," is there anything left to say?

In the face of such overwhelming information and with so many young lives in the balance, I believe that clergy have no choice but to teach as a way of preventing transmission of HIV/AIDS—whatever else all religions teach, the value of life is supreme. God would not want the means through which worship, ethics, and study is made purposeful to be a wasteland of irresponsibility. The transformative nature of the pandemic has forced clergy to consider a shift radically beyond the religious institution's tradition. Thus, the use of condoms, with an appropriate spermicidal lubricant, is a known factor in the prevention of HIV transmission. If premarital and extramarital sexuality and homosexual relations of any kind are all forbidden, does urging the use of a condom for all those who ignore this prohibition destroy the core of religious integrity even though it saves lives? If we can prevent the transmission of the virus by passing out clean needles are we also supporting or encouraging drug use? If clergy want to help educate (especially the young) about morality, responsibility, and the saving of lives, theirs and others, then clergy cannot simply repeat sacred verses of denial while overlooking the reality of condoms and clean needles. I offer no simple solution to this problem, only a warning, that a silent clergy, one that retreats behind the insular walls of tradition as if human lives were less important than doctrine, is a clergy that will bury those who "sin." It will be, in my view, the clergy who choose doctrine over human lives who will be responsible in part for these deaths, not a wrathful God. HIV/AIDS is not a divine punishment that clergy can use like a medieval threat regarding human behavior. HIV/AIDS is a virus that humans can and must control through behavior, especially when that behavior is outside the traditional bounds accepted by religious tradition. The prevention of HIV/AIDS transmission is a far-reaching transformative challenge for clergy. It is also the challenge that celebrates God's gift of life.

In future generations, others will judge how the servants of God treated God's creatures during this terrible period of suffering. Those of us who are called by God's presence to work for the time of divine fruition, a Messianic fulfillment, cannot turn our backs on the suffering in our midst. I know of no greater challenge facing the meaning and value of religious tradition than the HIV/AIDS pandemic. I am increasingly certain that God's loving compassion will embrace those who add caring and sanctity to life by insuring the dignity of all and by saving lives no matter how this is achieved.

Notes

1. Johann Baptist Metz, *The Emergent Church* (New York: Crossroads 1981), p. 28.

2. Joseph A. Edelheit, "The Rabbi and the Mandatory HIV Blood Test," *Journal of Reform Judaism* (Summer 1989): 1–9.

3. J. David Bleich, "AIDS: A Jewish Perspective," *Tradition* 26, no. 3 (1992): 49–80; David Novak, "AIDS: the Jewish Perspective," in *Frontiers of Jewish Thought*, ed. Steven Katz, (Washington, D.C.: Bnai Brith, 1992), pp. 141–156. Both of these are examples of very traditional conservative religious perspectives that approach the issue of HIV/AIDS *only* within the "sinful" behavior through which it is transmitted.

4. Charles Gerkin, *The Living Human Document: Re-visioning Pastoral Counseling in a Hermeneutical Mode* (Nashville: Abingdon, 1984), p. 38.

5. Ibid., p. 26.

6. Ibid., p. 14.

7. Suzanne C. Ouellette Kobasa, "AIDS Volunteering: Links to the Past and Future Prospects," in *A Disease of Society*, ed. Dorothy Nelkin, David P. Wills, and Scott V. Pavles (Cambridge: Cambridge University Press, 1991), pp. 186–187.

8. Ibid., p. 186.

9. Ibid., p. 187.

10. Mary Katherine Bateson, *Thinking AIDS* (Reading Mass.: Addison-Wesley, 1988), pp. 120–121.

10

Journalistic Responsibilities and AIDS

Michael Pritchard

The emergence of AIDS as a major threat to public health raises fundamental questions about the responsibilities of journalists. Any major threat to public health is sufficiently newsworthy to warrant extensive media coverage. The public depends on the media for reliable, comprehensive, and comprehensible information about such threats. Also, insofar as it is available, the media should provide information that will help the public take preventive measures to minimize such threats. All of this, we might say, is part of the public's "right to know," correlative to which is a journalistic duty vigorously to seek out information to which the public has a right.

At the same time, concern about AIDS within the professions, the workplace, government, and the public at large has given rise to a number of complex ethical issues that need informed public discussion and resolution. So journalists have a responsibility to assist their readers in coming to grips with these issues. This responsibility is complicated by both the difficulty of obtaining reliable, useful information and the challenge of dealing with very sensitive personal and moral issues with fairness and understanding.

That such concerns cannot be responsibly avoided is affirmed by journalists' codes of ethics. The code of ethics of the Society of Professional Journalists, Sigma Delta Chi, affirms that journalists have a duty to "serve the truth."[1] The code's statement on journalistic responsibility emphasizes the media's role as serving "the public's right to know of events of public importance and interest." Journalists are characterized as serving the general welfare as "carriers of public discussion and information." Freedom of the press, an inalienable constitutional right of the people, "carries with it the freedom and the responsibility to discuss, question, and challenge actions and utterances of our government and of our public and private institutions."

In addition, the code has statements on conflicts of interest; the need for accuracy and objectivity; respect for the dignity, privacy, rights, and well-being of others (fair play); and the importance of maintaining "the bond of mutual trust and respect between American journalists and the American people."

The Statement of Principles of the American Society of Newspaper Editors contains a similar set of provisions.[2] However, it makes a somewhat stronger statement on journalistic responsibility.

> The primary purpose of gathering and disturbing news and opinion is to serve the general welfare by informing the people and enabling them to make judgments on the issues of the time. Newspapermen and women who abuse the power of their professional role for selfish motives or unworthy purposes are faithless to that public trust.
>
> The American press was made free not just to inform or just to serve as a forum for debate but also to bring an independent scrutiny to bear on the forces of power in the society, including the conduct of official power at all levels of government.

Stephen Klaidman and Tom L. Beauchamp capture the basic values of these codes within a set of journalistic virtues: seeking the truth insofar as it is attainable, avoiding bias, avoiding harm, serving the public, maintaining trust, escaping manipulation, and inviting criticism and being accountable.[3] Each of these presents considerable challenge to journalists in addressing the problems of AIDS. This chapter focuses especially on problems of seeking truth, avoiding bias, avoiding harm, and serving the public.

Providing Needed Information

While it is hard to contest basic journalistic responsibilities in the abstract, real-world issues can bring them into tension, if not conflict, with one another. For example, while the responsibility to serve the public may generally be enthusiastically embraced by journalists, this is not always the case. For example, news media dependence on advertising support from the tobacco and alcohol industries may dampen enthusiasm for pursuing information that will discourage the use of the products of these industries. Such dampened enthusiasm invites conflict-of-interest charges from critics, and it raises serious questions about the ability of the news media to maintain independence and objectivity in reporting when vested interests are at stake. A related, but distinct, problem is satisfying customers. If newspapers and news magazines do not sell, journalists are out of business.[4] This problem invites two other problems: (1) the avoidance of thorough coverage of matters that are perceived to be of limited interest, or even distasteful or offensive, to readers; and (2) the pursuit of sensationalistic stories. AIDS coverage has suffered on both counts.

The 1976 outbreak of legionnaire's disease received considerably more press coverage when it first became known as a health threat in the United States than AIDS did.[5] Yet, there were far fewer known victims of legionnaire's disease. Unlike AIDS, legionnaire's disease was not believed to be communicable. Unlike the reported AIDS cases, the cause of legionnaire's disease was unknown and a highly speculative matter. In the case of both diseases, it was believed that significant, but limited, numbers of people were at real risk. Unlike AIDS, however, legionnaire's disease provided little evidence for determining who might be at greatest risk—or what might be done to lower that risk. So stated in the abstract, it would seem that AIDS would have received much greater attention from the press. How, then, is this contrasting coverage to be explained?

One possible explanation is that legionnaire's disease was deemed of more interest precisely because less was known about it. This made it more mysterious and intriguing—a group of men from diverse geographic areas attending a convention of Legionnaires in Philadelphia, seemingly having nothing more in common than staying in the same hotel, were suddenly struck down by a noncommunicable, fatal disease. Added to this were rare, but seemingly random, victims elsewhere. In the absence of further knowledge, this added an element of widespread fear to the intrigue—*anyone* could be victimized, and it was not known what, if anything, anyone could do to avoid becoming a victim.

But this explains only why the news media showed intense interest in legionnaire's disease. It does not explain why the initial coverage of AIDS was, by comparison, so low. If the portion of the public apparently at greatest risk was readily identifiable, and if preventive measures were also readily identifiable, why was the coverage so comparatively low? It will not do to say that when only some identifiable *part* of the public is thought to be at risk, journalistic interest can be expected to be lower. Toxic shock syndrome threatened a significant number, but by no means the vast majority, of women. The combined number of deaths from legionnaire's disease and toxic shock syndrome was less than the known number of deaths from AIDS by 1982.[6] Yet, from the standpoint of sheer numbers, toxic shock syndrome received disproportionately greater coverage.

The most plausible explanation of the contrasting coverage is in precisely who was believed to be at risk and why they were believed to be at risk. In the initial coverage of AIDS in the United States, the primary population considered to be at high risk consisted of gay men and intravenous drug users. Individuals in the first group engage in behavior that many regard as distasteful, offensive, and even "deviant" or "unnatural." Sexual behavior is also regarded by many as essentially private and not appropriate for detailed public discussion or scrutiny. Individuals in the second group engage in illegal behavior and are, therefore, regarded by many as marginal members of society. Both groups are viewed by many as behaving immorally and as, therefore, being at least partially responsible for their own fate. Some may even believe that such victims deserve their fate.

As harsh, unfair, and discriminatory as such attitudes may be, journalists are certainly aware of their existence. Insofar as some journalists may themselves share such attitudes, their lack of enthusiasm for AIDS coverage can be expected (as distinct from *justified*). But in the early years of AIDS coverage, even those journalists who did not share these attitudes may have been less than enthusiastic about aggressively pursuing information about a disease unlikely to be given a sympathetic understanding by those not clearly at risk.

In his review of the vast critical literature, Matthew Paul McAllister identifies several basic kinds of criticism leveled against early journalistic coverage of AIDS.[7] Journalists were criticized for relying on medical sources of information to the virtual exclusion of other important sources, especially the perspectives of the very people claimed to be at risk. Thus, there was no check on the overt or hidden distortions and biases that medical professionals and researchers might convey to journalists.[8] The further charge is that this was reflected in the early characterization of AIDS as a "gay plague" and as associated with "deviant" behavior. Groups already discriminated against and marginalized in society were now being stigmatized as transmitters of a fatal disease of their own making—another, more dramatic, case of "blaming the victim."

Regardless of the extent to which these criticism can actually be supported, they point to key ethical concerns that journalists should bear in mind. First, journalists should strive for objectivity. But this is as much a matter of fairness as of informational accuracy. Particularly in areas where vital human interests are at stake, objectivity requires taking carefully into account all relevant perspectives. This requires value sensitivity rather than the "value neutrality" so often linked with the idea of objectivity. Second, especially in areas of such sensitivity as AIDS, journalists need to exercise great care to avoid reinforcing prevailing social stereotypes and prejudices. This is both a matter of fairness and of not causing harm. Third, journalists have a responsibility to benefit the public, but "public" must be understood to include all members of society, not just the "mainstream" majority. It should not be necessary for a disease like AIDS to be perceived as a potential threat to virtually anyone for the press to give it more attention than something like legionnaire's disease.

When it became evident that virtually anyone is at risk of contracting AIDS, news coverage changed. Although coverage may not be totally immune from the above sorts of criticisms, the issues are now addressed with greater sensitivity and they occupy center stage in the media. Still, the challenges to responsibly providing reliable, useful information are no less formidable. The severity of risk posed by AIDS naturally raises three fundamental questions to which answers are needed: First, what are the risks of contracting AIDS? Second, how can the risks be minimized? Third, what can be done to help those who have tested HIV-positive or who actually have AIDS?

The first two questions cannot be completely separated. The level of risk varies with the context under consideration, and what happens within these contexts can be altered in ways that alter the risks. For example, the use of condoms lowers risk in sexual behavior. Improved methods of checking blood banks reduces the risk of having blood transfusions. But the general public is not accustomed to sophisticated discussions of risk levels. Although it should be evident to all that wearing a helmet reduces the risk of severe head injury when riding a bicycle, not many are prepared to discuss the *extent* to which the risk is reduced. Even though most of us realize that "safe" does not mean "risk-free," few are accustomed to talking about risk in quantitative terms. So, how should journalists communicate information about risk? Consider two examples.

The first example is from an Ann Landers column entitled "Heed the Warning: The Only Safe Sex Is Abstinence."[9] She replies to a letter from a man who says he is worried because he has learned that a man with whom he had sexual relations has tested HIV-positive:

> Your letter should serve as a reminder to everyone who is sexually active—straight, gay or bisexual—that there is always a risk involved. Today there is no such thing as safe sex. Condoms reduce the risk of AIDS, but they cannot provide 100 percent protection. Condoms can break or leak and they don't always stay on.

Remember this column when you feel yourself heading toward
a passionate encounter. Ask yourself, "Is this worth dying for?"

Ann Landers writes an advice column. Is this useful advice? The
first paragraph quoted is quite straightforward. It is unhelpful in two
respects, however. First, since she apparently equates "safe" with
"100 percent risk-free," her claim that there is no such thing as safe
sex with another person is uninformative for most. Second, informing
readers that condoms are not foolproof does not give any indication of
how reliable or unreliable they are.

The second paragraph provides the actual advice. Is it helpful?
Combined with the title of the column, it seems intended to discourage
sexual relations entirely. Asking "Is this worth dying for?" she seems
to suggest, will lead us to conclude that if the answer is no, that we
should say no to sex. But suppose we apply the same question to other
activities, like walking across the street or even walking down the
sidewalk. Are these activities worth dying for? Are they more or less
risky than having sexual relations? Unfortunately, the column provides
no comparative information. Assuming that readers will not take
seriously the option of giving up sex, walking, and virtually everything
else, they are left with no particular advice at all.

The second example is from a *New York Times* article, "Researchers List Odds of Getting AIDS in Heterosexual Intercourse."[10] Unlike
the Ann Landers column, this article provides plenty of numbers. It
contains a chart that divides sexual partners into categories: high- and
not-high-risk groups that do or do not use condoms, and that have or
have not tested HIV-positive. Odds that persons in these categories are
infected are presented, along with the odds of becoming infected after
1 sexual encounter with such persons as compared with 500 sexual
encounters with them. As might be expected, the odds at either
extreme are radically different (1 in 5 billion for 1 encounter with
someone who has tested negative and is using a condom; 2 in 3 for 500
encounters with someone who is infected with the AIDS virus and
without a condom). Clearly, the worst odds are grim indeed. What
about 1 chance in 5 billion? How does this compare with 1 chance in
500 million with the same person but without a condom? Or with 1
chance in 11 million for 500 times using a condom? Or 1 chance in 1.6
million for 500 times not using a condom? For most people, these
numbers mean little by themselves. There is nothing else with which
to compare them. (How is it with jogging and fatal heart attacks,
driving 300 miles on a holiday trip and having a fatal accident?) Even
pointing out that the risk is about ten times greater without condoms

is of little help unless we can attach meaning to 1 chance in 1.6 million, and so on.

The typical reader (even of the *New York Times!*) needs help interpreting the significance of such numbers. Fortunately, the author, Philip M. Boffey, provides some. He cites the various qualifications offered by the scientists who originally presented their projections in the *Journal of the American Medical Association*. They emphasize the incompleteness of their data, and they identify some important variables that they were unable fully to take into account. Boffey also cites what the scientists call their report's most important recommendation, namely, that heterosexuals restrict their sexual partners to those they know are at low risk of infection. What is not made clear is how the data drove them to this conclusion rather than, say, that the use of condoms, avoidance of certain kinds of sexual activities, or reduction of the number of sexual partners are equally, if not more, critical factors. Readers are left to accept these conclusions on authority or compare them with those of others (assuming that other studies have been reported)—which themselves pose similar problems of authority for all but possibly some statisticians. So journalists need to know how to present the results of studies such as this to lay readers, and they need to have some means of ascertaining that the researchers they cite have enough credibility that their work merits citing.

Boffey does not simply leave the numbers uninterpreted for readers. Unlike Ann Landers, he does offer some specific comparisons:

> In a middle category, one-time sex with someone who is not in a high risk group but whose infection status is unknown carried a 1 in 5 million risk of infection without a condom. That is about the same as the risk of being killed in a traffic accident while driving 10 miles on the way to that sexual encounter. The odds of winning the current Lotto game sponsored by the New York State Lottery are 1 in 13 million.

These comparisons are helpful. However, many more kinds of comparisons are needed if the typical reader is to acquire a sufficient grasp of risk factors to make confident judgments about reasonable risk. So although journalists should not be expected to be researchers themselves, there is much they can do to help lay readers interpret the practical significance of the research they summarize for their readers.[11]

Articles like Boffey's also help readers with the question of how risks might be minimized. Even if readers have some difficulty interpreting the significance of the numbers presented, they can see that various measures are likely to reduce risk somewhat. In the early years of AIDS coverage, reluctance to talk straightforwardly about sexual behavior was an obstacle to answering this question. McAllister cites a 1983 David Brinkley story indicating that apparently AIDS can be transmitted by "contact" between heterosexuals.[12] The vague reference to "contact" apparently resulted in many worried phone calls to AIDS research organizations. As Klaidman and Beauchamp point out, explicit mention of anal intercourse as higher-risk sexual behavior was even slower to appear in the media:[13]

> By late 1985 (especially after [Rock] Hudson announced that he had AIDS), more and more editors decided that taste should give way to explicit, potentially life-saving information involving blunt language. Even Ann Landers referred directly to "the receiving partner in anal sex" in her syndicated column, which is undoubtedly common fare at breakfast tables around the country. Her sister, Abigail Van Buren, was even more explicit. She wrote: "How is AIDS transmitted? The most significant route is by anal sex, oral sex and 'old fashioned' sexual intercourse with a person who has been infected by the AIDS virus."[14]

In retrospect, the choice between possibly saving lives and risking offending some readers seems obvious. However, no doubt this breakthrough took some courage, as it overrode a longstanding practice of avoiding explicit discussion of what heretofore was regarded as too private to be mentioned in the press.

According to George Will, the reluctance to discuss sexual behavior candidly was based on more than concerns about privacy. Writing in 1987, Will comments:[15]

> Earnestly, and with applause from journalists, politicians are saying about AIDS: candor, regardless of the cost.
> But truths are being blurred because they inconvenience a political agenda and shock sensibilities. The agenda is to avoid giving offense to certain factions and to avoid something more terrifying than AIDS—the accusation of "discrimination."

Claiming that fewer than 4 percent of AIDS cases have been caused by heterosexual contact, Will urges the press candidly to zero in on the central problem:

> Journalism seems reluctant to clarify that the primary reason for the AIDS epidemic is that the rectum, with its delicate and

absorptive lining, is not suited to homosexual uses. The nation needs unsparing journalism of the sort found in the *Chicago Tribune Magazine* of April 26: "81.5 percent of the second cluster of AIDS patients had engaged in the practice called 'fisting,' which causes rectal trauma, in the years before they fell ill. The researchers defined fisting as the insertion of a portion of the hand—or even the entire fist—into the anus of another person. The 27 men studied had a median of 120 sexual partners during the year before the onset of symptoms, with one man reporting up to 250 sexual partners in each of the three years before symptoms."

Will quickly adds, "Of course, not all homosexuals are promiscuous or given to high-risk behavior." Still, he acknowledges, many who are not strongly object to the publication of articles like that in the *Chicago Tribune Magazine*. But, Will concludes, "insufficient information about homosexual practices has impeded understanding of the epidemic."

In the same article Will attributes the rising incidence of heterosexual transmission of AIDS primarily to "black and Hispanic teenagers whose sex partners are intravenous drug users." Citing statistics that, in the United States, New York City has one-third of all AIDS cases, and that more than one-third of these cases are intravenous drug users, Will concludes his article by rejecting the idea that the most pressing need is funding research for a vaccine: "Of course research should be funded generously, but dollars spent getting addicts off needles and onto methadone will do more good, as will journalism that does not trim the truth to spare our feelings." Insisting that AIDS victims deserve care and compassion, Will urges that more important is getting on with the task of prevention.

As it is becoming evident that ever larger portions of the population are at risk, Will might wish to modify somewhat his statements of more than five years ago. It is doubtful, however, that he would modify his call for candor. Perhaps he should. His endorsement of candor is made in the name of AIDS prevention, not simply the value of "truth." So, we must ask whether the sort of candor he supports is likely to make a significant contribution to that end—and even if it is, whether other more acceptable means could accomplish the same end. The concern about other, more acceptable means is important, given the harm that might result from the sort of candor he supports.

Why would gays be disturbed by the publication of material like the *Tribune* passage Will cites? No doubt they worry about further stereotyping and stigmatization of gays. How many readers are likely to make special note of the fact that although 81.5 percent of the patients had engaged in "fisting" and the median number of sexual partners in the past year was 120, the entire group consisted of only 27 men—and that this was a "second cluster" of patients? Nothing is said in Will's article about the first group of patients or any other groups; and no indication is given of how representative of gays any of the groups might be. It is doubtful that many readers bothered to consult the original *Tribune* article to see if these questions are answered. Probably few asked them.

Immediately following the cited passage from the *Tribune*, Will concludes: "Without here adding details about dildos and enemas, suffice it to say that the data suggest that receptive anal intercourse is the major, if not the only, important exposure by which homosexuals acquire the infection." This is the sum of the evidence Will provides to support his conclusion. Unfortunately, this is the sum of the evidence that many who nod their heads in agreement with Will possess. Those already inclined to think stereotypically of gays are unlikely to be moved much by Will's disclaimer that, "Of course, not all homosexuals are promiscuous or given to high-risk behavior." So we need to ask whether there is good reason to think that the degree of candor Will advocates really does promote the sort of understanding that is likely to result in lowering the incidence of AIDS. All that seems clear is that the *other* problems gays face (e.g., being stereotyped, stigmatized, and discriminated against) are worsened.

The third question, that concerning what can be done to help those who have tested HIV-positive or who have actually contracted AIDS, is particularly difficult to answer, since so far no cures have been found and it is not clear to what extent the full effects of AIDS can even be temporarily arrested. Those at high risk or who already are infected are naturally anxious to hear some good news. Researchers are anxious to provide it. However, research takes time and perseverance, and good science and government regulations require caution. At the same time, experimental testing is sometimes done in other countries before being permitted here. Journalists must tread a thin line between recklessly raising false hopes by prematurely reporting promising research and reassuring a concerned populace that promising research is going on. They must also resist the lure of sensationalism when they hear that a breakthrough may be imminent.

Addressing the Moral, Legal, and Public Policy Issues

So far the focus of this chapter has been on responsibilities journalists have to seek out and report information about AIDS. However, as public concern has increased, a variety of controversial issues have arisen in regard to professional practice, the workplace, and public policy. Patients worry about whether doctors, dentists, nurses, and attendants have AIDS. Many ask whether such professionals should be restricted in their practice if they are infected, and some urge mandatory testing of medical professionals. In turn, medical professionals worry about whether their patients have AIDS. Some show reluctance to treat those who do, and some favor mandatory testing of patients. Self-regulation is prized by most professions. The problems posed by AIDS, however, press for public resolution.

Related concerns are present in the workplace. Workers may fear working with colleagues who have AIDS. Employers may not want to employ people with AIDS. Patrons may not want to be served food prepared by those with AIDS, and so on. Again, the question of mandatory testing arises, along with related concerns about discrimination and rights to privacy.

Journalists have an important role to play in these controversies. In addition to helping the public understand information relevant to the resolution of the problems (e.g., assessments of the risks of patients and professionals), journalists have a responsibility to facilitate understanding of the moral and legal issues at stake. This involves more than providing information. It requires sensitivity to the value issues themselves.

These value issues often are quite complex, both morally and legally. To assist the public in understanding what policies should be formulated concerning HIV testing, for example, it is necessary to raise relevant questions about rights, freedom, privacy, fairness, and the public interest. Students in journalism have opportunities to prepare for this task by taking classes in philosophy, political science, sociology, and other areas that address such concerns. Those who are already practicing journalists can consult some of the vast literature available in periodicals and books. Much of this is written for specialized audiences (legal scholars, philosophers, sociologists) rather than the general public. Even interdisciplinary publications such as the *Hastings Center Reports* are written more at an academic and professional level than the general public is accustomed to. So journalists need to find ways of communicating relevant and important ideas to a lay audience.

In short, just as journalists need to work hard in gathering factual information and making it understandable to the public, they need to do some homework on value issues as well. But they need not do this alone. They can talk with scholars and professionals who have developed views on these matters. They can talk with hospital ethics committees and policy-making boards, political officials, social workers, health-care professionals, activist groups, and, of course, those who are suffering from AIDS. Equally important, journalists can consult with one another, either in workshops and study groups, or informally in the newsroom.

In addition, journalists can examine existing AIDS policy statements that themselves address ethical concerns. For example, in September 1992 the Michigan Department of Public Health published a set of recommendations for health-care workers infected by hepatitis B (HBV) and HIV.[16] The document begins with statistics about the comparative risks of HIV transmission from dental procedures (1 of every 263,100 to 2,631,000) and from surgical procedures (1 of every 41,600 to 416,000). These figures are then compared with undergoing general anesthesia (1 of every 10,000 die) and being treated with penicillin (1 to 2 of every 100,000 with an adverse reaction resulting in death). The conclusion drawn is that the HIV risk is at an acceptable level. Neither mandatory testing of health-care workers nor mandatory disclosure to patients of health-care workers' HIV infection is recommended.

How are these recommendations supported? The document points out that the intent of mandatory testing and disclosure is to limit the practice of HIV-infected health-care workers. It then identifies four adverse consequences of such mandatory policies.[17] First, these policies would discourage health-care workers who are not HIV-infected from treating patients who are. They may even discourage some from entering the health-care field, since their practice could be limited should their patients' HIV infection be transmitted to them. Second, the loss of HIV-infected health-care workers means a loss of services to society. Third, fear of contracting HIV infection from patients would likely mean a reduction of needed services to HIV-infected patients. Fourth, those testing false positive would suffer socially, psychologically, and financially.

After discussing these four adverse consequences, the document asks, "Doesn't the patient have the right to know?"[18] It replies: "A patient certainly has the right to know anything that might reasonably be expected to affect his or her health status. In general, the HIV infection status of HCW's [health-care workers] does not meet this criterion because of the extremely low risk of HIV transmission from the HIV-infected HCW." Added to this is the claim that if patients are given the right to know if their health-care providers are HIV-infected, and they exercise this right, this would, in effect, be a mandatory disclosure policy. The likely consequence would be mandatory testing, resulting in the adverse consequences already described.

So the argument presented against mandatory testing and disclosure is broadly utilitarian. Left undiscussed is what the Michigan Department of Public Health would recommend if the risks to patients ever turn out to be significantly higher. The adverse consequences of mandatory testing and disclosure mentioned above would remain. Should these be outweighed by a consideration of patients' right to know (since now they might reasonably expect their health status to be affected), or should the utilitarian considerations still prevail?

Given the current estimates of risk, perhaps it is unnecessary for the Michigan Department of Health to speculate about when, if ever, the right to know regarding health-care workers should be given more serious consideration. Even if this is so, however, there are other policy areas in which the right to know needs to be more fully addressed, along with other rights, such as the rights to privacy and freedom. The workplace, the schools, and the athletic arena, for example, are also areas in which clear policies are needed.

Journalists can assist the public in addressing these policy concerns. Yet it is surprising how little media attention has been given to the Michigan Department of Public Health recommendations. The report indicates that its recommendations came from the department's Ad Hoc Committee on HIV-infected Health Care Workers. Committee members included representatives from a variety of health-care areas, as well as "ethical, legal, and public health disciplines."[19] No mention is made of committee efforts to interact directly with the wider public while deliberating about its recommendations. The recommendations have been endorsed by the major health-care associations in Michigan, as well as the Medical Ethics Resource Network of Michigan and the National Commission on AIDS.[20] The report indicates that the Michigan Department of Public Health is "widely disseminating" its recommendations "to all health care facilities, local public health agencies, and all health care–related professional organizations within the state."[21] However, no mention is made of the importance of informing the general public of its recommendations, and thus far the media have largely ignored the report.

So there is much in the policy area that journalists can bring to public attention. This does not mean that journalists themselves should be expected to adopt one position rather than another on particular issues. However, they should strive to make sure that open and fair consideration of the issues is made available to the public. This cannot be done without exercising judgment about what the morally and legally significant aspects of the issues are.

Of course, news coverage most often focuses on some particular set of circumstances rather than on general policy issues concerning rights, privacy, fairness, discrimination, public safety, and the like. Nevertheless, these more general concerns of the journalist may frame how more particular circumstances are presented. Open and fair consideration of controversial issues requires journalists to be as aware of this as they can.

If the public is to reflect meaningfully on issues of risk, safety, and responsibility, it must be given more than information. It must also be helped in relating this information to the more general value questions in terms of which the issues are debated. Providing further assistance in understanding underlying value issues is an important journalistic responsibility regardless of where journalists themselves happen to come down on particular issues. Editorial writers and syndicated columnists, of course, often explicitly do take stands on issues. As Article V of the American Society of Newspaper Editors makes clear, this is not an objectionable departure from requirements of impartiality. "To be impartial does not require the press to be unquestioning or to refrain from editorial expression. Sound practice, however, demands a clear distinction for the reader between news reports and opinion. Articles that contain opinion or personal interpretation should be clearly identified."[22] With writers like Ann Landers and George Will this is always clear, as it is with editorial pages of newspapers generally. When a news magazine lists authors at the end of an article without indicating clearly whether the article is meant strictly as a news report or partly as opinion, matters may be less clear.

A Danger of Excess

Despite the crisis proportions of the AIDS problem, there is a danger of journalistic excess. Two illustrations are offered here. The first is fictional. The Rex Morgan, M.D., comic strip has taken on the task of portraying some of the difficult ethical issues surrounding AIDS. It explores the plight of a surgeon who has just learned that she is HIV-positive. She shares this with her young daughter, who, in turn, shares this with her teacher. Her teacher inadvertently reveals this to her boyfriend, Bob, who happens to be a television reporter. Operating on the pretext that the public has a right to know that a local surgeon has AIDS, Bob shares this information with his viewers. No doubt many viewers are interested in learning such things. Some may use this information and refuse to be treated by the surgeon. But at least two questions need to be considered. First, do the interests of viewers provide grounds for their having a right to know that the surgeon has tested HIV-positive? Second, even if the answer is yes, does this show that it is the reporter's responsibility (or even right) to provide it?

In regard to the first question, without further information it is not at all clear that the public has a right to know that the surgeon is infected. Whether surgeons who test positive for HIV place patients at unacceptable risk is itself a matter of some controversy. But even if it is agreed that the surgeon should not continue doing surgical work, this is normally something that would be taken care of within the hospital rather than in the glare of the public eye. There is no need for the public to know that she is infected. If there is evidence that the matter is not being handled properly, the case for public revelation is strengthened. But even then, as in whistle-blowing, other avenues might better be explored first (such as notifying hospital authorities of the concern). This could accomplish the desired end (removal of the surgeon from practice) without causing her and others unnecessary harm or suffering.

In this case, however, the reporter seems more determined to have a sensational "scoop" than to serve the public interest. He has made no detailed investigation into the surgeon's circumstances, what her hospital does or does not intend to do, and so on. Apparently indifferent to the harm or suffering he may be causing the surgeon, Bob simply seems determined to gain credit for a "big story."

A further feature of this example is that even if it were the case that Bob had a responsibility to reveal that the surgeon is HIV-positive, this would not be because of his special occupation as news reporter. Normally, as already indicated, all responsibilities would be handled within the medical community. If someone outside that community observes a breakdown in responsibly handling such a matter, it would be unusual that their special occupational role would determine their own responsibility. In the case of illegal behavior (although there is no indication this is such a case), lawyers and law enforcement officers may have special responsibilities. Bob said he had to make the revelation because, "I'm a reporter." But this seems no more relevant than if the daughter's teacher had insisted she had to reveal the story because, "I'm a teacher." The crucial difference in this case between a reporter and others who might know about the surgeon's condition (e.g., a teacher, waiter, tax driver, or friend) is that a reporter has a ready *opportunity* to publicize the information. But merely having such an opportunity does not distinguish personal ambition (sensationalist "scoop") from responsible reporting.

The second case is not fictional. Arthur Ashe, 1975 Wimbledon tennis champion, tested HIV-positive in 1988. His infection resulted from a blood transfusion he had received in 1983. A very private person, it was Ashe's strong desire to keep knowledge of his infection out of the public eye. His privacy was respected for four years even though his condition was apparently known by several journalists.[23] Although there is no doubt that the story would greatly interest the public, this does not establish the public's right to know about Ashe's condition. Even if telling the story might benefit others in some way, this alone does not establish either that its revelation would be in the "public interest" or that it would be appropriate for any reporter to bring it into the open. Furthermore, the possible suffering it could cause Ashe seems to override any interest others might have in bringing it to public attention.

Sportswriter Frank Deford (and apparently several other journalists) was convinced that Ashe's wishes should be respected:

> The injustice was not that a disease would take his life. *That's the way it is.* The injustice was that someone had to "rat on me" and thereby discolor the rest of his life. Ashe wasn't naive. "Realistically," he told me a couple of months ago, "I'm afraid someone will blow the whistle on me soon." But he yearned for the secret to be kept. He grew up in the public eye being officially an apposition: "Arthur Ashe, the first Negro to . . ." And he knew that, once the news was out, he would have a new label forever after: "Arthur Ashe, AIDS sufferer."[24]

Nowhere in Deford's article is there even a hint that knowing Ashe's condition put journalists in a difficult position. (Directly under the title of Deford's article is the line, "He built a protective cocoon around the fact he had AIDS. And why not?") Yet, even some who agree with Deford's conclusion apparently see matters differently. A *Kalamazoo Gazette* sports editorial entitled "A Tough Call" comments:

> We've been asked what our personal decision would have been if we'd been in the position of USA Today's Gene Policinski. It's a no-win situation of course and the media, both print and electronic, have the responsibility to keep the public informed.
>
> But where does that responsibility end? Tough question. We defer to the comment of Randolph Murray, editor of the Anchorage, Alaska, Times, who said: "I guess if I had to choose, I'd

come down on his (Ashe's) side on this one. We have to be courageous enough sometimes to be decent.''[25]

This is the right conclusion. But the comments preceding it leave something to be desired. It is a "no-win" situation only if the media's responsibility to keep the public informed can be shown to have some relevance to the present case. The editorial makes no attempt to show this, and it is not clear how this could be done. Instead, it apparently assumes that the responsibility does apply here but is overriden by considerations of decency. What decency seems to override here, however, is the temptation to cause suffering to someone for the sake of sensationalism and the financial profits that go with it.

That it takes courage to resist such a temptation is sad but, unfortunately, apparently true. Although Klaidman and Beauchamp refer to courage at several points in *The Virtuous Journalist*, they do not do so in the context of upholding decency. In fact, "decency" does not appear in their index. Perhaps the addition of one more item to their list of journalistic virtues is in order.

Conclusion

This discussion has offered only an introduction to problems journalists face in attempting responsibly to address the AIDS crisis. The general standards of responsible journalism can be stated rather succinctly. Each of the two codes mentioned in this chapter takes up only a few pages of text. Interpreting and attempting to live up to these standards is another matter entirely. As some of the illustrations in this chapter show, it is sometimes easy to see how matters might be handled badly. Much more difficult is seeing how they might be handled well. The problems associated with AIDS are growing rather than diminishing. Not only are the numbers of people infected increasing at a frightening rate, with no known cures, baffling new kinds of cases continue to surface. Responsible journalistic coverage will continue to face difficult, sensitive, but essential tasks in helping us understand and cope effectively with these problems.

Notes

1. See Rena A. Gorlin, ed., *Codes of Professional Responsibility*, 2d ed. (Washington, D.C.: Bureau of National Affairs, 1990), p. 141.

2. Ibid., pp. 137–138.

3. Stephen Klaidman and Tom L. Beauchamp, *The Virtuous Journalist* (New York: Oxford University Press, 1987).

4. The focus here is on print media. Television journalists, however, face the same problems.

5. "Gay Disease Outbreak Gets Meager Attention, Critics Say," *Medical World News*, (May 10, 1982): 13–15. Cited in Klaidman and Beauchamp, *Virtuous Journalist*, p. 147. Headlining bias (AIDS as a "gay disease") will be discussed later in the chapter.

6. Ibid.

7. Matthew Paul McAllister, "Medicalizations in the News Media: A Comparison of AIDS Coverage in Three Newspapers," doctoral diss., University of Illinois at Urbana–Champaign, 1990.

8. McAllister cites sources claiming that some medical researchers referred to prostitutes as "reservoirs of infection," intravenous drug users as constitutionally lacking in will and "uneducatable," and gay men as "sexual addicts" ("Medicalizations," p. 135). He also points out that in the early years AIDS was given the informal label "WOGS" ("wrath of God syndrome") in some New York hospitals (p. 138).

9. Ann Landers, "Heed the Warning: The Only Safe Sex Is Abstinence," *Kalamazoo Gazette*, August 7, 1992, p. B5.

10. Philip M. Boffey, "Researchers List Odds of Getting AIDS in Heterosexual Intercourse," *New York Times*, April 12, 1988, sec. 1.

11. The difficulty of this task should not be underestimated, however. S. Holly Stocking and Paget H. Gross discuss recent psychological findings about our tendencies toward error and bias in processing information. "Understanding Errors and Biases That Can Affect Journalists," in Elliot Cohen, ed., *Philosophical Issues in Journalism* [Oxford: Oxford University Press, 1992], pp. 223–236). For example, they note our tendency to favor anecdotal presentations of the news over drier, more abstract statistical information. Journalists need to be aware of such tendencies, not only in their readers, but in themselves.

12. McAllister, "Medicalizations," p. 160. McAllister is citing J. Kinsella's account of this in *Covering the Plague: AIDS and the American Media* (New Brunswick, N.J.: Rutgers University Press, 1989), p. 22.

13. Klaidman and Beauchamp, *Virtuous Journalist*, p. 149.

14. Klaidman and Beauchamp are citing Ann Landers, "Methods of Protection Against AIDS," *Oakland Tribune*, October 29, 1985, p. C6; and Abigail Van Buren, "Getting the Facts Straight on AIDS," *Chicago Tribune*, August 12, 1985, sec. 5.

15. George F. Will, "True or False: AIDS Is a Democratic Disease That Perils Us All—FALSE," *Kalamazoo Gazette*, June 5, 1987, p. 7.

16. *Michigan Recommendations on HBV-infected and/or HIV-infected Health Care Workers*, Michigan Department of Public Health, September 1992. Copies of this document are available from the HIV/AIDS Prevention and

Intervention Section, Michigan Department of Public Health, P.O. Box 30195, Lansing, Mich. 48909.

17. Ibid., pp. 3–4.

18. Ibid., p. 4.

19. Ibid., p. 1.

20. Ibid. The associations include, for example, the Michigan Association for Local Public Health, the Michigan State Medical Society, the Michigan Association of Public Health Physicians, the Michigan Dental Association, and the Michigan Nurses Association.

21. Ibid., p. 9.

22. Gorlin, *Codes of Professional Responsibility*, p. 138.

23. Frank Deford claims to have known about Ashe's condition for several years. See Deford, "Arthur Ashe's Secret," *Newsweek* (April 20, 1992): 62–63.

24. Deford, "Arthur Ashe's Secret," 62.

25. Jack Moss, "A Tough Call," *Kalamazoo Gazette*, April 4, 1992, p. H1.

11

AIDS and a Politician's Right to Privacy

Vincent J. Samar

For my sister, Ninette

What are a politician's privacy rights in this AIDS crisis? What are his or her duties? These questions have become prominent as more and more of the public have begun to ask politicians and other persons to disclose their HIV status. On the one hand, politicians have an interest in determining what personal information is presented to the public. On the other hand, the public has an interest in learning about the health and potential influences that may affect political judgments and about how these judgments should be made. These divergent interests often come into conflict in either of two ways: first, when the public seeks direct disclosure of information through the enactment of laws such as campaign-financing statutes, and, second, when the press is about to publish the results of an investigative report.

In the first situation, one should ask whether the public's interest in the information is sufficiently compelling to impinge on individual privacy. In the second case, one needs to delimit the relative importance of individual privacy and freedom of the press, and their respective scopes and limits. Although both situations raise serious issues for a democratic society that takes autonomy as a fundamental end, it is the second that will occupy our attention since it is here that the issues of HIV-status disclosure and HIV-policy choices are most likely to become entangled. The bottom line will be to show how freedom of the press and a politician's right to privacy can be made consistent and what duties this places on both groups.

Because the law (let alone philosophy) in this area is complicated, I take the following approach toward unraveling it. First, I examine the interests of both the politician for privacy and the public to learn a good deal about a politician's life. Next, I explain why both these interests should be protected: the first as a right, and the second as either a compelling state interest or a legitimate aspect of freedom of the press. I then discuss what happens when interests conflict: how one decides the conflict and what role the politician's status as a public figure or public official should play in making that decision. Next, I apply these principles to what the public has a right to learn regarding the politician who has AIDS and the politician who is seropositive for HIV. Finally, I have some comments about a politician's obligation to educate the public about AIDS and HIV and the role that relevant health information should have in the creation and promotion of AIDS policies.

The Politician's Privacy Interest

Everyone wants to be seen in certain ways. Politicians qua politicians want to appear strong, in charge, and decisive. Consequently, politicians have an interest in ensuring that information published about them carries a favorable "spin."

Information about anyone can have a chilling effect on their behavior. This is particularly true of politicians, who measure their actions by how the public's perception of their decisions will affect their electability. Politicians have an interest in not having information published about them that the public will construe negatively. In some instances, the information will be downright false; in other cases, it will be true or partially true. Even if the information is fully true, the politician may properly not want the information known because it is likely to be misunderstood.

Information can be misleading because it is incomplete. It can also be misleading when certain facts are emphasized because of their appeal to social prejudice. Public education might help to avoid a politician's necessary attentiveness to this problem, but that takes time. Education is simply slow at changing ingrained public attitudes, so for the short run, the concern about perception will continue to dominate. This point is especially poignant when the issue appears more related to a politician's personal interest than to a legitimate concern of the public. In that case, a politician's claim to selectively disclose information is strongest.

This claim is based on the fact that the information involved is of no relevance to the performance of public responsibilities but has a high likelihood of chilling performance of private actions.[1] For example, if the politician were a cross-dresser, he or she would probably not feel comfortable with the way the public would respond to this information, and, therefore, informational leaks to that effect might discourage the politician from cross-dressing even in the confines of his or her own home. Other more controversial examples could easily be thought of, but this one illustrates an activity that might be prejudicial even though it has no obvious effect on the formulation or carrying out of public policy or public responsibilities. (I avoid discussion of indirect effects such as role modeling since the concern here is with politicians who choose to remain inside a personal informational closet and whether that should be allowed.) In short, the politician who is seeking or serving in public office has (at least) a prima facie case to selectively disclose information of a strictly private nature.

The Public's Interest

A democratic society in the Western sense takes as fundamental the right to vote based on individual interests. By doing so, the society affirms a deeper commitment to a principle of autonomy in which the people practice the art of self-rule. This end is different from that of Marxist countries (of which there are now very few) to seek the good of the collective based on some prearranged social conception. In the Western democratic model, the choice of what good to seek is left to the individual and is subject only to a similar right of choice in others.[2]

To effectuate their right to vote fully, citizens need to know the positions and character of the people who will represent them. Positions are important, as these might affect individual interests. Character is also important as it is related to the credibility of persons seeking public office.

When elected office involves a lengthy term or great distance from the day-to-day events, the positions that one can expect to learn about will necessarily be limited. Here, the politician will need to talk more about the basic principles that will guide the decision making rather than the decisions themselves. Character becomes particularly important in these contexts as a means of assessing the trustworthiness of the candidate to follow his or her own principles. If democratic government is to be secure, this evaluative process must provide satisfactory preelection answers to such questions as what will this candidate, if elected, count as a reason for adopting a particular policy and how will he or she assign weight to different and presumably conflicting reasons.

This does not mean that elected officials should never change their minds from whatever preelection policy position they might have taken. It does mean, however, that their decision should be controlled by clear principles at a not-too-abstract level publicly articulated in the preelection process. It also means that society will suffer a loss of autonomy in respect to an individual's ability to vote on her or his own interests when relevant information regarding positions and character is not made available at the preelection stage. Therefore, society has a direct interest in information about a politician's life and conduct as might bear on future policy decisions. To this extent, then, the interest of the public to learn a good deal about a politician's life and conduct is directly related to its interest in autonomy as a fundamental end of Western democratic society.

The Right to Privacy and the Right to Know

A society that takes autonomy (even in the narrow sense of the right to vote on one's interest) as a fundamental end must also take privacy as a fundamental right. Nevertheless, it will also take the public's need for information about the positions and character of its politicians as a compelling reason that will in some instances override individual privacy. The rationale for both these positions (albeit related) is different.

In the case of privacy, the concern is primarily with acts and only secondarily with information. This is because privacy traces out a boundary within which the holder of the right is free to act. It does this by identifying certain autonomous actions that a government bent on fostering individual autonomy should want to protect. These acts are self-regarding in that the mere description of the act without the inclusion of any additional facts or causal theories would not suggest a conflict with another's interest in the comparison group.[3] (The inclusion of additional facts or causal theories with respect to private *action* relates to a type of compelling state interest we need not be concerned with here.) Privacy in this sense is direct protection of autonomy, since such cases of privacy are aspects of autonomy a priori.

In the case of the politician whose self-interest lies in selectively disclosing information, private acts are not directly at stake. That is because the object to be protected is not an act per se but information. Like most people, politicians often feel constrained in acting by the possibility that information about those activities might become public. This suggests a causal link between the protection of private acts and the protection of private information. That link is formed by the very real concern that voters may turn away from a politician if certain information about the politician becomes known, even though the information is, strictly speaking, irrelevant to the politician's policies or character. Therefore, to promote autonomy generally, privacy in the sense of guaranteeing the selective disclosure of information must also be protected. Privacy in this second sense is indirect protection of autonomy in that it is valued not for itself (as part of autonomy), but as a means to guaranteeing autonomy a posteriori.

Of course, it might be argued that this second sense of privacy is counterproductive to the end of promoting autonomy generally, that the autonomy of all individuals would be more secure if they were less concerned about what other people thought. This objection, however, overlooks the fact that for the politician his or her livelihood is dependent on the opinions of others. A better variation of the objection starting from the same premise might argue for impinging on a politician's privacy from the standpoint of making better voters and more stalwart politicians. While appealing at first hearing, this variation too is quickly attenuated as one moves from learning about actions that bear on public policy toward those in the realm of private activity.

Like the right to privacy, the public's need for information bearing on the positions and character of its politicians also arises out of the protection of autonomy. The public's interest here relates to the right to vote in that citizens need to discover how the politician truly stands on the issues and whether he or she can be trusted. Consequently, the public's interest in information protects autonomy by helping the citizen to become a better voter.

A particularly difficult issue arises when the politician asserts a claim to privacy on a matter about which the public seeks information. The latter interest may be asserted directly by a proposed campaign disclosure law or indirectly by the press investigating a story. When the interest is asserted indirectly, it is usually accompanied by a rights claim for freedom of the press. (As will be seen in the next section, freedom of the press shares a common justificatory basis with the right to privacy.) Whichever way the issue comes about, a decision must be made regarding the relative strength of the politician's right to privacy versus the public's interest in the information in question. Of special importance is the means adopted for determining the correct balance.

Conflict of Rights and Compelling State Interest

We begin here by noting that the right to privacy as described above is a prima facie right. It arises out of a democratic concern to protect individual autonomy generally. Other active rights, including the right to a free press, also promote individual autonomy generally as, for example, when the press disseminates information about a politician's positions and character. Indeed, it is because freedom of the press also promotes autonomy that a conflict of rights between freedom of the press and privacy can be decided on the basis of which right, under the circumstances, will better promote maximal autonomy. Here, promoting autonomy requires that we accept no less for our citizens in the range of possible choices than the maximum our democratic institutions could support without loss or conflict.

A somewhat different analysis governs the case of campaign disclosure laws. Here the point is to determine whether the public has a compelling interest for overriding individual privacy. Society's concern in this context is the protection of the integrity of the campaign process as a means for gathering relevant information on which a voter can make an electoral decision. That process is harmed when a candidate misuses the campaign environment to wrongly accuse his or her opponent of some failing or when the candidate withholds information about character defects or potential biases that should be made available to the public. Whatever the harm, the test to be applied when deciding on the propriety of disclosure laws is to determine whether enactment of the proposed statutes or protection of individual privacy will better protect autonomy generally. If privacy is the answer, then the public interest in enacting such laws (however strong it is) is not compelling;[4] if disclosure laws are the answer, then privacy is overridden.

Even when privacy is overriden, it does not drop out of the picture. This is because the right to privacy is still a fundamental right, fundamental in the sense that it too is necessary for the protection of autonomy generally. Consequently, even when the right to privacy is overriden, privacy continues to regulate the degree to which the dominant interest governs the case. Here the guiding principle is that the maximum allowable intrusion on privacy is the minimum needed to achieve the state's compelling interest.

In the case of politicians, privacy plays a somewhat more subservient role than it does for private citizens because no one is required to seek public office either for themselves or the good of the community. Even so, society has an interest not to discourage good people from entering public life by requiring too high a price in the sacrifice of their private lives. And voters have an interest in avoiding a loss of their own autonomy because relevant information is not available in time to make intelligent choices among candidates. When taken together, these considerations create a presumption in favor of the public interest in information over the politician's right to privacy. This does not mean that the public interest will always win out, but it does mean that the politician who would seek protection for a privacy claim has an uphill battle to show that autonomy is better served by protecting privacy in the given instance than by allowing the information to be disclosed. Indeed, it is the law's recognition of just this presumption that is at the heart of the distinction between public person and private citizen.

The Public Person/Private Citizen Distinction

Since 1964 the law has come to recognize that persons in public life (be they government officials or celebrities such as movie and television actors, politicians, or sports stars) stand in a significantly different relation to the public than do private citizens, who even though they have the same rights do not command the same media attention with which to influence others. Public officials and public figures have substantially more media access and can command (by virtue of who they are or the position they hold) more of the public's attention to get their messages across. Consequently, the law has developed different standards of protection for persons in these two groups than for private citizens.

For private citizens, the law prohibits the publication of defamatory statements[5] or statements that invade personal privacy[6] unless the individual is part of a current news story.[7] For example, in the celebrated case *Melvin v. Reid*,[8] Gabrielle Darley, a former prostitute, decided to give up her life of prostitution and move to a different part of the country after becoming involved in a murder trial. In her new environment, she married and became a respected member of her new community. Seven years later, the movie *The Red Kimono* was made, portraying Darley's early life. The California appellate court held that Darley had a claim for invasion of privacy under California's constitution, which, according to the court, guarantees to each person an inalienable right to pursue and obtain happiness. Noting the need to protect against irrationality and prejudice, the court determined that privacy must be part of that inalienable right.

In contrast, *Time v. Hill*[9] involves a story published about the Hill family's experience in being held hostage in their home by three escaped convicts. The story had previously inspired a novel and a play. *Life* magazine chose to do a feature on the incident, in which it depicted violence being inflicted on the hostages. In fact, no violence had occurred. Under a New York statute that allowed for suits where the article lacks newsworthiness or is substantially and materially false, The Hills won a lawsuit against the magazine. In reversing a lower court's affirmance of the Hill judgment, however, the Supreme Court, per Justice William Brennan, stated: "The constitutional protections for speech and press preclude the application of the New York statute to redress false reports of matters of public interest in the absence of proof that the defendant published the report with knowledge of its falsity or in reckless disregard of the truth."[10] In his concurring opinion, Justice William O. Douglas offered the comment that "such privacy as a person normally has ceases when his life has ceased to be private."[11]

Thus, *Time* established the proposition that publishing statements about a public figure is not an invasion of privacy unless the statements are known to be false or are published despite serious doubts regarding their truth. This actual malice standard clearly holds the press to a lower standard of care when discussing persons in public life than when discussing private persons. The rationale for the principle's application to public officials is the need to encourage scrutiny of those who hold public office.[12] Similarly, the rationale for application to public figures is to hold those who present themselves to the public (presumably to have an influence over what the public does or believes) to a higher degree of scrutiny than ordinary citizens.[13] In both cases, a further rationale from the standpoint of fairness would note the public person's greater accessibility to media to rebut inaccuracies and distortions than is possessed by private citizens.

Still, the fact that a person is a public official or a public figure does not mean that all doors are opened on their private life.[14] No doubt even the most liberal view of the above standard would find it hard to justify invading the bedroom of Bill and Hillary Clinton. The question is where to draw the line. Here is where the residual regulatory character of the privacy right becomes important.

For politicians, information irrelevant to their positions or character (including the attitudes they are trying overtly to create) bears a prima facie claim to privacy. Consequently, when seeking to uncover such information, one should ask whether the information would allow citizens to become better voters (where "better" is understood to mean more aware of their own interests or how a particular candidate will promote or lessen those interests). This question has two parts. The first part concerns relevance; the second, materiality or the appropriate weight to be assigned the information. Under the above analysis, only information related to the performance of the duties and responsibilities of public office and the setting of public policy should be discoverable. Otherwise, we give up the possibility of politicians having any private life. The rationale is particularly strong in the case of statutory disclosure laws since such laws rely on the police power of the state, which can become menacing to those the dominant political opinion views as dissidents. With respect to the second concern, voters should be able to determine for themselves what weight to give the information once the information is determined likely to affect (if it has not done so already) the public interest. This latter limitation is discussed more fully in the next section.

These two requirements do not mean that there cannot be legal criteria set by a majority of the elected representatives for determining whether a person is fit to hold public office: for example, whether they are a convicted felon or underage. Certainly, this would reflect an appropriate assignment of weight to widely held concerns that are relevant to holding public office. What it does mean, however, is that the importance of information related to fitness for public office is ultimately for the voters to determine, provided there is good reason to believe that the information in question is relevant to the carrying out of public responsibilities and will likely affect the manner in which those responsibilities are carried out.

This then brings us to the question of how these standards might apply in the context of AIDS. Since I presume that the answer might vary depending on whether the information sought concerns being symptomatic for AIDS or merely seropositive for HIV, I treat each of these issues separately. Although I focus on the press in this part of the discussion and not on statutory disclosure laws, it is fair to say that the approach that I suggest for the press to follow traces very closely the method adopted by the Supreme Court in reviewing statutory disclosure laws.

AIDS and the Politician's Obligation to Release Health-Related Information

When seeking information about whether a politician has AIDS, the question is not about spread of the virus. Rather, it is about whether the candidate will be able to perform the duties of office if he or she is already symptomatic for the disease.

Here the concern is the public's interest in knowing the state of health of the person running for public office prior to an election. By analogy with what I say here regarding elected politicians, a similar argument could be made for persons seeking appointment to public office, including federal judgeships, cabinet positions, and various other bureaucratic offices, with which voters are not directly involved. To make this assessment, one begins by asking whether the information in question is relevant to persons being able to vote on their interests. If the answer is affirmative, then the further question needs to be asked: Are there any limits on what information can be gained?

This latter question arises because privacy retains the regulatory function of ensuring that the maximum amount of intrusion on the private interest of the politician is the minimum necessary to meet the state's compelling interest.

A comment on methodology is in order. Earlier I noted that in conflicts-of-rights situations, the test is the promotion of maximal autonomy. Since the health status of candidates for public office will likely become an issue in contexts where the press asserts a right to disclose and the politician a right to privacy, it might be supposed that one should decide the case based on an appeal to maximal autonomy.

The difficulty with this conclusion is that it misconstrues the true nature of the dispute. The problem here is not to determine whether the press's right to disclose relevant information about a politician overrides the politician's right to privacy; we have already said that it does on maximal autonomy grounds reflecting the status of the politician as public figure/public official (depending on whether he or she is currently in office). Rather, the question here is whether these two rights are in conflict when applied to AIDS disclosure. To decide this question, one must discover whether the interest to be protected is relevant to what the public needs to know to be able to make an informed decision about a candidate's fitness for public office. A subtlety arises because a judgment about relevance cannot be content neutral; that is, there is always the interposition of the values of the one judging.[15] Still, reporters and others who have to make these judgments should always be aware of personal biases, as opposed to public needs, that may be motivating their decisions.

Obviously, if a true conflict of rights exists between privacy and freedom of the press, then the courts should hold the press liable only when there is a knowing falsity or reckless disregard of the truth. But what about questioning the press's initial judgment regarding whether the information relied on in the story is relevant to the public's ability to make an electoral decision? The difficulty is that different people undoubtedly have very different ideas about what qualities relate to carrying out public responsibility, and these differences in outlook cannot be precisely harmonized under a hard-and-fast rule. Still, at the extreme, the courts could allow liability when the publication relates to actions that are both fully private in that they fall under the above definition and have no causal connection to the responsibilities of the office. Admittedly, this is a very hard test to meet in practice given the multiple ways in which the causal connection might be established and the compelling interest that would then exist to allow such information to be made known to the public. Nevertheless, the approach does (at least) set the boundary line for court intervention on the question of relevance by avoiding the problem of specific content and treating the matter along the lines of an adjustment to the existing malice standard.[16] Most important, nothing in the approach limits the press from imposing a higher standard on itself.

In a democratic society, where autonomy necessitates giving deference to the press, it also necessitates that the press take on a substantial role in policing itself. This is essential if the privacy of public officials and public figures is to be protected. Under this view, then, the press has the dual role of first protecting society's compelling interest to learn of a politician's actions, attitudes, character, and beliefs that bear on the function of public office, and second of seeing to it that the *private* information presented to the public is no broader than the minimum necessary to meet the public's compelling interest. That the press should be thought to have these dual functions follows from why we protect freedom of the press to start with, namely, to guarantee autonomy by making sure that voters have adequate information on which to make electoral decisions.

In the case of persons with AIDS, we discover a wide variability in their ability to perform different kinds of tasks at different times. For example, a person who succumbs to HIV-related dementia may not be able to function even to the same extent that a person with Kaposi's sarcoma is able to function. And the latter may not be able to function at times when the disease becomes most intrusive in the operations of life. Consequently, learning whether a candidate is able to perform the functions of office is relevant to an assessment of that candidate's fitness for public office. At least to this extent, the issue of AIDS is similar to the issue of any other deadly or debilitating disease. A difference does lie, however, with what goes along with knowledge of HIV disease.

Here it is naive not to notice that HIV carries with it a social stigma related, unfortunately, to misconceptions. HIV disease is often thought to be related to being a gay man or an intravenous-drug user. While these groups are at risk for the disease, gay white males over twenty years old have been able to reduce the rate of infection through education programs, although the infection rate among teenage males has jumped.[17] Additionally, there remains the stigma that part of society still associates with being gay, which at this point can be viewed only as a prejudice.[18] Therefore, given these social realities, the public interest in discovering the health status of politicians must be considered in the context of these other concerns.

What is needed is a formula that would satisfactorily balance both the public's legitimate interest to know the health and well-being of a candidate for public office and the politician's interest in privacy. That formula is for the press to report the general health status of the candidate, including how it bears on job performance without reporting either the name of the disease or more of a description of it than is necessary to explain how it will affect job performance. In the case of AIDS, in particular, the press should not speculate on possible effects of every opportunistic infection that may come about but only on the infections that currently exist or (in light of the candidate's current medical condition) are highly likely to come about within the term of office. For example, the press could report that the candidate suffers a potentially fatal disease that will affect the candidate's ability to perform the duties of office in certain definite respects and at various times without labeling the disease or providing any more of a description than that. So long as this is done generally to protect the legitimate privacy interests of all politicians with respect to health care, it would not be as if the press were trying to pick out certain individuals for special protection. Other diseases, including tuberculosis and cancer, also have their stigmas. It would then be up to the candidate whether to explain further. Needless to say, the public in this instance would receive the health information it needed to evaluate fitness for the job without directly intruding on the candidate's privacy.

It might be objected that the argument presented is overinclusive, that because it mandates that we not reveal the cause of a health injury, it would, in a different context, prevent an identification when the cause was a police officer's bullet during an escape from a robbery. The objection, however, ignores the fact that different situations may present different reasons for informing the public of the events surrounding an injury. That one should not be able to discover the cause merely because it is appropriate to discover the effect does not mean that in a context where both cause and effect are independently relevant to voters making an informed electoral judgment (as in a case when one has engaged in criminal behavior) that both should not be discoverable.

A variation on this objection is that voters are entitled to knowledge of the cause in the case of AIDS just because there may be a connection to sexual orientation or intravenous-drug use. While intravenous-drug use might be relevant were it to involve a violation of criminal statute[19] or an addiction, the status of being gay clearly is not. Still, it might be argued that this argument is too narrow and that the status issue would also fall within the public purview in states where homosexual sodomy is a crime. Let us treat each of these two claims in turn.

Clearly, the claim that an addiction is something that the public should be made aware of is relevant to voting on one's interest if the addiction would likely affect performance or lead to violations of local law while in office. This justification is undercut, however, if the individual is enrolled in a drug or alcohol treatment program and there are no current indications (violations of law, etc.) that he or she has "fallen off the wagon." Granted, such treatment programs are sometimes accompanied by checkered responses, and in these instances judgment is called for to know whether the circumstances surrounding a lapse are sufficient to pose serious questions regarding the politician's fitness for public office. Because this is an area of judgment regarding the importance rather than the relevance of the information in question, the standard to be applied is the materiality standard I discuss in the next section.

Similarly, if the jurisdiction in question has a sodomy statute that makes homosexual activity criminal, this may be a reason to report actual conduct in violation of that statute but is certainly not a reason to report on one's status as gay or to assume that HIV disease was acquired in the context of committing a crime or even, for that matter, in the context of being gay. (Gay men can also receive infected blood transfusions.) Moreover, there is good reason to question both the morality and constitutionality of such statutes despite the Supreme Court's decision in *Bowers v. Hardwick*[20] to allow states to enact them.[21] Indeed, many states that have such legislation do not regularly enforce it. Consequently, in those states where the people seem uncertain about the propriety of making such acts illegal, the press should be especially circumspect in publishing the names of any persons who have been found guilty of such offenses if no one was harmed and no party was a minor.[22]

A similar ban would not apply to situations where evidence shows that a politician who knew that he or she was HIV-positive had unsafe sex with another person without disclosure of his or her health status. In that instance, the information is both relevant and material to the character of the politician and is therefore discoverable.

No doubt, even with these safeguards there will be plenty of times when the public will suspect AIDS. Even more obvious may be the effect of the disease on the politician's campaign performance. Still, by treating all life-threatening or performance-affecting health risks similarly, we acknowledge (at the level that we acknowledge race to be irrelevant without failing to know the race of the candidate) the legitimate privacy interest involved and illegitimacy of prejudice in choosing people for public office.[23] While this is no surefire guarantee that the social bias against AIDS will be eliminated, it nevertheless creates an environment in which such bias is tainted with illegitimacy, much like racism is today. The long-term consequential effect of doing this should be to erode the misconceptions and prejudices surrounding this disease.

Other objections might be raised to the conclusion drawn here. However, since these objections would apply equally well to the disclosure of a politician's nonsymptomatic HIV status, I place them under that category.

The Politician's Obligation to Release HIV Status

Given the current state of medical treatment for HIV disease, it must be concluded that being seropositive for the virus reduces to some extent the probability of living a long and healthy life. Moreover, being seropositive for HIV disease raises the same issues of prognostic health prediction that attend genetic susceptibility to heart and other diseases.

These facts bear on the issue of whether the press should or should not disclose a politician's HIV status to the public. The issue here is again one of relevance. It cannot be assumed that since there is some alteration of health status the information would necessarily be relevant. The issue is whether the knowledge gained by such a disclosure is sufficiently related to performance in office so as to warrant the consequent intrusion on individual privacy. The issue cannot be resolved by a mechanical formula. A reporter faced with the issue must exercise his or her own judgment based on what is known. This means the reporter must take into account the frequency with which HIV infection leads to full-blown AIDS. He or she must also take into account that the triggering mechanism is not known and that the time factor is quite variable. Finally, the reporter must balance this information along with information about the current health status of the politician. Unless it appears (as determined by all the relevant data, including T-cell count) that the politician will not be able to perform the duties of office during the assigned term, the disclosure should not be made. In short, there would simply be no story. (Obviously, the standard by which fitness is judged will vary with the current state of health information about HIV disease.)

It might be argued that learning about a politician's HIV status is like learning about his or her financial investments. To the extent that such investments or status might influence how the politician makes public policy decisions once in office (whether, for example, he or she will seek a personal benefit over a benefit for the general public), the public has a right to know about the existence of these investments and financial status in advance of the election. Consequently, it is relevant for the press to report on the HIV status of a politician during a political campaign.

This criticism applies only to those politicians whose job it is to effect public health policy. It would not, for example, justify publishing the IIIV status of the director of the CIA since there the matter would not be relevant. However, it might justify publishing the HIV status of a great many other persons (including members of congress, and state and local representatives) who effect public health policy through a variety of means, not the least of which is voting on budget allocations. This issue of potential bias is especially poignant for health-care issues because, as yet, there is no overall scheme for determining as a matter of social justice what the proper allocation of scarce resources to health care should be. Nor is there a clear view within the health-care field of what the proper allocation of limited health-care resources to eradicating various diseases should be. Were there such a scheme, a politician's HIV status would be irrelevant (unless he or she sought to deviate from the pattern), since the scheme would determine how resource allocations should be made. Unfortunately, the current environment in which health-care policy is determined in the United States does not include such a model. Consequently, a politician's HIV status may be thought relevant.

Saying this, however, does not mean that disclosure of a politician's HIV status is always or even often material to an electoral decision. Even aside from offices that do not effect health-care policy (where the issue would be one of relevance), there may be a whole set of objective reasons for why a public official might prefer one allocation of resources for health care over another. Consequently, one should not draw from the fact that a politician has to decide a question of resource allocation to or within health care the conclusion that his or her own health will bias these decisions. Not to recognize this is to imply that there can never be an objective basis for a decision over which one has a personal interest.

Still, the fact that there can be an objective basis may not remove the uncertainty that a particular decision was made from a self-benefiting motive. What it does remove is the presumption that when politicians make decisions in this area, everything that *may* influence them should be made known to the public prior to the election. For this reason, when reporting a politician's views about health care, if the reporter knows of the possibility of a personal bias, the reporter should first assess the particular views independent of possible influences. In essence, the reporter should determine if the politician really was being biased by assessing the credibility of the politician's own argument on its merits.

The reporter should seek to learn the reasons why the politician believes as he or she does or why the politician voted in a particular manner. If after reviewing the arguments proffered the reporter still cannot decide whether the controlling factor was the adequacy of reasons or personal bias, then the reporter should let the public decide by publishing the fact that both possibilities exist. The public can then decide for itself the materiality of the information disclosed to performance in public office.

In this context, the failure to be convinced may arise because the arguments are inadequate to establish either the position being advocated or the degree of advocacy involved. In respect to the former, the problem may be one of evidence or deduction. Here the question concerns the weight of the evidence and whether it would likely lead any rational person to the same result. If the answer is no, then the possibility of bias is on hand and should be reported. In respect to the latter, one is reminded of that immortal line in Shakespeare's Hamlet: "The lady doth protest too much." Here, the question is why is the politician devoting a disproportionate amount of time to one project over others. If the answer cannot be found within the politician's job description (for example, committee work assignments), or the degree of concern of his or her constituency (as expressed in mail received, etc.), then bias should be suspected. Note that in neither case is bias proved, but that should be for the public to decide. If the situation is one in which the reporter's judgment is not clear-cut, the rule to be followed is: the greater the difficulty the reporter has in deciding the issue of bias, the greater the reason for letting the public decide. This democratic criterion applies to cases in which what is at stake is a conflict between publishing private information about a public figure or a public official and not publishing information relevant to citizens being able to vote on their interests. It requires that the reporter exercise discretion with a view to protecting autonomy generally.

As long as the reporter's judgment is controlled by a set of principles that seeks to balance the legitimate interests of the public against the private interests of the politician, the judgment cannot be seen as arbitrary or undemocratic. This latter point is made on the ground that democracy requires that citizens (including public persons qua citizens) be able to discover their own interests and that such discovery is more likely to take place when a realm of privacy exists that protects against intrusions that do not affect the public interest.[24] Neither can the reporter's judgment be subject to a mechanical formula in which the result in every case is uncontroversially determined. For this reason, courts would still be held only to application of the malice standard governing publications about public officials and public figures suitably adjusted to take account of the issue of relevance as suggested above. Again, that standard applies only at the outer boundary of proper conduct, when the press has failed to police itself and a court needs to step in to avoid an egregious violation of rights. Of course, this may mean that an occasional unscrupulous reporter gets away with publishing information solely on the basis of its tantalizing nature in spite of its irrelevance or its bearing little importance to public service. Nevertheless, it does recognize that in a democracy every institution including the press must do its part to guarantee the balance of rights. As a check on this responsibility, courts can secure the perimeter, but within that perimeter other institutions must also play a role.

Duty of Politicians

So far this analysis has focused on the privacy rights of politicians and the correlative duties these rights impose on the press and on legislatures passing disclosure legislation. The remainder of this chapter focuses on the duty of politicians to help change public opinion, especially in the context of AIDS.

When the Kimberly Bergalis case (which involved a young woman who contracted AIDS from a dental procedure) first surfaced, many members of Congress and many state legislators introduced and supported legislation that was truly repressive, discriminatory, unreflective, and mostly responsive to public hysteria. Such a response might have been expected from Senator Jesse Helms, who seems to believe that AIDS is a punishment from God and that he is God's legislative servant. For most politicians, however, the issue was one of simply reading the polls and caving in to public hysteria, primarily for self-interested (political survival) reasons. So the question arises, What are a politician's moral responsibilities both with respect to AIDS legislation and with respect to public education about AIDS?

It may be recalled that earlier I noted that a government bent on fostering individual autonomy should seek to provide the maximum degree of autonomy consistent with a similar autonomy for all. From this arises a positive duty to provide legislation that rationally and compassionately promotes the fundamental autonomy of persons with

AIDS (PWAS) and other persons as yet uninfected. This positive duty means that the goals of AIDS legislation must take into account relevant knowledge about the etiology of HIV disease and how it is spread. It also means that legislation must be provided to adequately deal with the pandemic of AIDS in all its many facets, including education, prevention, research, and treatment. When this obligation is combined with the further condition that the maximum allowable intrusion on a person's privacy rights is the minimum necessary to achieve the state's compelling interest, it becomes apparent that the legislation must also balance the rights of PWAS and non-PWAS so as to guard against measures that might be unduly repressive or discriminatory toward either group. As I have dealt with these matters elsewhere, let me summarize two points from that discussion that most concern the relationship between education and prevention on the one hand and the role of government on the other, while offering at the same time comment on the Bergalis case.[25] I will then argue that every politician who can influence AIDS health policy has a duty to educate the public about HIV disease so as to maximize the possibility that appropriate legislation will be enacted.

To begin with, good public health-care policy should not rely solely on abstinence from sex, even if this may be the safest choice. First, most people will not accept this degree of limitation, especially if they are unknowledgeable about the transmission of AIDS or believe that there exist other, less intrusive means for self-protection. Neither is it likely to be effective at least in the long run to present false information in the hopes of scaring people into a level of risk reduction beyond what they otherwise might accept. Such misleading information, if later discovered, creates the possibility of rejection of correct information and suspicion about government intentions generally. Second, both parties to a sexual act can choose to take medically prudent steps (such as using condoms and spermicides containing Nonoxynol-9) to protect themselves against HIV infection. Thus, lying under these circumstances does not advance autonomy generally, since the individuals are capable of making reasonable choices. Of course, all this presupposes that relevant and material health information is available throughout the society at large. Since no other institution is as capable of establishing such a practice as government, government has a duty to ensure that society is adequately informed about the AIDS pandemic.

One particular place where this duty might be met (and by no means the only one) is in the public schools. Here the responsibility of government is to recognize the legitimate interests of children with HIV disease to live as normal a life as possible, children without AIDS to be free of the disease, and all parties to be provided with a good education that includes learning how to both protect oneself and accept other people with different infirmities. Hence, restrictions on the child with HIV that have no bearing on spreading the disease should not be allowed. Moreover, an atmosphere of compassion and understanding for all persons with HIV should be promoted. Finally, adequate sex education should be provided so that students can learn what AIDS is, how it is spread, and what can be done to prevent getting infected.

With respect to the Bergalis case, many legislators and some of the citizenry have drawn the wrong conclusion. When understood in the context of privacy's regulatory function, this case does not point to a need for widespread testing of physicians and dentists for HIV but to funding universal health-care precautions such as those recommended by the Centers for Disease Control (CDC), including the use of gloves of proper-gauge plastic to prevent inadvertent cuts from needles, drills, or other sharp objects. Clearly, the use of such precautions raises health-care costs, but such costs may be offset if the results, as might be expected, lead to a reduction in the spread of other diseases like hepatitis and allow those who are trained in the various health-care fields to continue to contribute to society's well-being. Perhaps there are a few instances in which even in spite of CDC guidelines a patient would not be protected. I have in mind situations in which the guidelines do not take into account (let alone protect against) real risks to the patient. Perhaps cutting in an area where the surgeon cannot see poses this kind of threat if the surgeon's gloves are not designed to avoid scalpel cuts in this sort of operation. In these few instances, some legal standard would seem to be a reasonable response, provided the legislation applies to all health-care risks of comparable gravity and further provided that such standards are properly circumscribed by the scientific evidence available.

This, then, brings me to the last issue: Do politicians have an obligation to educate the public about the policy implications of a disease like AIDS? The issue arises because in a democracy the content of most laws is determined by its attractiveness to a favorable majority in the legislature. Consequently, if government is morally obligated to provide a certain kind of legislative response to a disease like AIDS, how well it succeeds in satisfying that obligation will be determined by how much support any particular piece of legislation can muster among individual legislators. The latter, of course, turns on what these same politicians anticipate to be the electoral response to their decision.

In political-science terminology, there is the distinction between the trustee role and the delegate role. The trustee role is that in which the particular legislator or politician gains expertise about a field and applies that expertise to legislative decision making without seeking in advance a great deal of consultation with his or her constituents. Politicians who come from safe districts (districts where politician's reelection is virtually assured) are regarded as playing a trustee role. In contrast, the delegate role is that in which the politician has far more contact with constituents; consequently, the politician follows their views when making legislative decisions. Politicians who come from unsafe districts are regarded as following this path.

While helpful as a description, when applied to public policy-making the trustee/delegate distinction presents a real threat that politicians, to insure their own reelection, will undo what government may be morally obliged to do. Even so, our concern here need not cause us to question our faith in the moral correctness of democracy. For while democracy may open up this sort of problem, it also provides us with the normative grounds for closing it. This it does by reminding us that autonomy is a fundamental end and the best way to insure autonomy generally is by encouraging widespread education and deliberation about issues, especially those over which the public is strongly concerned.

Here politicians have a special obligation to provide the background expertise in which controversial public policy issues should be considered. At the point between having to make decisions and having to respond to public pressure, politicians (like teachers) stand at least initially in the unique role of being able both to capture public attention and to mold that attention to a discussion of issues based on relevant information. Since the public has a compelling interest to know what might affect its overall autonomy (especially in the health area) and since politicians sometimes are in the best position to gather the results of testing and to provide to the public this information, politicians have a duty to ensure that the public is informed about the implications of various policy alternatives and to encourage the public to consider without fear or hysteria those alternatives. Moreover, in cases where the policy choice cannot wait for the outcome of a long deliberative process, politicians have both an interest and a moral obligation to ensure that their constituents understand the choices after the fact.

Thus, from a normative perspective, a politician always functions as a trustee for ensuring that the public is fully informed, especially on matters over which public opinion can affect policy outcomes. (The only possible exception—which does not apply here—is a case in which the information would add little to the public debate, such as information about the making of nuclear weapons, and might itself be used by third parties to seriously threaten the public safety.) In this sense, then, the positive duty of government to provide against repressive and discriminatory AIDS legislation and to provide for legislation that meets the needs of all the citizenry implies a corresponding duty on the part of politicians to create the necessary deliberative environment in which the former duty can be satisfied.

Conclusion

The responses by various public officeholders (and those who would seek public office) to the AIDS crisis provide a startling reminder of how far politicians have to go if democracy is to work for the good of all the people. It is also a reminder that a legitimate starting point for the press in evaluating a politician's fitness for public office is to what extent the politician is willing to live up to the clearly relevant leadership responsibilities that attend that office. To the degree that politicians fail in this task, the press should make note and the public should hold them to account. Failing this, democracy itself will be lost.

Notes

Acknowledgments: I wish to thank Michael Davis, Elliot Cohen, and John Kvedaras for their editorial suggestions on an earlier draft of this chapter.

1. Vincent J. Samar, *The Right to Privacy: Gays, Lesbians and the Constitution* (Philadelphia, Pa.: Temple University Press, 1991), pp. 99–101.

2. Here I do not take up the question of how social conditions may affect individual choices.

3. Samar, *Right to Privacy*, pp. 66–76.

4. When rights are not considered fundamental, the Supreme Court has followed a weaker standard such as the rational-relationship test. Under this test, a right is overriden if the state can show any rationally related legitimate reason for doing so. In contrast, the compelling-state-interest test is the strongest standard and applies when privacy is a consideration. I have argued that a compelling state interest exists only when the interest at stake is such that autonomy generally will be undercut if privacy is allowed to override the interest. See ibid., pp. 79, 112–115.

5. See William Prosser, *Handbook of the Law of Torts*, 5th ed. (St. Paul, Minn.: West, 1971), p. 778.

6. It should be noted that William Prosser identifies four types of informational privacy not related to the gathering of evidence of a crime. They include seclusion and solitude, not being placed in a false light, not having embarrass-

ing facts told about oneself, and finally, not having one's name or likeness taken for commercial purposes without permission. With respect to the matters concerning this essay, embarrassing facts and false light are what is at issue (ibid., pp. 851–866).

7. Ibid., pp. 862–866.

8. *Melvin v. Reid*, 112 Cal. App. 285, 297 (1931).

9. *Time v. Hill*, 385 U.S. 374 (1967).

10. Ibid., at 394.

11. Ibid., at 401 (Douglas concurring).

12. *See New York Times v. Sullivan*, 376 U.S. 254, 278 (1964), involving a case of libel against a public official.

13. *Gertz v. Robert Welch Inc.*, 418 U.S. 323, 345 (1974).

14. In *Nixon v. Administrator of General Services*, 433 U.S. 425, 465 (1977), the Supreme Court acknowledged that public officials have (at least) a legitimate privacy interest in personal communications. See Laurence Tribe, *American Constitutional Law*, 2d ed. (Mineola, N.Y.: Foundation Press, 1988), pp. 889–890, noting that there may come a point where personal control over information outweighs the value of uninhibited public discussion.

15. In *Monitor Patriot Co. v. Roy*, 401 U.S. 265, 276–277 (1971), the Supreme Court stated: "A standard of care 'can be neutral with respect to the content of the speech involved, free of historical taint, and adjusted to strike a fair balance between the interests of the community in free circulation of information and those of individuals seeking recompense for harm done by the circulation of defamatory falsehood.' A standard of 'relevance,' on the other hand, . . . is unlikely to be neutral with respect to the content of speech and holds a real danger of becoming an instrument for the suppression of those 'vehement, caustic, and sometimes unpleasantly sharp attacks,' which must be protected if the guarantees of the First and Fourteenth Amendments are to prevail [citations omitted]." In contrast, see Cass R. Sunstein, *The Partial Constitution* (Cambridge, Mass.: Harvard University Press, 1993), pp. 226–228.

16. The proposed adjustment to the malice standard is consistent with the statement made in *Monitor Patriot Co. v. Roy* (401 U.S. at 275): "Given the realities of our political life, it is by no means easy to see what statements about a candidate might be altogether without relevance to his fitness for the office he seeks. The clash of reputations is the staple of election campaigns, and damage to reputation is, of course, the essence of liable. But whether there remains some exiguous area of defamation against which a candidate may have full recourse is a question we need not decide in this case."

17. For statistics on the number of new AIDS cases reported worldwide as based on a World Health Organization report, see "46,600 New AIDS Cases Worldwide," *Chicago Tribune*, October 6, 1991, sec. 1.

18. See Richard D. Mohr, *Gays/Justice: A Study of Ethics, Society, and Law* (New York: Columbia University Press, 1988), pt. 4, which deals with ethics in the context of AIDS; see generally Michael Ruse, *Homosexuality*

(New York: Blackwell, 1988), which examines the foundational suppositions for why people hold different views on homosexuality.

19. In *Monitor Patriot Co. v. Roy*, 401 U.S. at 277, the Supreme Court held "as a matter of constitutional law that a charge of criminal conduct, no matter how remote in time or place, can never be irrelevant to an official's or a candidate's fitness for office for purposes of application of the 'knowing falsehood or reckless disregard' rule of *New York Times v. Sullivan*" 376 U.S. 254, 279–280 (1964).

20. *Bowers v. Hardwick*, 478 U.S. 186 (1986).

21. For an analysis of the analytic and normative problems with *Bowers*, see Samar, *Right to Privacy*, pp. 82, 167–172.

22. Having written this article when I did, I cannot help but notice the role of the press in reporting on the sexual harassment charges of Professor Anita Hill against Supreme Court nominee Judge Clarence Thomas. An important question arises over whether the press should have broken a story on such a criminal charge after the statute of limitations has run. Here I would note two conflicting considerations: in support of reporting the story is the view that the Senate inquiry was not a criminal trial but a political inquiry into the qualifications of the nominee; against this position is the concern that the statute of limitations protects against a failure to discover all relevant evidence because of failed memories or loss of witnesses. In the Thomas hearing, the concerns behind the statute of limitations were not at stake since no important witnesses were unavailable. As a general rule, however, the press should consider the purposes and concerns behind the statute as a relevant factor in deciding in the future whether to report the story.

23. In *School Board of Nassau County v. Arline*, 480 U.S. 273 (1987), the Supreme Court held that a schoolteacher who contracted tuberculosis was protected against discharge under Section 504 of the Rehabilitation Act of 1973, 29 U.S.C. sec. 794 (1982). The Court stated that in most cases there should be an individualized inquiry with appropriate findings of fact so that "504 [may] achieve its goal of protecting handicapped individuals from deprivations based on prejudice, stereotypes, or unfounded fear, while giving appropriate weight to such legitimate concerns of grantees as avoiding exposing others to significant health and safety risks" (*School Board v. Arline*, p. 1131). The decision has since been applied in AIDS cases. See, for example, *Chalk v. United States District Court*, Cent. Dist. of Calif. 840 F. 2d 701, 704–706 (9th Cir. 1988).

24. See Samar, *Right to Privacy*, pp. 88–89, 90–103.

25. See Samar, *Right to Privacy*, pp. 157–167; idem, "Privacy and AIDS," *University of West Los Angeles Law Review* 22 (1991): 1.

A Bibliography on AIDS and Professional Ethics

Sohair W. ElBaz and William Pardue

This bibliography is a brief survey of titles available as of March 1993 on the topic of AIDS/HIV infection and its ethical implications for the professions. The bibliography is intended for those readers wishing to do introductory research on the topic. In cases for which relatively few articles directly about ethical issues exist, citations concerning legal issues have been included.

The bibliography begins with two short lists, one of readings on AIDS/HIV in general, and introductions to professional ethics. Following that is a list of general material on AIDS and ethics (not necessarily professional ethics). The remainder of the bibliography is divided into three sections: "AIDS, Ethics, and the Non–Health Professions," "AIDS, Ethics, and the Health Professions," and a final section on videos about AIDS and ethics. When a citation is relevant to more than one subject, it is listed under all relevant subjects.

Researchers intent on finding the most recent material available on AIDS and professional ethics may need to examine materials published later than those listed in this bibliography. Several resources would be well worth browsing for articles on the topic. *The Bibliography of Bioethics*, edited by LeRoy Walters and Tamar Joy Kahn (Washington, D.C.: Kennedy Institute of Ethics) is by far the most important of the bibliographic resources on AIDS and ethics, covering all aspects of the topic, not just professional issues. *AIDS and Public Policy Journal* (Frederick, Md.: University Publishing Group) is an important journal with frequent articles on issues directly related to professional ethics. Other sources include the *Journal of Medical Ethics* (London: British Medical Association), *The Hastings Center Report* (Briarcliff Manor, N.Y.: Hastings Center), *Milbank Quarterly* (Port Chester, N.Y.: Cambridge University Press), and the *Journal of the American Medical Association* (Chicago: American Medical Association).

General Material on AIDS

Barouh, Gail. *Support Groups: The Human Face of the HIV/AIDS Epidemic.* Huntington Station, N.Y.: Long Island Association for AIDS Care, 1992.

Bartlett, John G., and Ann K. Finkbeiner. *The Guide to Living with HIV Infection: Developed at the Johns Hopkins AIDS Clinic*. Baltimore, Md.: Johns Hopkins University Press, 1991.

Dalton, Harlon L., Scott Burris, and the Yale AIDS Law Project. *AIDS and the Law: A Guide for the Public*. New Haven, Conn.: Yale University Press, 1987.

Edison, Ted, ed. *The AIDS Caregiver's Handbook*. New York: St. Martin's Press, 1988.

Faison, Brenda S. *The AIDS Handbook: A Complete Guide to Education and Awareness*. Durham, N.C.: Designbase Publishing, 1991.

Hubley, John. *The AIDS Handbook: A Guide to the Prevention of AIDS and HIV*. London: Macmillan, 1990.

General Material on Professional Ethics

Bayles, Michael D. *Professional Ethics*. Belmont, Calif.: Wadsworth, 1989.

Callahan, Joan C., ed. *Ethical Issues in Professional Life*. New York: Oxford University Press, 1988.

Camenish, Paul F. *Grounding Professional Ethics in a Pluralistic Society*. New York: Haven, 1983.

Goldman, Alan H. *The Moral Foundations of Professional Ethics*. Totowa, N.J.: Rowman and Littlefield, 1980.

Kultgen, John H. *Ethics and Professionalism*. Philadelphia, Pa.: University of Pennsylvania Press, 1988.

General Material on AIDS and Ethics

"AIDS: The Emerging Ethical Dilemmas." *Hastings Center Report* 15, no. 4 (suppl.) (August 1985): 1–32.

Almond, Brenda, ed. *AIDS: A Moral Issue*. New York: St. Martin's Press, 1990.

Bayer, Ronald. "As the Second Decade of AIDS Begins: An International Perspective on the Ethics of the Epidemic." *AIDS* 6, no. 6 (June 1, 1992): 527–533.

Bayer, Ronald, Daniel M. Fox, and David P. Willis, eds. *AIDS: The Public Context of an Epidemic*. New York: Cambridge University Press, 1986. This volume is also published as *Milbank Quarterly* 64 (suppl.). See other listings below for specific articles.

Cahalan, Kathleen A. *AIDS: Issues in Religion, Ethics and Care*. (A Park Ridge Center bibliography.) Park Ridge, Ill.: Park Ridge Center, 1988.

Center for the Study of Law, Science and Technology. *Responding to the AIDS Epidemic: Constitutional, Legal and Social Policy Issues*. Tempe: Center for the Study of Law, Science and Technology, Arizona State University College of Law, 1986.

Daniels, Norman. "Duty to Treat or Right to Refuse?" *Hastings Center Report* 21, no. 2 (March/April 1991): 36–46.

Fineberg, Harvey V. "The Social Dimensions of AIDS." *Scientific American* 259, no. 14 (October 1988): 128–134.

Freedman, Benjamin. "Health Professions, Codes and the Right to Refuse to Treat HIV-infectious Patients." *Hastings Center Report* 18, no. 2 (suppl.) (April/May 1988): 20–25.

Gostin, Lawrence. "The AIDS Litigation Project: A National Review of Court and Human Rights Commission Decisions—Discrimination." *Journal of the American Medical Association* 263, no. 15 (April 18, 1990): 2086–2093.

Hastings Center. *AIDS: An Epidemic of Ethical Puzzles*. Brookfield, Vt.: Dartmouth University Press, 1991.

Humber, James M., and Robert F. Almeder, eds. *Biomedical Ethics Reviews: 1988*. (Special issue: "AIDS and Ethics.") Clifton, N.J.: Humana Press, 1989.

Ide, Arthur Frederick. *AIDS Hysteria*. Dallas, Tex.: Monument Press, 1986.

Illingsworth, Patricia. *AIDS and the Good Society*. New York: Routledge, 1990.

Kirp, David L., and Ronald Bayer. *AIDS in Industrialized Democracies: Passions, Politics and Policies*. New Brunswick, N.J.: Rutgers University Press, 1992.

Kleinig, John. "The Ethical Challenge of AIDS to Traditional Liberal Values." *AIDS and Public Policy Journal* 5, no. 1 (Winter 1990): 42–48.

Lang, Norris G. "Difficult Decisions: Ethics and AIDS." *Journal of Sex Research* 28, no. 2 (May 1, 1991): 249–262.

Leonard, Arthur S. "Ethical Challenges of HIV." *Notre Dame Journal of Law, Ethics and Public Policy* 5, no. 1 (special issue: "Symposium on AIDS") (1990): 53–74.

Manuel, C. "The Ethical Approach to AIDS: A Bibliographical Review." *Journal of Medical Ethics* 16, no. 1 (March 1, 1990): 14–27.

McKenzie, Nancy F., ed. *The AIDS Reader: Social, Political and Ethical Issues*. New York: Meridian, 1991.

National Center for Social Policy and Practices. *AIDS and Ethics: A Bibliography*. Silver Spring, Md.: National Center for Social Policy and Practice, Information Center, 1990.

Newton, David E. *AIDS Issues: A Handbook*. Hillside, N.J.: Enslow Publishers, 1992.

Overall Christine, ed. *Perspectives on AIDS: Ethical and Social Issues*. New York: Oxford University Press, 1991.

Pierce, Christine, and Donald VanDeVeer, eds. *AIDS: Ethics and Public Policy*. Belmont, Calif.: Wadsworth, 1988.

Prior Jonson, Elizabeth. *AIDS: Myths, Facts and Ethics*. New York: Pergamon Press, 1988.

Reamer, Frederick G., ed. *AIDS and Ethics*. New York: Columbia University Press, 1991.

Schwalbe, Michael L., and Clifford L. Staples. "Moral Reasoning and Rhetoric: The Acceptability of Arguments About AIDS-related Dilemmas."

Journal of Applied Social Psychology 22, no. 15 (August 1, 1992): 1208–1221.

Smith, Joseph Wayne. *AIDS, Philosophy and Beyond: Philosophical Dilemmas of a Modern Pandemic.* Avebury Series in Philosophy. Brookfield, Vt.: Avebury, 1991.

AIDS, Ethics, and the Non–Health Professions

Business Ethics in General

Brockhoeft, John E. "AIDS in the Workplace: Legal Limitations on Employer Actions." *American Business Law Journal* 26, no. 2 (Summer 1988): 255–303.

Katz, Mark A. *Understanding AIDS: A Personal Handbook for Employees and Managers.* Washington, D.C.: Employee Benefits Review, 1988.

McDonald, Martha. "How to Deal with AIDS in the Work Place." *Business and Health* 8, no. 7 (July 1990): 12–22.

Myers, Phyllis Schiller, and Donald W. Myers. "AIDS: Tackling a Tough Problem Through Policy." *Personnel Administrator* 32, no. 4 (April 1987): 95–108.

O'Riley, Kathleen Keri. *AIDS in the Workplace: A Literature Review.* Position paper. Educational Research Information Clearinghouse (ERIC), ED334489, 1991.

Trebilcock, Anne M. "AIDS and the Workplace: Some Policy Pointers from International Labour Standards." *International Labour Review* 128, no. 1 (1989): 29–45.

Advertising

Drohn, Franklin B., and Laura M. Milner. "The AIDS Crisis: Unethical Marketing Leads to Negligent Homicide." *Journal of Business Ethics* 8, no. 5 (October 1989): 773–780.

Clergy

Cahalan, Kathleen A. *AIDS: Issues in Religion, Ethics and Care.* (A Park Ridge Center bibliography.) Park Ridge, Ill.: Park Ridge Center, 1988.

Crowther, Colin E. *AIDS: A Christian Handbook.* London: Epworth Press, 1991.

McCloughry, Roy, and Carol Bebawi. *AIDS: A Christian Response.* Grove Ethical Studies series. England: Grove, 1987.

National Conference of Catholic Bishops. *Called to Compassion and Responsibility: A Response to the HIV/AIDS Crisis.* Office for Publishing and Promotion Services Publication no. 327-2. Washington, D.C.: United States Catholic Conference, 1990.

Place, Michael D. "The Church, AIDS and Public Policy." *Notre Dame Journal of Law, Ethics and Public Policy* 5, no. 1 (special issue: "Symposium on AIDS") (1990): 75–88.

Education

Anderson, Gary R. *Courage to Care: Responding to the Crisis of Children with AIDS*. Washington, D.C.: Child Welfare League of America, 1990.

Jones, Nancy Lee. *AIDS and the Public Schools: Legal Issues Involved in the Education of Children*. Washington, D.C.: Congressional Research Service, Library of Congress, 1988.

Kirp, David L. *Learning by Heart: AIDS and Schoolchildren in America's Communities*. New Brunswick, N.J.: Rutgers University Press, 1989.

Manning, D. Thompson, and Paul M. Balson. "Policy Issues Surrounding Children with AIDS in the Schools." *Clearing House* 61, no. 3 (November 1987): 101–104.

McGee, Jerry C. *AIDS in Schools*. Educational Research Information Clearinghouse (ERIC), ED298618, 1988.

Siebert, Jeffrey M., and Roberta A. Olson, eds. *Children, Adolescents and AIDS*. Children and the Law series. Lincoln: University of Nebraska Press, 1990.

Strope, John L., Jr., and Cathy Allen Broadwell. *Students with AIDS: A Legal Memorandum*. Educational Research Information Clearinghouse (ERIC), ED310521, 1989.

U.S. Department of Education, Office for Civil Rights. *Placement of School Children with AIDS*. Washington, D.C.: U.S. Department of Education, Office of Civil Rights, 1991.

Welker, Matthew, and Sarah W. J. Pell. *The Formulation of AIDS Policies: Legal Considerations for Schools*. NOLPE Monograph/Book Series, no. 44. Topeka, Kans.: National Organization on Legal Problems of Education, 1992.

Insurance

Childress, James F. "An Ethical Framework for Assessing Policies to Screen for Antibodies to HIV." *AIDS and Public Policy Journal* 2, no. 1 (Winter 1987): 28–31.

Daniels, Norman. "Insurability and the HIV Epidemic: Ethical Issues in Underwriting." *Milbank Quarterly* 68, no. 4 (1990): 497–525.

Hammond, J. D., and Arnold F. Shapiro. "AIDS and the Limits of Insurability." *Milbank Quarterly* 64 (suppl. 1) (1986): 143–167.

Nelson, David K. "AIDS and Life Insurance: A Look Behind the Testing Issue." *AIDS and Public Policy Journal* 2, no. 3 (Summer/Fall 1987): 26–28.

Oppenheimer, Gerald M., and Robert A. Padgug. "AIDS and Health Insurance: Social and Ethical Issues." *AIDS and Public Policy Journal* 2, no. 1 (Winter 1987): 11–14.

Schatz, Benjamin. "The AIDS Insurance Crisis: Underwriting or Overreaching?" *Harvard Law Review* 100, no. 7 (May 1987): 1782–1805.

Vculek, James, ed. *AIDS One: Legal, Social and Ethical Issues Facing the Insurance Industry*. Chatsworth, Calif.: NILS, 1988.

Waymack, Mark H. "AIDS, Ethics and Health Insurance." *Business and Professional Ethics Journal* 10, no. 3 (Spring 1991): 73–84.

Journalism
Deni, Elliott. "Identifying AIDS Victims: The Destruction of Dr. Huse." *WJR* 10, no. 10 (October 1988): 26–29.
Gersh, Debra. "Unclear Boundaries." *Editor and Publisher, the Fourth Estate* 125, no. 16 (April 18, 1992): 7–10. Debate on the ethics of publishing details of Arthur Ashe's case of AIDS.
Kinsella, J. *Covering the Plague: AIDS and the American Media.* New Brunswick, N.J.: Rutgers University Press, 1989.
Nelkin, Dorothy. "AIDS and the News Media." *Milbank Quarterly* 69, no. 2 (1991): 293–307.

Law
Begg, Robert T. "Legal Ethics and AIDS: An Analysis of Selected Issues." *Georgetown Journal of Legal Ethics* 3, no. 1 (Summer 1989): 1–56.
Haines, Bruce. "The Moral Challenge of AIDS: A Lawyer's Perspective." *Canadian Family Law Quarterly* 4, no. 3 (October 1989): 349–363.
Lambda Legal Defense and Education Fund. *Living with AIDS: A Guide to the Legal Problems of People with AIDS.* New York: Lambda Legal Defense and Education Fund, 1987.
Nichols, Julie. " 'What Lawyers Do Best': The AIDS Crisis." *Human Rights* 15, no. 3 (Fall 1987): 49, 50–51.
The Truth About AIDS: Why Do Lawyers Have a Special Duty to Understand the Disease?" *Human Rights* 15, no. 3 (Fall 1987): 46–51.

AIDS, Ethics, and the Health Professions

The Health Professions in General
Bader, Diana, and Elizabeth McMillan. *AIDS: Ethical Guidelines for Health-care Providers.* St. Louis, Mo.: Catholic Health Association of the United States, 1987.
Cooke, Molly. "Occupational Transmission of HIV: The Ethics of Physician Risk and Responsibility." In *AIDS Clinical Review 1990*, ed. Paul Volberding and Mark A. Jacobson, pp. 1–10. New York: Marcel Deklar, 1990.
Feldblum, Chai R. "A Response to Gostin, 'The HIV-infected Health Care Professional: Public Policy, Discrimination and Patient Safety.' " *Law, Medicine and Health Care* 19, no. 1/2 (Spring 1991): 134–149. See listing for Gostin under "Physicians."
Loewy, Erich H. "Risk and Obligation: Health Professionals and the Risk of AIDS." *Death Studies* 12, no. 5/6 (September/December 1988): 531–545.
Medical Ethics and AIDS. Atlanta, Ga.: American Health Consultants, 1988. Sponsored by the monthly newsletter *Medical Ethics Advisor.*
Milbank Quarterly 68 (suppl. 2) (special issue: "A Disease of Society: Cultural

Responses to AIDS'') (1991). A collection of articles on the responses and obligations of society and various health practitioners (including nurses).

Nolan, Kathleen, and Ronald Bayer. *AIDS: The Responsibilities of Health Professionals*. Briarcliff Manor, N.Y.: Hastings Center, 1988.

North, Richard L., and Karen H. Rothenberg. "The Duty-to-Warn 'Dilemma': A Framework for Resolution." *Aids and Public Policy Journal* 4, no. 3 (1989): 133–141.

Schobel, Deborah A. "Management's Responsibility to Deal Effectively with the Risk of HIV Exposure for Healthcare Workers." *Nursing Management* 19, no. 3 (March 1988): 38–42.

Shin, Diana M., and Jo-Anne Avers, eds. *AIDS/HIV Reference Guide for Medical Professionals*. Los Angeles: Center for Interdisciplinary Research in Immunology and Disease at UCLA, 1988.

Tuohey, John F. *Caring for Persons with AIDS and Cancer: Ethical Reflections on Palliative Care for the Terminally Ill*. St. Louis, Mo.: Catholic Health Association of the United States, 1988.

Dentistry

American Dental Association. *Report of Council on Ethics, Bylaws and Judicial Affairs Regarding Ethical Ramifications of Refusing to treat Patients with AIDS or Patients Who Are HIV Seropositive*. Chicago, Ill.: American Dental Association, 1988.

Cohen, Leonard A., and Edward G. Grace, Jr. "Attitudes of Dental Faculty Toward Individuals with AIDS." *Journal of Dental Education* 53, no. 3 (March 1989): 199–202.

Gerbert, Barbara, Victor Badner, and Bryan Maguire. "AIDS and Dental Practice." *Journal of Public Health Dentistry* 48, no. 2 (Spring 1988): 68–73.

Hazelkorn, Herbert M. "The Reaction of Dentists to Members of Groups at Great Risk of AIDS." Ph.D. diss., University of Illinois—Chicago, 1990.

Karp, Mitchell. *AIDS Discrimination and the Dental Professional: A Presentation from the New York City Commission on Human Rights, AIDS Discrimination Unit*. New York: New York City Commission on Human Rights, 1988.

Koelbl, James J. "AIDS at the Medical College of Georgia: A Study in Institutional Ethics." *Journal of Dental Education* 55, no. 4 (April 1991): 235–237.

Peterson, L. M. "AIDS: The Ethical Dilemma for Surgeons." *Journal of Law, Ethics and Dentistry* 2, no. 2 (April/June 1989): 78–84.

Rogers, V. C. "Dentistry and AIDS: Ethical and Legal Obligations in Provision of Care." *Medicine and Law* 7, no. 1 (January 1988): 57–65.

Nursing

American Nurses' Association. *Personal Heroism, Professional Activism: Nursing and the Battle Against AIDS*. Kansas City, Mo.: American Nurses' Association, 1988.

Boland, Barbara K. "Fear of AIDS in Nursing Staffs." *Nursing Management* 21, no. 6 (June 1990): 40–44.

Downes, J. "Acquired Immunodeficiency Syndrome: The Nurse's Legal Duty to Serve." *Journal of Professional Nursing* 7, no. 6 (November/December 1991): 333–340.

Flaskerud, Jacquelyn H., ed. *AIDS/HIV Infection: A Reference Guide for Nursing Professionals*, 2d ed. Philadelphia, Pa.: Saunders, 1992.

Laufman, Janet K. "AIDS, Ethics and the Truth." *Journal of Nursing* 89, no. 7 (July 1989): 924–931.

Lippman, Helen. "HIV and Professional Ethics: Nurses Speak Out." *RN* 55, no. 6 (June 1992): 28–32.

Rogers, Bonnie. "AIDS and Ethics in the Workplace." *Nursing Outlook* 37, no. 6 (November/December 1989): 254–255, 290.

Sim, J. "AIDS, Nursing and Occupational Risk: An Ethical Analysis." *Journal of Advanced Nursing* 17, no. 5 (May 1992): 569–575.

Occupational Therapy

Hansen, Ruth Ann. "The Ethic of Caring for Patients with HIV or AIDS." *Journal of the Occupational Therapy* 44, no. 3 (March 1, 1990): 239–243.

Physicians

"AAFP Position Statement: Ethical 'Need to Know' Considerations in HIV Infection." *American Family Physician* 42, no. 4 (October 1990): 1117.

"AIDS: The Emerging Ethical Dilemmas." *Hastings Center Report* 15, no. 4 (suppl.) (August 1985): 1–32.

"AIDS and the Ethics of Medical Care and Treatment." *Quarterly Journal of Medicine* 83, no. 302 (June 1, 1992): 419–426.

"AIDS Symposium." *Journal of Medical Ethics* 15, no. 2 (June 1989): 61–81.

Angoff, N. R. "Do Physicians Have an Ethical Obligation to Care for Patients with AIDS?" *Yale Journal of Biology and Medicine* 64, no. 3 (May 1991): 207–246.

Bayer, Ronald. "The HIV-infected Clinician: To Exclude or Not to Exclude?" *Trustee* 44, no. 5 (May 1991): 16–17.

Brazier, M., and M. Lobjoit. "AIDS, Ethics and the Respiratory Physician." *Thorax* 45, no. 4 (April 1, 1990): 283–286.

Chipman, Lauchlan. "Philosophical and Ethical Aspects of AIDS." *Australian Journal of Forensic Sciences* 18, no. 1 (September 1985): 25–32. Transcript of paper presented at National Symposium on AIDS, University of New South Wales, June 8, 1985.

Clarke, Oscar W., and Robert B. Conley. "The Duty to 'Attend upon the Sick.'" *Journal of the American Medical Association* 266, no. 20 (November 27, 1991): 2876–2877.

Cleveland, Henry C., III, and Barbara L. Crawford. "When Physicians Refuse to Treat Patients Who Have AIDS." *Trustee* 41, no. 3 (March 1988): 18–19.

Daley, J., and L. Forrow. "Ethical Issues." *Primary Care* 19, no. 1 (March 1992): 203–216.

Daniels, Norman. "Duty to Treat or Right to Refuse?" *Hastings Center Report* 21, no. 2 (March/April 1991): 36–46.

Dunbar, Scott, and Susan Rehm. "On Visibility: AIDS, Deception by Patients and the Responsibility of the Doctor." *Journal of Medical Ethics* 18, no. 4 (December 1992): 180–185.

Emanuel, Ezekiel J. "Do Physicians Have an Obligation to Treat Patients with AIDS?" *New England Journal of Medicine* 318, no. 25 (June 23, 1988): 168–169.

Freedman, Benjamin. "Health Professions, Codes and the Right to Refuse to Treat HIV-infectious Patients." *Hastings Center Report* 18, no. 2 (suppl.) (April/May 1988): 20–25.

Gostin, Lawrence. "HIV-infected Physicians and the Practice of Seriously Invasive Procedures." *Hastings Center Report* 19, no. 1 (January/February 1989): 32–39.

Hirsch, Harold L. "Medical Dilemma, Legal and Ethical Quagmire." *Medical Trial Technique Quarterly* 37, no. 4 (Summer 1991): 417–450.

Howe, Edmund G. "Military Physicians' Legal and Ethical Obligations to Third Parties When Treating Servicepersons Infected with Human Immunodeficiency Virus." *AIDS and Public Policy Journal* 2, no. 3 (Summer/ Fall 1987): 46–62.

Imperato, Pascal James. "Historical Precedent and the Obligation to Treat AIDS Patients." *Journal of Community Health* 14, no. 4 (Winter 1989): 191–195.

Lo, B. "Ethical Dilemmas in HIV Infection." *Journal of the American Podiatric Medicine Association* 80, no. 1 (January 1990): 26–30.

Pelligrino, Edmund D. "Altruism, Self-interest and Medical Ethics." *Journal of the American Medical Association* 258, no. 14 (October 9, 1987): 1939–1940.

———. "Ethics." *Journal of the American Medical Association* 263, no. 19 (May 16, 1990): 2641–2642.

Picone, John. "Caring for HIV-infected Patients Should Not Be Required." *Journal of the American Medical Association* 261, no. 9 (March 3, 1989): 1359.

Piorkowski, Joseph D. "Between a Rock and a Hard Place: AIDS and the Conflicting Physician's Duties of Preventing Disease Transmission and Safeguarding Confidentiality." *Georgetown Law Journal* 76, no. 1 (October 1987): 169–202.

Ross, Michael W. "Psychosocial Ethical Aspects of AIDS." *Journal of Medical Ethics* 15, no. 2 (June 1989): 74–81.

Sheldon, M. "HIV and the Obligation to Treat." *Theoretical Medicine* 11, no. 3 (September 1990): 201–212.

Tegtmeier, James W. "Ethics and AIDS: A Summary of the Law and a Critical Analysis of the Individual Physician's Ethical Duty to Treat." *American Journal of Law and Medicine* 16, no. 1/2 (1990): 249–265.

Toomey, Kathleen E. "HIV Infection: The Dilemma of Patient Confidentiality." *American Family Physician* 42, no. 4 (October 1990): 955, 959.

Wein, Michael. "Ethics and AIDS: Duty to Warn." *Journal of the American Medical Association* 261, no. 9 (March 3, 1989): 1355, 1360.

Witt, Michael D., ed. *AIDS and Patient Management: Legal, Ethical and Social Issues*. Owings Mills, Md.: National Health Publishers, 1986. Papers from a conference sponsored by Public Responsibility in Medicine and Research.

Zuger, A., and R. Weitz. "Professional Responsibilities in the AIDS Generation." *Hastings Center Report* 17, no. 3 (June 1987): 16–23.

Zuger, Abigail. "AIDS on the Wards: A Residency in Medical Ethics." *Hastings Center Report* 17, no. 3 (June 1987): 16–20.

Zuger, Abigail, and Steven H. Miles. "Physicians, AIDS and Occupational Risk: Historic Traditions and Ethical Obligations." *Journal of the American Medical Association* 258, no. 14 (October 9, 1987): 1924–1928.

Psychology, Psychiatry, and Counseling

Adler, Gerald, and Alexandra Beckett. "Psychotherapy of the Patient with an HIV Infection: Some Ethical and Therapeutic Dilemmas." *Psychosomatics* 30, no. 2 (Spring 1989): 203–208.

American Psychological Association, Committee for Protection of Human Participants in Research, and Committee on Gay Concerns. "Ethical Issues in Psychological Research on AIDS." *Journal of Homosexuality* 13, no. 1 (Fall 1986): 109–116.

American Psychologist 43, no. 11 (November 1988). Special issue on psychology and AIDS, and includes coverage of ethical issues by such authors as Gary B. Melton.

Appelbaum, Paul S. "AIDS, Psychiatry and the Law." *Hospital and Community Psychiatry* 39, no. 1 (January 1988): 13–14.

Cohen, Elliot D. "Confidentiality, Counseling and Clients Who Have AIDS: Ethical Foundations of a Model Rule." *Journal of Counseling and Development* 68, no. 3 (January/February 1990): 282–286.

Dyer, Allen R. "AIDS, Ethics and Psychiatry." *Psychiatric Annals* 18, no. 10 (special issue: "Ethical Treatment of Patients with AIDS") (October 1988): 577–581.

Girardi, John A., Robert M. Keese, and Lynn Bonilla Traver. "Psychotherapist Responsibility in Notifying Individuals at Risk for Exposure to HIV." *Journal of Sex Research* 25, no. 1 (February 1988): 1–27.

Gray, Lizbethy A., and Anna K. Harding. "Confidentiality Limits with Clients Who Have AIDS." *Journal of Counseling and Development* 66, no. 5 (January 1988): 219–223. A reply to this article was written by Craig D. Kain (see citation below).

Kain, Craig D. "To Breach or Not to Breach: Is That the Question? A Response to Gray and Harding." *Journal of Counseling and Development* 66, no. 5 (January 1988): 224–225. Citation for article by Gray and Harding is above.

Kelly, K. "AIDS and Ethics: An Overview." *General Hospital Psychiatry* 9, no. 5 (September 1987): 331–340.

Knapp, Samuel, and Leon Van de Creek. "Application of the Duty to Protect to HIV-positive Patients." *Professional Psychology: Research and Practice* 21, no. 3 (June 1990): 161–166.

Melton, Gary B. "Ethical Judgements Amid Uncertainty: Dilemmas in the AIDS Epidemic." *Counseling Psychologist* 19, no. 4 (October 1991): 561–565.

Melton, Gary B., and Joni N. Gray. "Ethical Dilemmas in AIDS Research: Individual Privacy and Public Health." *American Psychologist* 43, no. 1 (January 1988): 60–64.

Morrison, Constance F. "Ethical Implications for Psychological Intervention." *Professional Psychology Research and Practice* 20, no. 3 (June 1989): 166–171.

Olson, Roberta A., Heather C. Huszti, Patrick J. Mason, and Jeffrey M. Siebert. "Pediatric AIDS/HIV Infection: An Emerging Challenge to Pediatric Psychology." *Journal of Pediatric Psychology* 14, no. 1 (March 1989): 1–21.

Perry, Samuel W. "Pharmacological and Psychological Research on AIDS: Some Ethical Considerations." *IRB: A Review of Human Subjects Research* 9, no. 5 (September/October 1987): 8–10.

Posey, E. Carol. "Confidentiality in an AIDS Support Group." *Journal of Counseling and Development* 66, no. 5 (January 1988): 226–227.

Psychiatric Annals 18, no. 10 (October 1988). Special issue on AIDS and psychiatry, with a number of articles dealing with issues of confidentiality, ethical treatment, and so on.

Ross, Michael W. "Psychosocial Ethical Aspects of AIDS." *Journal of Medical Ethics* 15, no. 2 (June 1989): 74–81.

Schwalbe, Michael L., and Clifford L. Staples. "Moral Reasoning and Rhetoric: The Acceptability of Arguments About AIDS-related Dilemmas." *Journal of Applied Social Psychology* 22, no. 15 (August 1, 1992): 1208–1221.

Simon, Robert I. "AIDS and the Psychiatrist's Ethical and Legal Duty to Stay Abreast." *Psychiatric Annals* 18, no. 10 (October 1988): 561–562.

Szasz, Thomas. "The Medicalization of Sex." *Journal of Humanistic Psychology* 31, no. 3 (Summer 1991): 34–42.

Totten, Georgina, Douglas H. Lamb, and Glen D. Reeder. "Tarasoff and Confidentiality in AIDS-related Psychotherapy." *Professional Psychology: Research and Practice* 21, no. 3 (June 1990): 155–160.

Wood, Gary James, Robert Marks, and James W. Dilley. *AIDS Law for Mental Health Professionals: A Handbook for Judicious Practice*. San Francisco, Calif.: AIDS Health Project, 1990.

Zonana, Howard, Michael Norko, and David Stier. "The AIDS Patient on the Psychiatric Unit: Ethical and Legal Issues." *Psychiatric Annals* 18, no. 10 (special issue: "Ethical Treatment of Patients with AIDS") (October 1988): 587–593.

Public Health

Adler, Michael W. "Debate at the Coalface: HIV, Confidentiality and 'a Delicate Balance.' " (A Reply to Leone Ridsdale.) *Journal of Medical Ethics* 17, no. 4 (December 1991): 196–198.

"AIDS: Public Health and Civil Liberties." (Symposium.) *Hastings Center Report* 16, no. 6 (suppl.) (December 1986): 1–36.

"AIDS and the Ethics of Medical Care and Treatment." *Quarterly Journal of Medicine* 83, no. 302 (June 1, 1992): 419–426.

Association of State and Territorial Health Officials (U.S.). *Guide to Public Health Practice: AIDS Confidentiality and Anti-discrimination Principles.* Public Health Foundation Publication no. 105. Washington, D.C.: Public Health Foundation, 1988.

Avins, Andrew L., and Bernard Lo. "To Tell or Not to Tell: The Ethical Dilemmas of HIV Test Notification in Epidemiologic Research." *American Journal of Public Health* 79, no. 11 (November 1989): 1544–1548.

Banks, Taunya Lovell. "AIDS and the Right to Health Care." *Issues in Law and Medicine* 4, no. 2 (Fall 1988): 151–174.

Bayer, Ronald. *Private Acts, Social Consequences: AIDS and the Politics of Public Health.* New Brunswick, N.J.: Rutgers University Press, 1991.

Bayer, Ronald, and Kathleen E. Toomey. "HIV Prevention and the Two Faces of Partner Notification." *American Journal of Public Health* 82, no. 8 (August 1992): 1158–1164.

Beauchamp, Dan E. "Morality and the Health of the Body Politic." *Hastings Center Report* 16, no. 6 (suppl.) (December 1986): 30–36.

Boyd, Kenneth M. (on behalf of the Institute of Medical Ethics Working Party). "HIV Infection and AIDS: The Ethics of Medical Confidentiality." *Journal of Medical Ethics* 18, no. 4 (December 1992): 173–178.

Charrel, J. M., P. Larher, and C. Manuel. "AIDS: The Rights of Patients." *AIDS and Public Policy Journal* 6, no. 1 (Spring 1991): 41–45.

Closen, Michael L., and Scott H. Isaacman. "Notifying Private Third Parties at Risk for HIV Infection: What Is the Role of Doctors and Other Health-Care Providers?" *Trial* 25, no. 5 (May 1989): 50–55.

Corless, Inge B. "Much Ado About Something: The Restriction of HIV-infected Health-Care Providers." *AIDS and Public Policy Journal* 7, no. 2 (Summer 1992): 82–88.

Crenshaw, Theresa L. "HIV Testing: Voluntary, Mandatory, or Routine?" *Humanist* 48, no. 1 (January/February 1988): 29–34.

Daley, J., and L. Forrow. "Ethical Issues." *Primary Care* 19, no. 1 (March 1992): 203–216.

Daniels, Norman. "HIV-infected Health Care Professionals: Public Threat of Public Sacrifice?" *Milbank Quarterly* 70, no. 1 (1992): 3–42.

DesJarlais, Don C., and Bruce Stepherson. "History, Ethics and Politics in AIDS Prevention Research." (Editorial.) *American Journal of Public Health* 81, no. 11 (November 1991): 1393–1394.

Dickens, Bernard M. "Legal Rights and Duties in the AIDS Epidemic." *Science* 239, no. 4840 (February 5, 1988): 580–586.

Dimas, James T., and Jordan H. Richland. "Partner Notification and HIV Infection: Misconceptions and Recommendations." *Aids and Public Policy Journal* 4, no. 4 (1989): 206–211.

Dourard, John. "HIV + Health-Care Workers: Ethical Problem or Social Problem?" *AIDS and Public Policy Journal* 6, no. 4 (Winter 1991): 175–180.

Dunbar, Scott, and Susan Rehm. "On Visibility: AIDS, Deception by Patients, and the Responsibility of the Doctor." *Journal of Medical Ethics* 18, no. 4 (December 1992): 180–185.

Fennell, R., and Beyrer, M. K. "AIDS: Some Ethical Considerations for the Health Educator." *Journal of American College Health* 38, no. 3 (November 1989): 145–147.

Gebbie, Kristine M. "HIV Testing Issues: The Context for Public Health Decision Making." *AIDS and Public Policy Journal* 2, no. 4 (Fall/Winter 1987): 31–34.

Glantz, Leonard H., Wendy K. Mariner, and George J. Annas. "Risky Business: Setting Public Health Policy for HIV-infected Health Care Professionals." *Milbank Quarterly* 70, no. 1 (1992): 43–79.

Gunderson, Martin, David J. Mayo, and Frank S. Rhame. *AIDS: Testing and Privacy.* Ethics in a Changing World series, vol. 2. Salt Lake City: University of Utah Press, 1989.

Hamblin, Julie, and Margaret A. Somerville. "Surveillance and Reporting of HIV Infection and AIDS in Canada: Ethics and the Law." *University of Toronto Law Journal* 41, no. 2 (Spring 1991): 224–246.

Imperato, Pascal James. "Historical Precedent and the Obligation to Treat AIDS Patients." *Journal of Community Health* 14, no. 4 (Winter 1989): 191–195.

Iosco, Robert C. *AIDS: Law, Ethics and Public Policy.* Washington, D.C.: National Reference Center for Bioethics Literature, Kennedy Institute of Ethics, Georgetown University, 1988.

Larhrer, M. P., J. Charrel, and P. Enel. "AIDS: A Storm Threatening Medical Confidentiality." *AIDS and Public Policy Journal* 6, no. 1 (Spring 1991): 28–31.

Levine, Carol, and Ronald Bayer. "The Ethics of Screening for Early Intervention in HIV Disease." *American Journal of Public Health* 79, no. 12 (December 1989): 1661–1667.

Lundy, Simon. "At the Coalface: HIV Testing and Mental Disorder." *Journal of Medical Ethics* 15, no. 2 (June 1989): 92–93.

Mann, Lee S., and Thomas N. Wise. "Privacy Rights and HIV Testing in the Hospital Setting: A Medicolegal Quagmire for the Administrators." *Health Care Supervisor* 8, no. 2 (January 1990): 57–63.

Manuel, C. P. Enel, and J. Charrel. "Ethics and AIDS: The Protection of Society Versus the Protection of Individual Rights." *AIDS and Public Policy Journal* 6, no. 1 (Spring 1991): 31–36.

Mitchell, Janet L. "Women, AIDS and Public Policy." *AIDS and Public Policy Journal* 3, no. 2 (1988): 50–52.

Moskop, John C. "AIDS and Hospitals: The Policy Options." *Hospital and Health Services Administration* 35, no. 2 (Summer 1990): 159–171.

Myers, Woodrow A., and Kristine M. Gebbie. *Guide to Public Health Practice: AIDS Confidentiality and Anti-discrimination Principles.* Washington, D.C.: Public Health Foundation, 1988.

North, Richard L., and Karen H. Rothenberg. "The Duty-to-Warn 'Dilemma': A Framework for Resolution." *AIDS and Public Policy Journal* 4, no. 3 (1989): 133–411.

Novick, Alvin. "Public Policy and AIDS." *AIDS and Public Policy Journal* 3, no. 1 (Winter 1988): 21–22.

O'Brien, Maura. "Needle Exchange Programs: Ethical and Policy Issues." *Aids and Public Policy Journal* 4, no. 2 (1989): 75–82.

O'Malley, Padraig, ed. *The AIDS Epidemic: Private Rights and the Public Interest.* Boston: Beacon Press, 1989.

Pierce, Christine, and Donald VanDeVeer, eds. *AIDS: Ethics and Public Policy.* Belmont, Calif.: Wadsworth, 1988.

Place, Michael D. "The Church, AIDS and Public Policy." *Notre Dame Journal of Law, Ethics and Public Policy* 5, no. 1 (special issue: "Symposium on AIDS") (1990): 75–88.

Ross, Judith Wilson. "AIDS: Rationing of Care and Ethics." *Family and Community Health* 12, no. 2 (August 1, 1980): 24–33.

Spece, Roy G., Jr. "AIDS: Due Process, Equal Protection and the Right to Treatment." *Issues in Law and Medicine* 4, no. 3 (Winter 1988): 283–344.

Walters, LeRoy. "Ethical Issues in the Prevention and Treatment of HIV Infection and AIDS." *Science* 239, no. 4840 (February 5, 1988): 597–603.

Whitaker, Rupert D., and Richard K. Edwards. "An Ethical Analysis of the U.S. Immigration Policy of Screening Foreigners with the Human Immunodeficiency Virus." *AIDS and Public Policy Journal* 5, no. 4 (Winter 1990): 145–156.

Witt, Michael D., ed. *AIDS and Patient Management: Legal, Ethical and Social Issues.* Owings Mills, Md.: National Health Publishers, 1986. Papers from a conference sponsored by Public Responsibility in Medicine and Research.

Yeide, Harry, Jr. "AIDS Policy and Ethics: Are We Using Enough Tools?" *AIDS and Public Policy Journal* 2, no. 4 (Fall/Winter 1987): 54–59.

Research Ethics

"AIDS, Ethics and Clinical Trials." *British Medical Journal* 305, no. 6855 (September 19, 1992): 699–701.

American Psychological Association, Committee for Protection of Human Participants in Research, and Committee on Gay Concerns. "Ethical Issues in Psychological Research on AIDS." *Journal of Homosexuality* 13, no. 1 (Fall 1986): 109–116.

Bayer, Ronald. "Beyond the Burdens of Protection: AIDS and the Ethics of Research." *Evaluation Review* 14, no. 5 (October 1, 1990): 443–447.

DesJarlais, Don C., and Bruce Stepherson. "History, Ethics and Politics in AIDS Prevention Research." (Editorial.) *American Journal of Public Health* 81, no. 11 (November 1991): 1393–1394.

Dixon, John Edward. *Catastrophic Rights: Experimental Drugs and AIDS.* Vancouver, B.C.: New Star Books, 1990.

Dubler, Nancy Neveloff. "Clinical and Epidemiologic Research on HIV Infection and AIDS Among Correctional Inmates: Regulations, Ethics and Procedures." *Evaluation Review* 14, no. 5 (October 1, 1990): 482–502.

Freedman, Benjamin. "Suspended Judgement—AIDS and the Ethics of Clinical Trials: Learning the Right Lessons." *Controlled Clinical Trials* 13, no. 1 (February 1, 1992): 1–5.

Fuenzalida-Puelma, Hernan, Ana Maria Linares Parada, and Diana Serrano LaVertu. *Ethics and Law in the Study of AIDS.* Washington, D.C.: Pan American Health Organization, Pan-American Sanitary Bureau, Regional Office of the World Health Organization, 1992.

Gostin, Lawrence. "Vaccination for AIDS: Legal and Ethical Challenges from the Test Tube, to the Human Subject, Through to the Marketplace." *AIDS and Public Policy Journal* 2, no. 2 (Spring/Summer 1987): 9–16.

Koff, Wayne C., and Daniel F. Hoth. "Development and Testing of AIDS Vaccines." *Science* 241, no. 4864 (July 1988): 426–432.

Kwitny, Jonathan. *Acceptable Risks.* New York: Poseidon Press, 1992.

Lang, Norris G. "Difficult Decisions: Ethics and AIDS." *Journal of Sex Research* 28, no. 2 (May 1, 1991): 249–262.

Levine, Carol. "Has AIDS Changed the Ethics of Human Subjects Research?" *Law, Medicine and Health Care* 16, no. 3/4 (Fall/Winter 1988): 167–173.

Melton, Gary B., Robert J. Levine, Gerald P. Koecher, Robert Rosenthal, and William C. Thompson. "Community Consultation in Socially Sensitive Research: Lessons from Clinical Trials of Treatments for AIDS." *American Psychologist* 43, no. 7 (July 1988): 573–581.

Perry, Samuel W. "Pharmacological and Psychological Research on AIDS: Some Ethical Considerations." *IRB: A Review of Human Subjects Research* 9, no. 5 (September/October 1987): 8–10.

Porter, Joan P., Marta J. Glass, and Wayne C. Koff. "Ethical Considerations in AIDS Vaccine Testing." *IRB: A Review of Human Subjects Research* 11, no. 3 (May/June 1989): 1–4.

Social Work

Khooper, Surjit S., David D. Royse, and Thanh V. Tran. "Social Work Practitioners' Attitudes Towards AIDS Victims." *Journal of Applied Social Sciences* 12, no. 1 (Fall/Winter 1987/1988): 108–123.

Reamer, Frederick G. "AIDS, Social Work and the 'Duty to Protect.' " *Social Work* 36, no. 1 (January 1991): 56–60.

Ryan, Caitlin C., and Mona J. Rowe. "AIDS: Legal and Ethical Issues." *Social Casework: The Journal of Contemporary Social Work* 69, no. 6 (June 1988): 324–333.

Wiener-Brawerman, Lori S. "An Attitudinal Study of Social Workers' Responses to the Acquired Immune Deficiency Syndrome (AIDS) Patient Population." Ph.D. diss., New York University, 1988.

Testing

Bayer, Ronald, Carol Levine, and Susan M. Wolf. "HIV Antibody Screening: An Ethical Framework for Evaluating Proposed Programs." *Journal of the American Medical Association* 256, no. 13 (October 3, 1986): 1768–1774.

Boyd, Kenneth M. "HIV Infection: The Ethics of Anonymised Testing and of Testing Pregnant Women." *Journal of Medical Ethics* 16, no. 4 (December 1990): 173–178. Institute of Medical Ethics working party report.

Childress, James F. "An Ethical Framework for Assessing Policies to Screen for Antibodies to HIV." *AIDS and Public Policy Journal* 2, no. 1 (Winter 1987): 28–31.

Crenshaw, Theresa L. "HIV Testing: Voluntary, Mandatory, or Routine?" *Humanist* 48, no. 1 (January/February 1988): 29–34.

Enel, Patricia. "Ethical Confusion: Detection of HIV Seropositives." *AIDS and Public Policy Journal* 7, no. 1 (Spring 1992): 42–49.

Faden, Ruth, Gail Geller, and Madison Powers, eds. *AIDS, Women and the Next Generation: Towards a Morally Acceptable Public Policy for Testing of Pregnant Women and Newborns.* New York: Oxford University Press, 1991.

Gebbie, Kristine M. "HIV Testing Issues: The Context for Public Health Decision Making." *AIDS and Public Policy Journal* 2, no. 4 (Fall/Winter 1987): 31–34.

Gunderson, Martin, David J. Mayo, and Frank S. Rhame. *AIDS: Testing and Privacy.* Ethics in a Changing World series, vol. 2. Salt Lake City: University of Utah Press, 1989.

Hamblin, Julie, and Margaret A. Sommerville. "Surveillance and Reporting of HIV Infection and AIDS in Canada: Ethics and the Law." *University of Toronto Law Journal* 41, no. 2 (Spring 1991): 224–246.

Hawthorne, William, and Larry Siegel. "Should There Be HIV Testing in Chemical Dependency Treatment Programs?" *Advances in Alcohol and Substance Abuse* 7, no. 2 (1987): 15–19.

Hirsch, Harold L. "Medical Dilemma, Legal and Ethical Quagmire." *Medical Trial Technique Quarterly* 37, no. 4 (Summer 1991): 417–450.

Hunter, Nan D. "AIDS Prevention and Civil Liberties: The False Security of Mandatory Testing." *AIDS and Public Policy Journal* 2, no. 3 (Summer/Fall 1987): 1–10.

Hurley, Peter, and Glenn Pinder. "Ethics, Social Forces and Politics in AIDS-related Research: Experience in Planning and Implementing a Household HIV Seroprevalence Survey." *Milbank Quarterly* 70, no. 4 (1992): 605–628.

Lundy, Simon. "At the Coalface: HIV Testing and Mental Disorder." *Journal of Medical Ethics* 15, no. 2 (June 1989): 92–93.

McAdam, Rhona. "AIDS and Confidentiality: The Records Manager's Dilemma." *ARMA Records Management Quarterly* 23, no. 3 (July 1989): 12–16.

Nelson, David K. "AIDS and Life Insurance: A Look Behind the Testing Issue." *AIDS and Public Policy Journal* 2, no. 3 (Summer/Fall 1987): 26–28.

Videos on AIDS and Ethics

A.I.D.S.: A Challenge to Health Care Professionals. Toronto: University of Toronto Faculty of Medicine, Instructional Media Services, 1983 (VHS, 30 min.). A little dated, but focuses strongly on ethics issues.

AIDS: A Matter of Corporate Policy. Alexandria, Va.: PBS Video, 1988 (VHS, 150 min.).

AIDS: Medical, Moral and Ministerial Dimensions. Dubuque, Ia.: Brown-Roa Publishing Media, 1989 (VHS, 30 min.).

AIDS and Ethics. Chicago, Ill.: Department of Biomedical Communications, Rush Presbyterian St. Luke's Medical Center., 1984 (¾ in, 72 min.).

AIDS and the Health Care Provider. Cleveland, Ohio: Care Video Production, 1988 (VHS, 25 min.).

AIDS and the Healthcare Worker (Videorecording.) Deerfield, Ill.: Coronet/MTI Film and Video, 1988 (VHS, 26 min.).

AIDS and the Law. Philadelphia, Pa.: American Law Institute, 1986 (VHS, 210 min.).

AIDS in the Healthcare Workplace: Fantasy, Fact and Ethics. Norfolk, Va.: PBS Adult Learning Service, 1992 (VHS, 120 min.).

Cox, Johnny. *AIDS and Healers: Ethical Concerns*. (Videotape.) Kansas City, Mo.: Sheed and Ward, 1988 (VHS, 40 min.).

Pellegrino, Edmund D., Lee J. Dunn, Jr., and Abigail Zuger. *Case Reports on the Ethics of AIDS*. Secaucus, N.J.: Network for Continuing Medical Education, 1988 (VHS, 30 min.).

Physicians and AIDS: The Ethical Response. Clinton, Tenn.: Carle Media, 1990 (VHS, 25 min.).

About the Contributors

JOAN C. CALLAHAN is associate professor of philosophy at the University of Kentucky, Lexington. Among her published works in applied and professional ethics are "The Fetus and Fundamental Rights," *Commonweal* (April 1986); *Ethical Issues in Professional Life* (Oxford University Press, 1988); and *Preventing Birth: Contemporary Methods and Related Moral Controversies*, with James W. Knight (University of Utah Press, 1989).

ELLIOT D. COHEN, professor of philosophy at Indian River Community College, Fort Pierce, Florida, is founder and editor-in-chief of *The International Journal of Applied Philosophy*. His recent books include *Philosophers at Work: An Introduction to the Issues and Practical Uses of Philosophy* (Holt, Rinehart and Winston, 1989); *Philosophical Issues in Journalism* (Oxford University Press, 1992); and *Caution: Faulty Thinking Can Be Harmful to Your Happiness*, self-help ed. (Trace-WilCo, 1992). Certified in rational-emotive therapy, he has conducted clinical research and published articles on counseling, including "Syllogizing RET: Applying Formal Logic in Rational-Emotive Therapy," *Journal of Rational-Emotive and Cognitive-Behavior Therapy* (Winter 1992).

HOWARD COHEN is presently dean of liberal arts at the University of Wisconsin, Parkside, and was formerly provost and associate professor of philosophy at the University of Massachusetts, Boston. His published works in applied and professional ethics include *Equal Rights for Children* (Littlefield-Adams, 1980); "Overstepping Police Authority," *Criminal Justice Ethics* (Summer/Fall 1987); and other works in the areas of police ethics and children's rights.

MICHAEL DAVIS is senior research associate at the Center for the Study of Ethics in the Professions, Illinois Institute of Technology, Chicago. He has published widely in ethics, political philosophy, and philosophy of law. His recent works include "On Teaching Cloistered Virtue: The Ethics of Teaching Students to Avoid Moral Risk," *Teaching Philosophy* (September 1991);

"Thinking Like an Engineer: The Place of a Code of Ethics in the Practice of a Profession," *Philosophy and Public Affairs* (Spring 1991); "The Moral Legislature: Contractualism Without an Archemedian Point," *Ethics* (January 1992); and *To Make the Punishment Fit the Crime: Essays in the Theory of Criminal Justice* (Westview Press, 1992).

JOSEPH A. EDELHEIT is senior rabbi of Temple Israel in Minneapolis and rabbinic co-chair of the Union of American Hebrew Congregations, Central Conference of American Rabbis Joint Committee on AIDS. He is the author of several published articles on AIDS, including "The Rabbi and the Abyss of AIDS," *TIKKUN* 4, no. 4 (July/August 1989), and "The Rabbi and the Mandatory Pre-marital HIV Antibodies Test," *Journal of Reform Judaism* (1989).

SOHAIR ELBAZ, director of libraries at the Illinois Institute of Technology, Chicago, has taught library science in Egypt and Saudi Arabia and is often a consultant to the Egyptian cabinet and to the United Nations. Among her many publications in Arabic and English is her doctoral dissertation on the motivational needs of librarians, which was recently published in *Advances in Library Administration and Organization* 9 (1991).

ALBERT FLORES is presently professor and chairperson of the department of philosophy and was formerly health professions coordinator at California State University, Fullerton. Among his works in applied and professional ethics are "On the Rights of Professionals," in *Business and Professional Ethics*, ed. Michael Pritchard et al. (Humana Press, 1983); *Professional Ideals* (Wadsworth, 1987); and *Ethics and Risk Management Engineering* (The University Presses of America, 1989).

AL GINI is associate professor of philosophy and adjunct professor at the Institute of Industrial Relations, Loyola University, Chicago. He is also managing editor of *Business Ethics Quarterly*. A consultant on corporate ethics and employee relations, he is regularly heard on National Public Radio's Chicago affiliate WBEZ–FM. His published works include *Philosophical Issues in Human Rights*, coedited with Patricia Werhane and David Ozar (Random House, 1986); *It Comes with the Territory: An Inquiry into the Nature of Work*, with David Sullivan (Random House, 1989); and *Case Studies in Business Ethics*, with Thomas Donaldson (Prentice Hall, 1989).

MARTIN GUNDERSON is associate professor of philosophy at Macalester College, Minneapolis, as well as an attorney in the state of Minnesota. Specializing in philosophy of law and biomedical ethics, his recent publications include *AIDS: Testing and Privacy*, coauthored with David Mayo and Frank Rhame (University of Utah Press, 1989); "Protecting Commercial Speech: Advertising and Advocating Illegal Activities," *Freedom, Equality, and Social Change*, ed. Creighton Peden and James Sterba (Edwin Mellen Press, 1989);

and "Justifying a Principle of Informed Consent: A Case Study in Autonomy-based Ethics," *Public Affairs Quarterly* (June 1990).

KENNETH KIPNIS, professor of philosophy at the University of Hawaii, Manoa, is the author of *Legal Ethics* (Prentice-Hall, 1986) and other works on professional ethics in the areas of pediatric intensive care, nursing, engineering, correctional health services, and education. With Stephanie Feeney, he is coauthor of the Code of Ethical Conduct and the Statement of Commitment of the National Association for the Education of Young Children.

WILLIAM PARDUE is librarian/information researcher at the Center for the Study of Ethics in the Professions, Illinois Institute of Technology, Chicago. He was previously departmental assistant, Melville J. Herskovits Library of African Studies, Northwestern University.

JILL POWELL is clinical nurse specialist at Eastern State Hospital, Lexington, Kentucky, where she developed and implemented an AIDS education program for the inpatient psychiatric population. As clinical coordinator for the Women's AIDS Project at the University of Kentucky, Lexington, she has also been involved in developing and implementing support services for HIV-positive women as well as facilitating a psychotherapy group for this population. Specializing in psychiatric mental health, she has written and lectured widely in this area.

MICHAEL PRITCHARD, professor of philosophy and director of the Center for the Study of Ethics in Society at Western Michigan University, is also an executive committee member of the national Association for Practical and Professional Ethics. He is coeditor of *Medical Responsibility* (Humana Press, 1978) and *Profits and Professions* (Humana Press, 1983); author of *Philosophical Adventures with Children* (University Press of America, 1985) and *On Becoming Responsible* (University Press of Kansas, 1991); and coauthor with James Jaksa of *Communication Ethics* (Wadsworth, 1988) and with C. E. Harris and Michael Rabins of *Ethics in Engineering: Cases and Concepts* (Wadsworth, 1993).

VINCENT J. SAMAR is instructor of law, Illinois Institute of Technology, Chicago/Kent, and adjunct professor of philosophy, Loyola University, Chicago. In 1990, he ran for alderman of Chicago's 46th Ward and later for delegate to the Democratic National Convention. A practicing attorney, he has had a longtime involvement in Chicago's gay and lesbian communities. His recent published works include *The Right to Privacy: Gays, Lesbians and the Constitution* (Temple University Press, 1991).

Index